Making Health Decisions

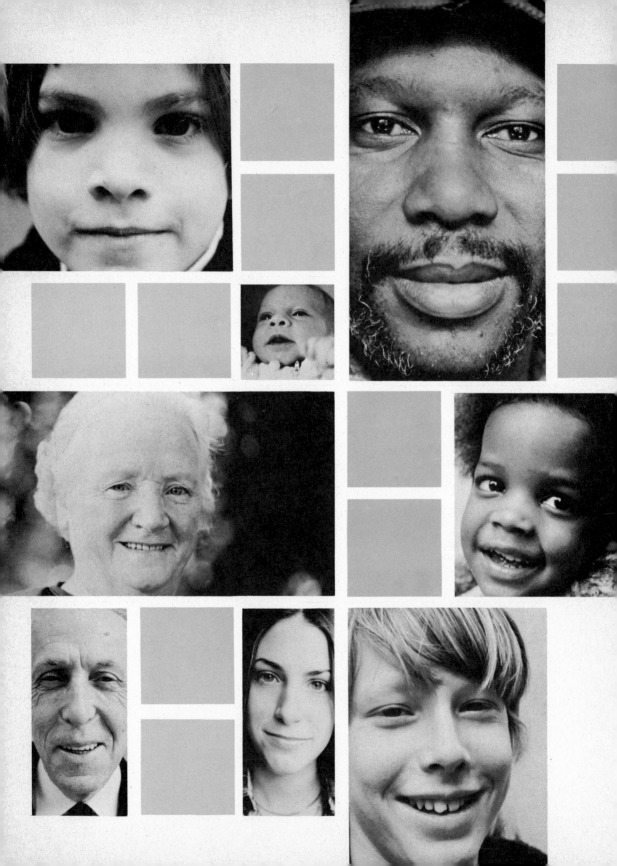

Making Health Decisions

Second Edition

Ben C. Gmur

Professor, Health Science and Safety Studies Department
California State University, Los Angeles
Los Angeles, California

John T. Fodor

Professor, Department of Health Science
California State University, Northridge
Northridge, California

L. H. Glass

Professor, Department of Health Science
California State University, Northridge
Northridge, California

Joseph J. Langan

Director of Instruction, Administrative Area L
Los Angeles City Schools
Los Angeles, California

Prentice-Hall, Inc., Englewood Cliffs, New Jersey

Supplementary Materials

Teachers Guide

Workbook

Tests

Making Health Decisions Second Edition

Ben C. Gmur
John T. Fodor
L. H. Glass
Joseph J. Langan

© 1975, 1970 by Prentice-Hall, Inc., Englewood Cliffs, New Jersey 07632

Printed in the United States of America
0–13–547927–4

10 9 8 7 6 5 4 3

Design by E. Peter Marcionetti

Prentice-Hall International, Inc., *London*

Prentice-Hall of Australia, Pty. Ltd., *Sydney*

Prentice-Hall of Canada, Ltd., *Toronto*

Prentice-Hall of India Private Ltd., *New Delhi*

Prentice-Hall of Japan, Inc., *Tokyo*

Health is a complex state. It involves the relationship between the physical, emotional, and social aspects of life. The most important component in this relationship is the individual.

The status of your health today and in the future is primarily your own responsibility. In our present society, with its medical and scientific advances, it is possible for you to live the healthiest, longest life of all time. But for you to achieve this potential you must make intelligent personal decisions. This book has been written to provide you with much of the information that must be analyzed and synthesized before making decisions that will affect your health.

You should be aware, too, that there are many unresolved health problems in your community, In our country, and, indeed, throughout the world. Finding ways of coping with these problems (such as water pollution and air pollution) can enhance your health even more in the years to come. Therefore, it is important for you to make decisions concerning your personal living which will contribute to and support efforts to control community problems. Ways in which you might actively support programs to resolve important health problems are discussed in this book.

In order for you to make intelligent health decisions there are important concepts or "big ideas" that you must fully understand. These concepts are clearly identified and explained in the chapters that follow. Study them carefully and when you understand them, let them guide you in your health behavior.

This is not a book in human anatomy or physiology. There is very little emphasis placed on memorization of body parts or systems and how they function. Instead, you will find that the focus is on health problems. Information about anatomy and physiology is provided only to the extent that it will help you understand and solve these health problems. In addition, for those who wish to study human anatomy and physiology in more detail, a series of anatomical drawings has been included near the middle of the book for your easy reference.

The writers wish to express their appreciation to the many people who contributed to the completion of this book.

To Fanny Mach we extend our utmost thanks for her graciousness and for her meticulous review of the manuscript and her technical assistance.

Grateful appreciation is also extended to Roslyn Barbash, M.D., member of the Clean Air Council of the New Jersey Department of Health, Chairman of the Air Pollution Committee of the Medical Society of New Jersey, and Founder and Clinical Director of the Allergy Clinic at Englewood Hospital in Englewood, New Jersey; Gus T. Dalis, Ed. D., Consultant in Health Education, Office of the Los Angeles County Superintendent of Schools; Dr. James A. Fikes, Professor in the Department of Health Science at Fresno State College, Fresno, California; Isidor H. Goldberg, Ph. D., Professor and Chairman of the Division of Health Sciences, Health, and Physical Education at Kingsborough Community College of the City University of New York; Herb Lewis, M.S., Supervisor of Health and Physical Education for the Jefferson County Public Schools, Louisville, Kentucky; Sister Clarice Lolich, M.S., Science Curriculum Chairman of the Western Catholic Education Association; and Mrs. Juanita S. Winn, Supervising Director for Elementary Schools, Washington, D. C. Public Schools, for their review of the manuscript and their invaluable suggestions.

Particular acknowledgement is given to Russell J. Purcey for developing the *Teachers Guide* for this textbook. We also appreciate the assistance of Eleda Grizzell and Dennis Snyder, who prepared the test booklet, and of Gordon Lebowitz and David Fried, who prepared the *Workbook.*

Very special thanks are extended to Ollie Stevener and Holly Levien for their major role in preparing the manuscript for submission to the publisher.

Finally, we warmly thank our wives, Lorraine J. Gmur, Mary J. Fodor, Rosalee E. Glass, and Phyllis R. Langan, for their devotion and support during the preparation of the text.

Although we, of course, assume full responsibility for the contents of this book, we appreciate the help these people have provided in its preparation.

Illustration Acknowledgments

AAHPER: Fig. 7-4 (bottom) ● American Basketball Association: p. 104 (bottom right) ● American Bowling Congress: Fig. 7-3 (bottom) ● American Cancer Society: p. 130; Fig. 12-6 (top); 12-11 (bottom right) ● The American Financial Corp., Cincinnati, Ohio: Fig. 2-2 (top right); Fig. 14-6 ● American Heart Association: Fig. 12-6 (top #5); (bottom #2, 3) ● American Lung Association: Fig. 9-6 ● American Machine Foundry/CUNO: Fig. 11-6 (water) ● American National Red Cross: Fig. 12-16 (volunteer); 14-11 ● American Telephone and Telegraph Co.: Fig. 4-3 ● Anderson/Monkmeyer: Fig. 10-2 (public health) ● Barton-Gillet Company: Fig. 1-1 (future) ● Bayer/Monkmeyer: Fig. 2-4 (2) ● Bergman Associates/DPI: Fig. 12-14; 15-5 (bottom left) ● Bijur/Monkmeyer: Fig. 10-5 ● Blanche/DPI: Fig. 10-2 (medical); 12-11 (radiation) ● Brown/Black Star: Fig. 10-2 (social) ● Browning/DPI: Fig. 15-9 (top left) ● Burlington House: Fig. 11-17 (sleep) ● Carolina Biological Supply Co.: Fig. 3-4; 11-4 ● Center for Disease Control, Atlanta, Ga.: Fig. 11-2 (rats); 11-6 (animals) ● Coplan/DPI: p. 188; Fig. 8-2 (bottom left); 12-16 (psychiatrist) ● Cynara: Fig. 2-1; 2-2 (center); 3-13; 5-5; 7-5; 7-6; 7-7; 11-7 (nail and cream); 12-15 ● Daniels/Documerica: Fig. 12-11 (bottom left) ● DiDio/NEA: p. 103 (top left) ● Disease Association of Los Angeles County: Fig. 12-4 (right) ● Dunigan/DPI: Fig. 11-6 (man) ● Dunn/DPI: Fig. 4-4 (beach) ● The DuPont Company: Fig. 2-4 (3) ● Eastman Kodak Co., Scholastic Photography Awards: Fig. 1-1 (you) ● EPA/DOCUMERICA: Fig. 12-11 (top left) ● Forsyth/Monkmeyer: Fig. 4-4 (family and ring); 8-2 (top right); p. 30; p. 104 (bottom right) ● General Electric Medical Systems: Fig. 12-6 (bottom #4); 12-8; 13-9; 15-5 (top left); 15-9 (top left) ● Girl Scouts of the U.S.A.: Fig. 11-2; 11-6 (host) ● Dr. Leonard H. Glassman, Mrs. Marcia C. Glassman: Fig. 12-18 ● Joel Gordon: Fig. 16-5 ● Greenberg/DPI: Fig. 11-6 (food); 12-11 (dental) ● Gritscher/DPI: Fig. 14-8 (left) ● Herman Heilman: Fig. 12-16 (clinical and therapist) ● Heron/Monkmeyer: Fig. 4-2 ● Hill-Rom Company, Inc.: Fig. 8-4 (mid-left); 11-9 ● Hospital Affiliates, Inc.: Fig. 8-2 (top left); 12-16 (nurse); 15-5 (top left and bottom right) ● William Huling: Fig. 3-8; 7-1; 8-7 ● Jefferson/Monkmeyer: Fig. 8-4 (top right) ● Karates/DPI: Fig. 10-2 (law) ● Kentucky Central Life Insurance Company: Fig. 2-4 (4); p. 103 (bottom right) ● Kraus/DPI: Fig. 15-5 (top right) ● Laping/DPI: Fig. 15-5 (bottom left) ● Lederle Laboratories, A division of American Cyanamid Co.: Fig. 15-5 (top left and bottom left) ● The Lee Company: Fig. 2-2 (mid-right) ● Lewis/French: Fig. 15-5 (bottom right) ● Lewis/Lambert: Fig. 2-2 (climate); 4-4 (at desk); 11-17 (exercise); 12-12; 15-5 (bottom right) ● Lewis/Vials: Fig. 11-2 (climate) ● Lieberman/Black Star: Fig. 10-2 (individual); p. 144 ● Los Angeles City Health Dept.: Fig. 11-10 ● L.A. City School districts: Fig. 16-6 ● L.A. County Air Pollution Control District: Fig. 13-1 ● L.A. County Health Dept.: Fig. 1-5; 11-11 ● L.A. County TB and Health Association: Fig. 12-3 ● Mahon/Monkmeyer: Fig. 10-2 (psychological) ● Manhattan Medical and Dental Assistants School: Fig. 15-9 (bottom left) ● Margolin/Black Star: Fig. 7-3 (top) ●

Making Health Decisions

One | Developing Your Concept of Health

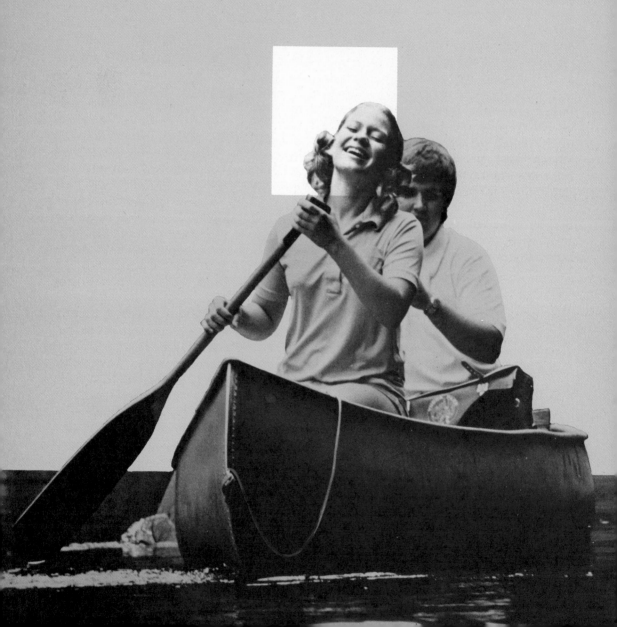

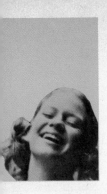

Human beings have always been concerned with health and how to combat illness. Through the years their attempts to fight disease have ranged from mysticism and magic to the latest scientific discoveries. These attempts and humanity's concept of health have been influenced by a number of factors.

Religion has been an important force in determining health practices. Even the most primitive people had some form of worship. In a rather simple fashion, they divided their spirits and gods into two categories, good and evil. Since they recognized that from time to time illness affected their tribe, it seemed only natural to blame this on evil spirits. Some groups attempted to control outbreaks of disease by rites designed to appease these spirits. These usually involved animal sacrifices. If illness involved only one person, it was commonly thought that the person was under the spell of an evil spirit. The treatment consisted of driving the evil spirit out of the body or banning the person from the group so that others would not become affected.

As people's religious thinking became more sophisticated, they transferred the responsibility for health to the so-called good gods or spirits. Disease was looked upon as punishment for sin. Those who somehow became ill were thought to have broken moral laws. Control measures were adopted to appease the offended god. During the Middle Ages, when a number of epidemics killed thousands of people, days of prayer, fasting, and sacrifice were established in an effort to control the outbreaks of disease. Many epidemics that took place during Colonial times were treated in a similar manner. Even today, we find many persons who sincerely believe that spiritual forces alone cause disease to develop.

Other theories on diseases and their control developed along with religious beliefs. People were constantly observing their environment. They noticed that the amount of disease, the kind of disease, and the severity of disease seemed to vary with the season of the year, the climate, the temperature, the amount of moisture, the geographic location of people, the degree of overcrowding, and the accumulation of filth. Many of their observations were accurate. However, when they tried to explain why these diseases were taking place, they developed wrong answers because they lacked the scientific knowledge we have today.

One of the most important concepts that resulted from observations of the environment was the miasma theory. This concept of ill health dates back to Hippocrates, a Greek physician in the pre-Christian era. People observed that those who lived near swamps had a higher incidence of fever than did those who lived away from these areas. They thought that these people were inhaling the mists that rose from the swamps and that these mists were poisonous. The fever was given the name malaria (*mala aria,* bad air). Not until the end of the 19th century could a better explanation be offered. At that time, the role of the mosquito in the transmission of malaria was discovered.

The miasma theory seemed to explain many types of health problem. All forms of decaying matter were thought to give off harmful or poisonous gases. These gases were then considered responsible for illness. During the Industrial Revolution, when cities became crowded, disease rates were high. When the environment was examined to discover the causes of disease, it was observed that conditions of extreme filth prevailed. Garbage and human waste were deposited in any place that was convenient. The spread of disease was blamed on the decaying of this organic matter.

Interestingly enough, the miasma theory was responsible for the development of many community sanitation programs. Efforts were made to dispose of decaying matter promptly and properly. Consideration was given to protecting water supplies from contamination. Thus what has since proved to be an incorrect explanation led to many modern health practices.

The work of Pasteur and others during the latter half of the 19th century did much to dispel the miasma theory. Pasteur demonstrated that certain diseases were caused by microscopic forms of life. This helped create the understanding that diseases could be spread from person to person and from animals to human beings. The breakthrough permitted the development of new measures of prevention and control. Additional research showed the role of insects as carriers of certain diseases. The concept of immunization was put into practice.

Over the years, a vast amount of medical knowledge has been accumulated. Much progress has been made in devising new approaches to the prevention and control of health problems. New concepts of health have been developed.

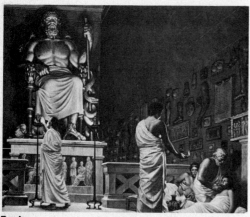

Past
Religious rites

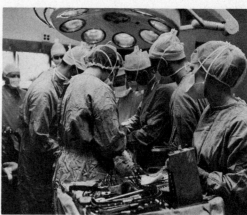

Present
Organ transplant

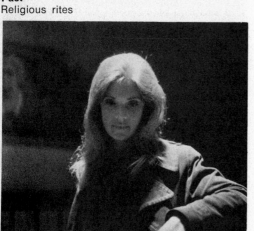

Figure 1-1 ● The past, present, and future have now and will continue to have an effect on your health.

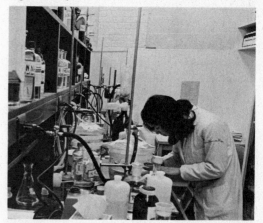

Future
Cures

Physical, Mental, Social Well-being

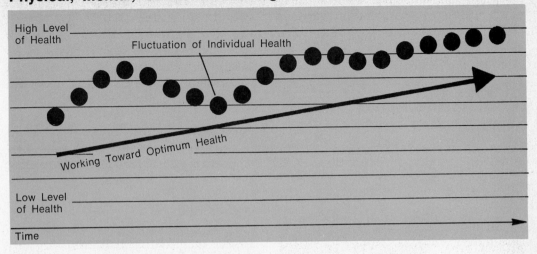

Figure 1-2 ● Your health will vary during any time span from optimal good health to poor health. This book should give you information to help you make decisions that will enable you to maintain a higher degree of health.

A Definition of Health

Health is more than the mere absence of disease or infirmity. Howard S. Hoyman, a prominent health educator, stresses the ecologic factors (that is, those affecting the pattern or total relationship of living things with their environment) in his definition of health, presented in his article "Our Modern Concept of Health" in *The Journal of School Health*. He states that health is concerned with

. . . the ecologic interaction of many complex factors and conditions such as:

■ Good hereditary endowment
■ A healthful, safe environment
■ An adequate standard of living
■ Adequate medical and dental care and public-health services and education
■ Resistance to communicable and non-communicable diseases

■ Optimum nutrition, growth, and development
■ Fitness and resistance to stress, fatigue, frustration, and boredom
■ Healing, repair, and recovery from injury or illness
■ Resistance to premature aging and death
■ A healthy, mature personality and healthful living
■ A will to live
■ Healthful attitudes, beliefs, and practices
■ Useful, satisfying work and creative achievement
■ Love and affectionate sharing and belonging
■ Enjoyable, constructive recreation and use of leisure
■ Opportunities for risks, challenges, adventures, and new experiences
■ Spiritual faith, ideals, values, and a search for meaning

This definition suggests that **people are whole individuals who function in a physical, ecologic, and social environment.** Many interrelated factors have an effect on an individual's health and in turn on the health of the community.

Factors Affecting One's Health

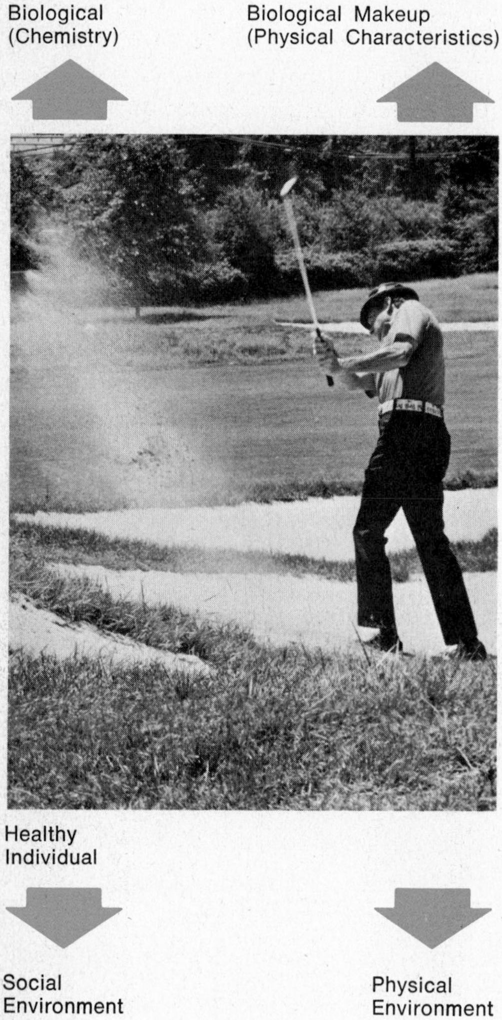

Biological
(Chemistry)

Biological Makeup
(Physical Characteristics)

Healthy
Individual

Social
Environment

Physical
Environment

Figure 1-3 ● How can you make the best use of the mental and physical capacities with which you were born?

Inherited Endowment

One of the influences affecting your health and your ability to function effectively is your inherited endowment. It plays a major role in determining your uniqueness. A basic inherited characteristic is your sex. The sexes have distinct internal chemical differences as well as the obvious external physical differences. Internal secretions (hormones) play an important role in determining an individual's sex characteristics, as well as in helping to influence that individual's overall behavior.

All aspects of your growth and development, including external characteristics as well as internal cell structure, are continuous. However, growth and development are not necessarily even, and they vary greatly among individuals.

Your total physical, mental, and social well-being is affected by your body size, body shape, general appearance, and internal cell structure and chemistry. All of these are partially influenced by what you have inherited. Each individual is different in this respect. In your uniqueness you should be aware of your potentials and limitations. You face the task of making the best use of the mental and physical capacities with which you were born.

Environment

The physical and social environment affects your daily living. Forces such as air pollution, radiation hazards, water pollution, noise, and inadequate waste disposal can be detrimental to your health. The number and accessibility of disease agents in your environment also affect your health.

Your social environment has a great influence on your health behavior. What you believe and how you act are determined to a great extent by your cultural values, customs, attitudes, and the patterns of behavior that are being practiced by the group to which you belong.

Life, and therefore health, involves a constant interaction between you and your environment. Consideration must be given to ways in which you can adjust to the environment or make changes that will provide favorable conditions.

Your Role

Much progress has been made in solving health problems and promoting the health of the individual. A number of health services are available to you. They include private health care by physicians and dentists, private and public hospital care, and private and public clinics for the treatment and prevention of a number of diseases and disorders. Through such services and our advanced technology, many infectious diseases have been controlled, and higher standards of medical practice have been established. This has resulted in a decline in death rate for certain diseases. In addition, suffering and disability from a number of illnesses have been diminished. Life expectancy, the average number of years an individual can expect to live, has increased.

These advances have led to new problems, such as the increased incidence of chronic disease, contamination of the environment, and problems of aging. The fact that more people live to maturity means that more people can, and probably will, have children, thus contributing to the population explosion with its ramifications.

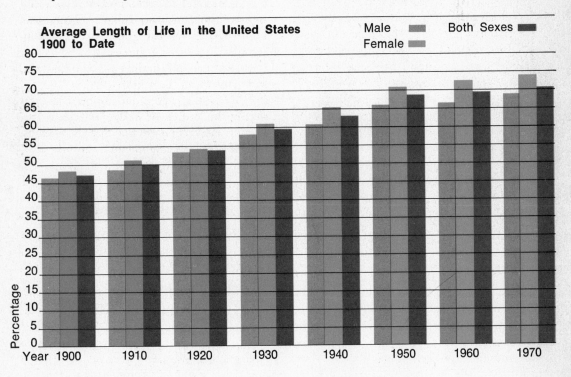

Figure 1-4 ● The chart shows the increase in average length of life in the United States since 1900. Can you think of any health problems with which you must deal because of this increased longevity?

The solutions for many of the new problems rest with the individual. **You can influence your health by the decisions you make and the actions you take.** You will have to decide how important health is to you. To cope with problems and make the best possible decisions, you will need to have accurate, scientific health information.

To this end President Nixon in 1971 appointed the President's Committee on Health Education. Its basic purpose was to establish a national policy that would help the people of the nation make wise decisions concerning the solutions to their health problems. The mechanism to be used to realize this goal would be effective health education in schools and in the community. The purpose of this text, too, is to enable you to make effective decisions regarding appropriate health behavior. Merely acquiring knowledge and being able to recall health facts or rules is not enough. For this information to be beneficial to you, you must apply it. As you read the various chapters, evaluate and apply the information to your own situation.

More and more people are becoming interested in health careers. There are many opportunities for careers in health. These careers are exciting and challenging. They also provide an opportunity to help others solve their health problems. You may want to consider the possibility of a health career yourself.

The Role of Others

Many organizations at the national, state, and local levels engage in activities that are closely related to your health. They carry on organized projects that protect your health and the health of the community. You should be aware of these activities and what you can do to help.

The Local Health Department

The fear of epidemics of disease helped bring about the establishment of many local health departments. Control of communicable diseases and improvement of community sanitation programs are still important health department functions. However, many other services are now included in the health department's program to protect and promote the health of the community.

Health departments perform such services as registering births and deaths; collecting reports of infectious diseases; offering consultation to physicians; providing examinations for tuberculosis and blood tests for venereal disease; inspecting restaurants, supermarkets, bakeries, and other food establishments; conducting studies of rheumatic fever, cervical cancer, and other diseases; inspecting public swimming pools, nursing homes, and hospitals; maintaining public-health nursing programs; providing care for infants and pregnant women; and carrying out sanitation, health information, and education programs.

The American Public Health Association points out in its policy statement *The Local Health Department—Services and Responsibilities* that:

> . . . Through daily contact with the public, the local health department obtains first-hand information concerning local health needs, and is responsible for providing its community with direct services. A unique combination of medical, dental, nursing, engineering, and other technical services, together with statistical, educational, managerial, and administrative skills, is made available through a full-time efficient and well-staffed local health department.

Health careers related to these services are: sanitarian, public-health statistician, public-health educator, public-health administrator, visiting nurse, home health aide, homemaker, health officer, and others.

Voluntary Health Agencies

In each community there are voluntary health agencies that are concerned with the health of people. These agencies are financially supported by voluntary contributions from individuals and groups.

There are three main types of voluntary health agencies: those that focus on specific diseases such as cancer, diabetes, epilepsy, and muscular dystrophy; those interested in safeguarding specific organs such as the heart, or functions of the body, like prevention of blindness; and those concerned with the health of special groups such as children or the aged.

The major functions of the voluntary health agencies include health education, exploring new fields of activity for research, demonstrating new ways of carrying out health programs, supporting health legislation, and assisting the local health department where necessary.

Examples of direct services provided by these agencies are: audiometer tests and speech correction (American Hearing Society); treatment and rehabilitation centers (National Society for Crippled Children); bedside nursing (Visiting Nurse Association); and casefinding by means of chest X-rays and skin test (American Lung Association).

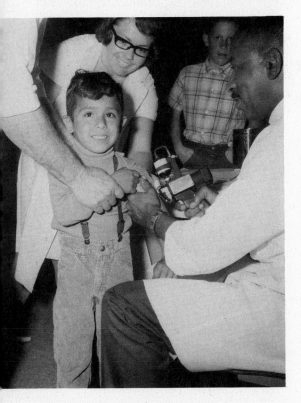

Figure 1-5 ● Your local health department provides many services that protect and maintain your health. What services does your local health department provide?

Private Medical and Dental Care

In your community private physicians and dentists are also concerned with your health. They help you and your family take care of your medical and dental needs. When you are not well, they can treat you. In addition, through regular medical and dental checkups, your doctor and dentist can help you prevent health problems from developing. Or, if a problem is found, they can treat it early and prevent more serious complications.

Industry and Labor

Industry and labor are very much interested in health and medical programs. The growth of health and welfare plans is one of the most significant developments in the promotion of community health in recent years. Both industry and labor are concerned with the healthy worker as an individual and as an important part of commerce.

Working together, management and labor have developed many industrial or occupational health programs. Some programs instituted by industry are in the field of preventive medicine. For example, chest X-rays, blood tests for diabetes, and flu shots are administered on company time and by company medical and nursing personnel. In many large firms, two nurses are always on duty, a physician comes in regularly to take care of sick employees, and there is an arrangement with a nearby hospital to handle on-the-job accidents. Many firms pay all or part of health-insurance plans for employees (Blue Cross, Blue Shield, Major Medical). Some industries have complete medical plans. Some unions have health plans that include complete medical-dental care, with diagnostic tests and other services.

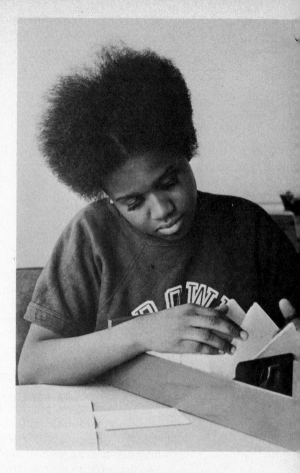

Figure 1-6 ● Voluntary health agencies provide services, education, and research for the protection and maintenance of your health.

Local Service Organizations

In many communities, service organizations such as Rotary, Lions, and Kiwanis include special health programs in their charitable work. Many other organizations, including parent-teacher associations and church groups, do the same. Under such programs eyeglasses, dental care, and other aids are provided to needy children and others.

Solving Personal Health Problems

This text is designed to help you solve critical health problems. Information about physiology, anatomy, and research findings

is included only to the extent that it helps in solving these problems. Try to understand the factors that influence your health. You can start by asking yourself such questions as:

■ Will I be able to accept myself for what I am?

■ How will I relate to others and adjust to the problems of everyday living?

■ How do my growth and development affect my well-being?

■ What types of food will I eat?

- In what kinds of physical activity will I engage?
- What will be my decision regarding cigarette smoking, the use of alcohol, and drugs?
- What action will I take to prevent or control communicable and chronic diseases?

- What action will I take to help my community solve such environmental health hazards as air pollution, water pollution, noise pollution, and radiation exposure?
- How will I prevent accidents?
- How will I utilize available medical, dental, and other health-related services and products?

Summary

As you consider specific health problems, try to think of the emotional and social implications of what might appear to be purely physical problems. For example, dental neglect may result in decayed and unsightly teeth which in turn may affect an individual's appearance. As a result, it might be more difficult for this person to make and keep friends or hold a job. This in turn can have a detrimental effect on this person's mental health.

There is no simple, magic formula that will ensure good health. Misconceptions have led people to try to solve health problems by treating symptoms rather than by getting at the underlying cause. In obesity control, for example, people have gone on crash diets rather than trying to understand their reasons for overeating. As a result, when they discontinue the diet, their weight problem returns. In addition, other health problems may have resulted from inadequate nutrition during the crash diet.

In other situations, the "magic formula" misconception has led to overemphasis of a specific practice as the solution to health problems. For example, there are those who believe that physical exercise or a particular type of food or vitamin supplement is all that is needed for good health. These individuals fail to recognize other factors, good or bad, that have a bearing on health. Health is dynamic. It is ever-changing. There is no simple formula that you can use to cope with the many forces affecting health.

Each chapter in this text is designed to help you determine the most significant health concepts that will enable you to function to your full potential effectively and productively. **These important concepts are highlighted throughout this text as in this sentence.** As a health-educated individual, you will be better equipped to evaluate health information. You will be able to discriminate between fact and fancy. You will be better qualified to avoid misconceptions that might lead you to make incorrect decisions concerning your health.

You can learn how to live healthfully and effectively. To do this, however, you must put into practice what you learn.

in making health decisions . . .

Understand These Terms:

biochemical factors	interrelated factors
concept	miasma theory
ecology	misconception
hazard	mysticism
health	physical environment
inherited endowment	social environment

Solve This Problem:

Assume you are the head of your household and are responsible for the health of the members of your family. What are some of the decisions you will have to make? Where might you find assistance?

Try These Activities:

1. Find out what agencies and organizations are working toward improving the health of your community.

2. Study the factors and conditions that influence your health (listed on Page 5). Evaluate your personal health on each of these points. Where do you excel? Where do you need improvement? How can you strengthen those areas in which you are weak?

3. In a class discussion, select two health authorities in your community (doctor, dentist, nurse, public-health worker, sanitarian, hospital administrator, etc.) and ask them what they think will be the major health problems in the 21st century. Try to get a variety of interviewees. In class, compare your findings with those of other students and be prepared to discuss them.

Interpret These Concepts:

1. Health is more than the absence of disease or infirmity.

2. People function in a physical, ecologic, and social environment.

3. You can influence your health by the decisions you make and the actions you take.

4. Many organizations at the national, state, and local levels help to protect your health and the health of your community.

Explore These Readings:

Brown, D., "Stories Behind Medicine's Most Dramatic Advances," *Today's Health,* 51:18–23 (April, 1973).

Furlong, W. B., "You and Your Dangerous Health Practices," *Today's Health,* 50:54–58 (October, 1972).

"Ignorance About Health," *Time,* 99:67 (Jan. 17, 1972).

Salk, Jonas, "What Do We Mean By Health?" *Journal of School Health,* 42:582–584 (December, 1972).

"Victories in an Endless War," *Story of Life,* Part I. London, England: Marshall Cavendish, Ltd., 1970, pp. 20–23.

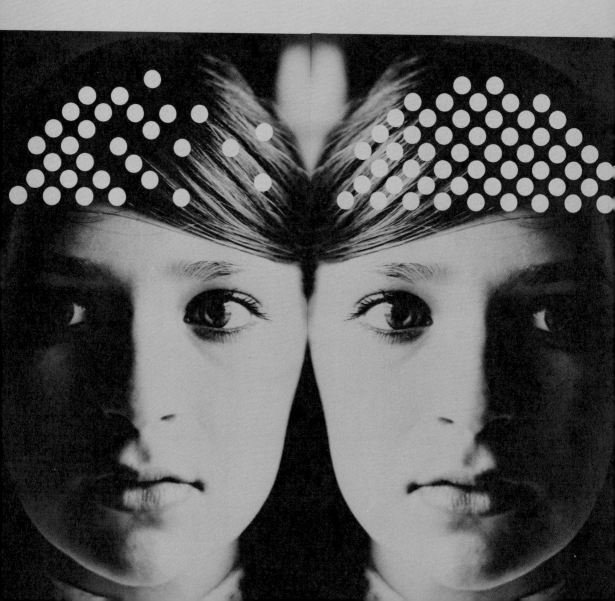

Two | Promoting Your Mental Health

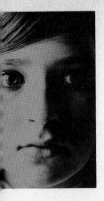

It seems that people have always searched for their "Shangri-La"—their peace of mind or good mental health. This has been an elusive target, for it is difficult to determine just what is good mental health. In addition, what we term mental health is influenced by many factors. Indeed, all that influences behavior influences mental health.

An individual's behavior is motivated in one way or another by the individual's needs. These needs may be biological, environmental, social, or emotional. People tend to behave the way they do in an attempt to satisfy their needs.

Individuals vary in their ability to adjust and adapt to life situations. Most people, however, satisfy their needs in socially acceptable ways. Poorly adjusted individuals also attempt to meet their needs, but their behavior frequently is not socially acceptable. Those who exhibit behavior that is not socially acceptable are often called abnormal or maladjusted.

Making a distinction between acceptable and unacceptable behavior is not a simple procedure. There is no universally accepted definition of normal behavior. Whether certain behavior is considered normal or acceptable depends upon the society in which one lives. Behavior that is acceptable in one society may not be acceptable in another. The following example illustrates this: Suppose you lived in a society in which the accepted behavior includes generosity and trust. If you showed characteristics of selfishness and distrust, you would be considered abnormal. However, if you moved to a society in which selfishness and distrust were the acceptable forms of behavior, as they are in some primitive cultures, you would be considered normal. The behavior of the individual does not change, but the expectations of the two societies are different.

It is easier to distinguish between normal and abnormal behavior in a small, primitive society in which behavior is more nearly homogeneous (uniform) than in a complex, heterogeneous (diverse) society such as ours. In our society, a wide range of behavior is both normal and acceptable. As a result, the process of defining good mental health becomes quite a bit more difficult.

Characteristics of Good Mental Health

Individuals who have good mental health exhibit some common characteristics. The characteristics of good mental health that are generally accepted in our society include understanding and liking one's self, understanding and getting along with others, and meeting the ordinary demands of everyday living.

Understanding and Liking One's Self

Take a close and honest look at yourself. Do you like what you see? Understanding and liking yourself means that you understand and accept both your strengths and your limitations. You recognize that you have emotions and use them appropriately. You have what psychiatrists call a healthy self-concept. This means that you do not belittle yourself or worry unnecessarily about your behavior, emotional balance, or physical well-being. You have self-respect and a sense of personal worth.

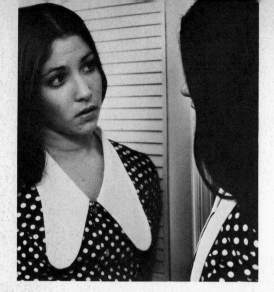

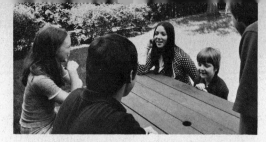

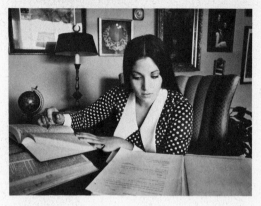

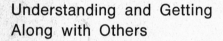
Figure 2-1 • Characteristics of good mental health. How do you measure up? (1) Understanding yourself. (2) Getting along with others. (3) Meeting the demands of daily living.

Understanding and Getting Along with Others

Getting along with others means that you understand and accept people for what they are. They need not be exactly like you. Their point of view and their behavior may be different from yours. Your ability to accept these differences and to establish relationships that are satisfying and lasting reflects how well you will get along with others.

Meeting the Demands of Daily Living

If you are able to meet the demands of daily living in a socially acceptable way, this is a good indication that you adjust to most situations as they arise. This type of adjustment also suggests that you get pleasure from everyday simple things. While special events increase your enjoyment of life, they do not have to take place every day.

Factors Influencing Mental Health

If you are to develop an understanding of your own mental health, it is important that you understand why you behave the way you do. Perhaps you can gain this understanding by reviewing the various factors that influence behavior and mental health.

Biological Factors

Biological factors influence one's mental health. Your cell structure, internal chemistry, and nervous system influence your reaction to stimuli in a particular way. Some experts feel that abnormal biochemical reactions are a basis for maladjusted behavior. That is, individuals may not adjust to a situation, or may act in a way that is not acceptable to society because certain chemicals manufactured in their body cause them to perceive their environment in a way quite different from the way others

Cell Structure

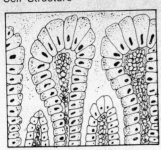

Environmental Factors

Housing

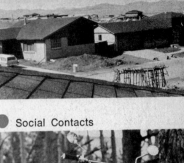

Biological Factors

Nervous System

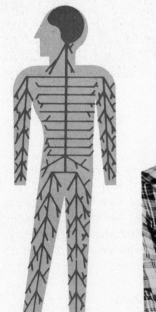

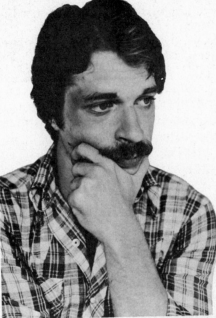

Social Contacts

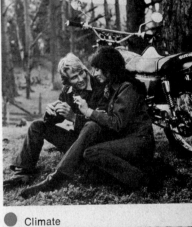

Climate

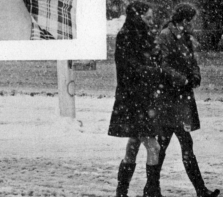

Biochemistry

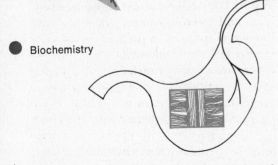

Figure 2-2 ● Factors that influence mental health.

perceive it. Other experts feel that one's environment causes changes in biochemical reactions which in turn affect behavior.

Much more research on the exact relationship between behavior and biochemistry is needed. Some relationship is known to exist. What is not clear is whether biochemical reactions cause behavior changes or behavior changes bring about biochemical changes, or both.

A person's appearance also affects behavior. Being very short or very tall, or being slight of build or obese may cause some individuals to feel different from others. In an attempt to compensate for their feelings, they tend to behave in ways that bring them into conflict with others. For instance, some short persons try to overcome their feelings of inferiority by being critical and domineering. People who are extremely tall for their age may become overly self-conscious around others and develop a stooped posture in an attempt to hide their height.

As you go through various stages of growth, you will experience certain chemical changes accompanied by moods of depression or exhilaration. Knowing that others have these same changes should help you to understand that many of your feelings are perfectly normal and are common to all.

Environmental Factors

The environment in which we live helps determine our mental health. Environmental factors may be classified as physical and social.

Physical Environment. The physical environment in which you live includes the air you breathe; the climate; the buildings in which you work, live, and play; the traffic in which you drive. All may have an effect on your behavior. Recent studies have shown that people driving during heavy traffic hours had an increase in pulse rate

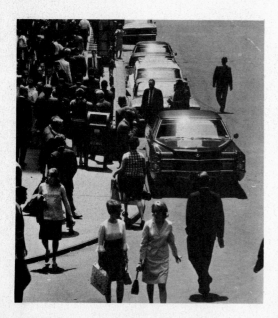

Figure 2-3 • Physical environment affects mental health.

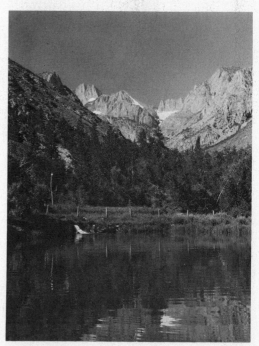

and blood pressure. This was due to increased production of adrenalin, a hormone produced in times of stress. Feelings of anxiety and apprehension were also noted. Other studies have shown that seeing something frightening can also trigger an increased secretion of adrenalin. This can cause a person to become distraught, emotional, panicky, or hysterical. Some people can adjust to changing environments more readily than others can.

Colors also affect the emotions of people in various ways. For some people, some shades of red and orange may cause uneasy and uncomfortable feelings; soft shades of blue and green may cause a peaceful feeling.

Crowded conditions and the fast pace of living in cities may also be related to emotional stress and poor mental health. Conversely, the serenity of the country or mountains may be conducive to good mental health. However, you should be cautious about making sweeping generalizations regarding physical environment and behavior. Some persons, for instance, might enjoy the city and thrive on the fast living pace. These persons might be very unhappy in the quiet of the country. Others might feel quite frustrated in the city and prefer rural life.

Foods eaten might also be considered an environmental factor influencing mental health. The nutrients derived from foods have a definite bearing on personality and behavior. Nutritional deficiencies can cause neurological disorders, irritability, weakness, and general poor health. Overeating can cause obesity, which in turn can bring about feelings of inferiority. On the other hand, overeating or not eating can be the direct result of unsatisfied emotional needs.

Social Environment. Social environment refers to your interactions with other people. You are a social being. The kind of behavior you exhibit is primarily learned from your contacts with other people. These contacts or social forces begin to affect you quite

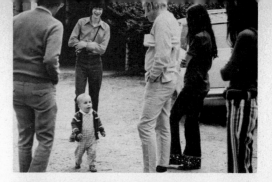

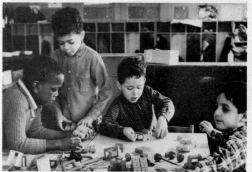

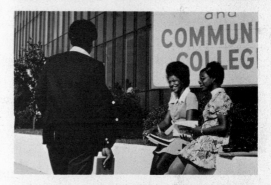

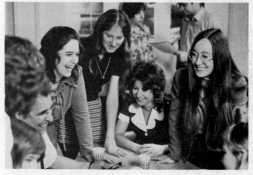

Figure 2-4 ● Your social contacts affect your mental health from infancy to adulthood. (1) Infancy. (2) At play. (3) With friends. (4) At work. Do you find social activities enjoyable and stimulating?

early in life. In early infancy, you are aware of only yourself. You are concerned with meeting your own needs. Very soon, however, you notice others. They react to you, and you react to them, and the process of learning behavior begins.

The love that individuals receive or do not receive from parents or other members of the family is thought to have a profound influence on their mental health as children and as adults. Other factors that may have a lasting influence on mental health are the ways in which punishment is given, how toilet training is achieved, and how physical needs of thirst and hunger are met. The degree to which children are allowed

to experiment and explore affects their behavior and the development of their personalities.

As the individuals grow, they begin to relate to people outside their family. Their earlier experiences within the family and their physical and biological makeup may help or hinder them as they try to establish these new relationships.

Gradually, individuals feel the need to try things on their own. They still need the security of the family, yet at times they need to act independently. Too many restrictions can completely thwart the individual and stifle initiative. However, too much independence without any restric-

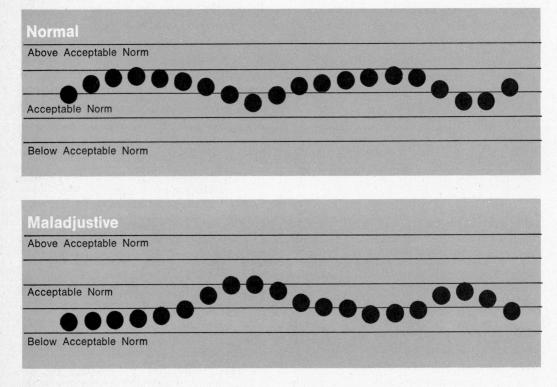

Figure 2-5 ● Difference between normal and maladjustive behavior patterns. The top drawing illustrates normal behavior. Note that normal persons are generally at or above the norm line in acceptable behavior, but occasionally show poor adjustment to stress. The lower drawing illustrates maladjustive behavior. Maladjusted persons generally display behavior below the accepted norm. However, they will occasionally respond to stress normally.

tions can create anxiety. Most people need the security of certain rules and limitations. The problem faced by most parents and their children is how to establish a proper balance between dependence and independence. Some parents find it difficult to let their children have more freedom. This may be a reflection of their own insecurity and fear of losing their loved ones.

As people mature, they begin to participate more in the social interaction of the community. Their behavior will continue to be influenced by their previous experiences of social interaction, their biological makeup, their physical appearance, and their physical environment. No one factor can be singled out as being more important than the others. **The interaction between biological and environmental factors influences one's mental health.**

Tensions and How to Deal with Them

Stress, an unavoidable product of our culture, can be either productive or detrimental. Stress and tension are not all bad. A certain amount is desirable and necessary. It is important, however, to distinguish between normal and chronic tension.

Normal Tension

All through your life, you can expect to have tensions. You should learn to live with them because they are a part of everyday life. Tensions are stimulating. They act as motivating forces. If the tension and stress are not overwhelming, they help you function at a higher level of efficiency. If you do not have any tension or stress, you are not reacting to the world around you. You tend to become complacent, listless, and unmotivated.

Feeling a little nervous from time to time or getting nervous or excited at a football game or some other occasion is perfectly normal. The ability to get nervous and excited, to feel and have emotions is what makes life worth living.

Chronic Tensions

Too much of anything can be harmful. Chronic tension, or tension that lasts for an extended period of time, can incapacitate, immobilize, or destroy you. It can make you ineffective in carrying out the simple tasks of everyday living. Continued or excessive nervousness, worry, and anxiety can take all the joy out of life.

Whether your tension is normal or chronic, your body initially reacts in the same way. Your brain interprets the stimuli it gets from the tension or stress and prepares your body to respond. Physiological responses that may occur include an increase in pulse, respiration, and blood sugar. Many other responses may also take place. Each response is normal and essential. Every response is preparing you to take action. More blood is being sent to the vital organs and muscles, and your intake of oxygen is increased.

As the physiological changes occur, they give rise to certain sensations or feelings. You might feel flushed when you are asked to make a presentation or when you are put in an embarrassing position. This is because of dilation of blood vessels. During moments of anger or stress, you might tremble. This is because of increased muscle tension. You might feel nauseated or might have the sensation of butterflies in the stomach before an athletic contest or a performance. This is due to changes that occur in the digestive tract. In these or in other situations you may suddenly become aware of your heart beating rapidly. You may feel as though there were a lump in your throat or your mouth may become very dry.

All these responses are normal. You probably have experienced them at one time or another. However, when you are suffering from chronic tension, there is a distinct difference. The same nervous and physiological responses take place, but they last longer. Your body does not have a chance to recuperate. As a result, there is a constant pressure on the various systems and organs of your body.

The stimuli causing chronic tension usually come from anxieties which involve a dread of the unknown or a fear of the future. The resulting uncertainty brings about a constant bombardment of the nervous system and the brain. This in turn causes prolonged adrenal gland activity, which in turn increases the duration of the physiological changes. The sensations and feelings that you have during these physiological changes sometimes add "fuel to the fire." Continued rapid pulse, indigestion, or a lump in the throat may give rise to further worry and anxiety and thus become an additional stimulus triggering more physical symptoms.

Chronic tension, if not checked or prevented, can incapacitate you. The emotional trauma may make you less alert as you become preoccupied with your anxiety. Continuous physiologic reactions to your anxiety may also bring about organic dis-

Possible Physiological Results of Tension

Normal (Temporary)	Chronic (Prolonged)
nausea	nausea
elevated blood pressure	hypertension
indigestion	colitis
headaches	migraine headaches
increased pulse rate	persistent rapid pulse
difficulty in swallowing	inability to swallow
poor appetite	loss of appetite
difficulty in sleeping	insomnia
muscle tremors	fatigue
lightheadedness	frequent dizziness
stomach spasms	ulcers
cold, clammy skin	
pale or flushed face	

Note the similarity of responses to normal and chronic tension. However, the results of chronic tension are prolonged and much more severe, and can incapacitate.

orders, such as high blood pressure, colitis (inflamation of the colon), ulcers, or migraine headaches. These physical disorders very often are the effect of the mind on the body. When such is the case, they are referred to as psychosomatic conditions (*psyche,* mind; *soma,* body). Other symptoms that indicate chronic tension include dizziness due to hyperventilation (forcing out too much carbon dioxide), weakness or numbness of the extremities, fatigue, light-headedness, and nausea.

Dealing with Tensions

You can handle your tensions so that they do not become chronic and incapacitating. The following measures have been suggested by George S. Stevenson, M.D., in the pamphlet, *How To Deal With Your Tensions,* published by the National Association for Mental Health.

- **Talk it out.** When something worries you, talk it out. Do not bottle it up. Confide your worry to some levelheaded person you can trust; your . . . father or mother, a good friend, your clergyman, your family doctor, a teacher, school counselor, or dean. Talking things out helps to relieve your strain, helps you to see your worry in a clearer light, and often helps you to see what you can do about it.

- **Escape for a while.** Sometimes, when things go wrong, it helps to escape from the painful problem for a while: to lose yourself in a movie or a book or a game or a brief trip for a change of scene. Making yourself "stand there and suffer" is a form of self-punishment, not a way to solve a problem. It is perfectly realistic and healthy to escape punishment long enough to recover breath and balance. But be pre-

pared to come back and deal with your difficulty when you are more composed, and when you and any others involved in the situation are in better condition to deal with the problem and solve it.

- **Work off your anger.** If you feel yourself using anger as a general way of behavior, remember that while anger may give you a temporary sense of righteousness, or even of power, it will generally leave you feeling foolish and sorry in the end. If you feel like lashing out at someone who has provoked you, try holding off that impulse for a while. Let it wait until tomorrow. Meanwhile, do something constructive with the pent-up energy. Pitch into some physical activity like gardening, cleaning out the garage, carpentry or some other do-it-yourself project. Or work it out in tennis or a long walk. Working the anger out of your system and cooling it off for a day or two will leave you much better prepared to handle your problem.

- **Give in occasionally.** If you find yourself getting into frequent quarrels with people, and feeling obstinate and defiant, remember that that's the way frustrated children behave. Stand your ground on what you know is right, but do so calmly and make allowance for the fact that you could turn out to be wrong. And even if you're dead right, it's easier on your system to give in once in a while. If you yield, you'll usually find that others will, too. And if you can work this out, the result will be relief from tension, the achievement of a practical solution, together with a great feeling of satisfaction and maturity.

- **Do something for others.** If you feel yourself worrying about yourself all the time, try doing something for somebody else. You'll find this will take the steam out of your own worries and—even better—give you a fine feeling of having done well.

■ **Take one thing at a time.** For people under tension, an ordinary work load can sometimes seem unbearable. The load looks so great that it becomes painful to tackle any part of it—even the things that most need to be done. When that happens, remember that it's a temporary condition and that you can work your way out of it. The surest way to do this is to take a few of the most urgent tasks and pitch into them, one at a time, setting aside all the rest for the time being. Once you dispose of these you'll see that the remainder is not such a "horrible mess" after all. You'll be in the swing of things, and the rest of the tasks will go much more easily. If you feel you can't set anything aside to tackle things this sensible way, reflect; are you sure you aren't overestimating the importance of the things you do—that is, your own importance?

■ **Shun the "Superman" urge.** Some people expect too much from themselves, and get into a constant state of worry and anxiety because they think they are not achieving as much as they should. They try for perfection in everything. Admirable as this ideal is, it is an open invitation to failure. No one can be perfect in everything. Decide which things you do well, and then put your major effort into these. They are apt to be the things you like to do, and hence those that give you most satisfaction. Then, perhaps, come the things you can't do so well. Give them the best of your effort and ability, but don't take yourself to task if you can't achieve the impossible.

■ **Go easy with your criticism.** Some people expect too much of others, and then feel frustrated, let down, disappointed, even "trapped" when another person does not measure up. The "other person" may be a wife, a husband or a child whom we are trying to fit into a preconceived pattern—perhaps even trying to make over to suit ourselves. Remember, people have their own virtues, their own shortcomings, their own values, their own right to develop as individuals. People who feel let down by the shortcomings (real or imagined) of their relatives, are really let down about themselves. Instead of being critical about the other person's behavior, search out the good points and help to develop them. This will give both of you satisfaction, and help you to gain a better perspective on yourself as well.

■ **Give the other fellow a break.** When people are under emotional tension they often feel that they have to "get there first"—to edge out the other person, no matter if the goal is as trivial as getting ahead on the highway. If enough of us feel that way—and many of us do—then everything becomes a race in which somebody is bound to get injured —physically, as on the highway, or emotionally and mentally, in the endeavor to live a full life. It need not be this way. Competition is contagious, but so is cooperation. When you give other people a break, you very often make things easier for yourself; if they no longer feel you are a threat to them, they stop being a threat to you.

■ **Make yourself "available."** Many of us have the feeling that we are being "left out," slighted, neglected, rejected. Often, we just imagine that other people feel this way about us, when in reality they are eager for us to make the first move. It may be we, not the others, who are depreciating ourselves. Instead of shrinking away and withdrawing, it is much healthier, as well as more practical, to continue to "make yourself available"—to make some of the overtures instead of always waiting to be asked. Of course, the opposite of withdrawal is equally futile: to push yourself forward on every occasion. This is often misinterpreted and may lead to real rejection. There is a middle ground. Try it.

- **Schedule your recreation.** Many people drive themselves so hard that they allow themselves too little time for recreation—an essential for good physical and mental health. They find it hard to make themselves take time out. For such people a set routine and schedule will help—a program of definite hours when they will engage in some recreation. And in general it is desirable for people to have a hobby that absorbs them in off hours—one into which they can throw themselves completely and with pleasure, forgetting all about their work.

Adjustment Mechanisms

Individuals vary in their ability to adjust to the demands of daily living. Adjustment mechanisms (escape mechanisms, safety valves) are used by everyone to help them handle the tensions and problems of everyday living. These mechanisms help people make temporary adjustments to situations that might threaten their security. They help people save face and preserve their self-image. A description of some of these adjustment mechanisms follows.

Fantasy

Fantasy is a means of escaping from reality by daydreaming. In your fantasies, you can do anything you want to do or be anyone you want to be. You can achieve imaginary goals and desires. To a point fantasy is beneficial and even constructive. But, when you use it continuously instead of facing reality, fantasy can be harmful.

Regression

Regression means reverting to childish behavior. The individual is seeking the security of the past. Examples of this mechanism in operation are a boy having a temper tantrum, a girl weeping so that she will get her way, or people pouting if they do not get what they want. Psychiatrists tell us that the person who uses this mechanism is trying to apply old solutions to present problems.

Repression

Repression is a means of pushing unpleasant memories into the subconscious. This is an important mechanism because it helps people control desires and feelings that might be socially unacceptable. It minimizes painful thoughts or experiences. Repression is a process of selective forgetting. It may be harmful when it is overused or when it keeps people from facing problems they should deal with in a realistic fashion. Repressed thoughts may show themselves in dreams, slips of the tongue, or amnesia (loss of memory).

Rationalization

Rationalization is finding reasons or explanations to justify one's behavior. It is a means of lessening the disappointment when people cannot achieve what they desire. In a sense, it is a preservation of self-image by means of self-deception. A person who fails to get a much-sought-after job might rationalize the failure by saying that the new job is not desirable after all because the chances for promotion are very slight. By rationalizing, the individual saves face. This makes up for the shortcomings.

Projection

Projection involves trying to blame others for our shortcomings or guilt feelings. The mechanism is similar to rationalization in that the individual wants to save face, does not want to admit failure. It differs in that the individual uses explanations that are not reasonable or logical. An individual may blame a teacher for the failure to pass an examination, hiding the fact of not studying. The use of projection as a defense mechanism can be very helpful in solving guilt feelings. When carried to an extreme, it can be a sign of emotional disturbance.

Identification

Identification is a form of hero worship. It is an attempt to improve one's self-worth by identifying with persons or institutions that represent ideal qualities. People who idolize a television star or an athlete and see themselves as having the same attributes are using identification. Most people use this mechanism at one time or another.

However, excessive or exaggerated use of identification to escape reality or to overcome one's own weakness may result in a loss of personal identity. Thus individuals who cannot adjust properly may escape reality by "becoming" the person with whom they have identified.

Compensation

Compensation is a means of reducing feelings of inferiority by emphasizing desirable traits. The individual compensates for an apparent weakness by developing another skill or by working harder on the area of weakness. For example, the individual who is not intellectually brilliant may make up for this by studying harder. The girl who has paralyzed legs may develop gymnastic skills that require the use of her arms rather than her legs. Compensation that leads to strong motivation in achievement is adjustive. When such motivation leads to increased anxiety, it may be harmful.

Substitution

Substitution is very similar to compensation. It is a means of capitalizing on one's strengths. A young man who desires to be an athlete, but lacks the necessary attributes, may capitalize on his writing ability and become a sportswriter.

Everyone uses adjustment mechanisms to a certain degree. This is considered normal behavior. When a person depends on these mechanisms too much, rather than facing the realities of life, the person may be considered maladjusted.

Fantasy or daydreaming, for example, is a perfectly normal and beneficial means of temporarily escaping unpleasant tasks or duties. Daydreaming also enables a person to reflect on past experiences and to plan for the future. It provides some people with an outlet for creative imagination. However, when people are always in a dream or fantasy world, they are protecting themselves, but in a maladjustive way. In this dream world they are neither functional nor productive individuals. Overuse or overdependency on any one of the adjustive mechanisms can be a sign or cause of maladjustive behavior. It is not the mechanisms themselves, but the extent to which they are used that makes them adjustive or maladjustive.

Maladjustive Behavior

Some authorities feel that the traditional classification of mental illness into categories such as psychoses and neuroses is artificial and unwarranted. They have replaced these categories with broader concepts such as "irresponsible behavior" or "maladjustive behavior."

While maladjustive behavior is briefly discussed here, a more extensive discussion of the traditional classification of mental illness is given in Chapter 12.

Maladjustive behavior varies in its impact on the individual and society. It manifests itself in a variety of ways. Individuals who cannot adjust may take refuge in an imaginary world. They will overuse the adjustment mechanism of fantasy to escape the problems of daily living. They may become another personality, a "Napoleon" or a "god." Others may be so obsessed with their own guilt feelings that they use projection in its extreme form to salvage their self-image. Others rather than they are the culprits. In their minds, everyone may be against them, and as a result, they may be suspicious of everyone.

Others may display their maladjustive behavior by reacting to an excessive fear (phobia) of places or things. Some individuals are able to learn to control this fear so that it does not rule their life. Others are so overwhelmed that their behavior is converted into a physical abnormality such as inability to see, or hear, or talk, or move certain parts of the body. This is called conversion hysteria.

There is a very real difference between conversion hysteria and psychosomatic illness. You will recall from the discussion of chronic tensions that psychosomatic illnesses are true physical illnesses that are triggered by mental situations or moods or aggravated by emotions. The body actually undergoes a functional change. Conversion hysteria is also related to mental and emotional situations, but is without actual physical disorder. In other words, there is a mental block.

Illustrations of maladjustive behavior are unending. It is important to remember that such behavior can stem from a variety of factors and take on many forms. Understanding this can help you comprehend your own behavior as well as the behavior of others.

Qualified help is available for those with maladjustive behavior. It is important for you to understand that behavioral problems are not a disgrace and that they can happen to anyone. It is necessary, however, to get help when it is appropriate. Whenever you feel that you cannot adjust to the problems of daily living, seek the advice of your parents, school nurse, counselor, religious leader, or family physician. If these people cannot help you sufficiently, you may need the services of a psychologist (a scientist who has studied the mind and the way people behave) or a psychiatrist (a medical doctor who specializes in the treatment of mental ill health).

Summary

Mental health is an integral part of total health. They cannot be separated. Your mental health can be affected by the foods you eat, and in turn your eating habits may be a means of satisfying emotional needs.

Good mental health is essential to making satisfying and mature adjustments. The decisions you make about smoking, drinking, and the use of drugs are related to your mental well-being. These decisions must be made carefully. You must consider their impact upon your physical and mental well-being as well as your social relationships.

The ability to handle tensions can have profound effects on your physical and mental health. Psychosomatic conditions resulting from an inability to handle tensions can result in heart and circulatory disorders, digestive disorders, and endocrine imbalances. Mental health and physical health are interrelated.

You should understand the characteristics and influencing factors of good mental health. It is important for you to understand the causes of tensions and how to deal with them. In this way, you will be able to gain insight into your own behavior and the behavior of those around you. Through this understanding, you should be able to improve and maintain your own mental health.

in making health decisions . . .

Understand These Terms:

adjustment mechanisms
chronic tension
maladjustive behavior
mental health

psychosomatic
social environment
stress

Solve This Problem:

From time to time everyone has a problem to adjust to or solve. Identify a problem that is troublesome to you. See whether you can solve this problem by doing the following:

1. Make a list of advantages or assets you have to help solve the problem.
2. Make a list of obstacles that make it difficult to solve the problem.
3. Make a list of possible solutions or courses of action you can take to help solve the problem.
4. Now choose a course of action that is most appropriate for you.

Try These Activities:

1. Write a paper entitled "How Do I Stack Up?" In this paper describe your assets and liabilities. Then indicate how you think you can make the most of your assets and minimize your liabilities. In writing the paper you may want to seek the advice of parents, friends, or others.

2. Make a list of the biological and environmental factors that have influenced your mental health and personality. Indicate which of these factors you can alter.

3. Survey your community to determine what mental-health facilities and services are available. In class, be prepared to discuss whether such services are adequate and what improvements might be made.

Interpret These Concepts:

1. Individuals who have good mental health exhibit some common characteristics.

2. The interaction between biological and environmental factors influences one's mental health.

3. Stress, an unavoidable product of our culture, can be either productive or detrimental.

4. Individuals vary in their ability to adjust to the demands of daily living.

Explore These Readings:

"Answers to Anxiety," *Story of Life,* Part I. London, England: Marshall Cavendish, Ltd., 1970, pp. 16–19.

Connant, M. M., "Learning to Be a Boy, a Girl, or a Person," *P.T.A. Magazine,* 66:18–21, 32 (March, 1972).

Gaylin, Willard, "What's Normal?" *New York Times Magazine,* VI:14–15 (Apr. 1, 1973).

Mead, Margaret, "Mental Health in Our Changing Culture," *Mental Hygiene,* 56:6–8 (Summer, 1972).

Safran, Claire, "How Some Busy People Let Off Steam: Relieving Tensions," *Today's Health,* 51:26–30 (February, 1973).

Three | Growing Toward Maturity

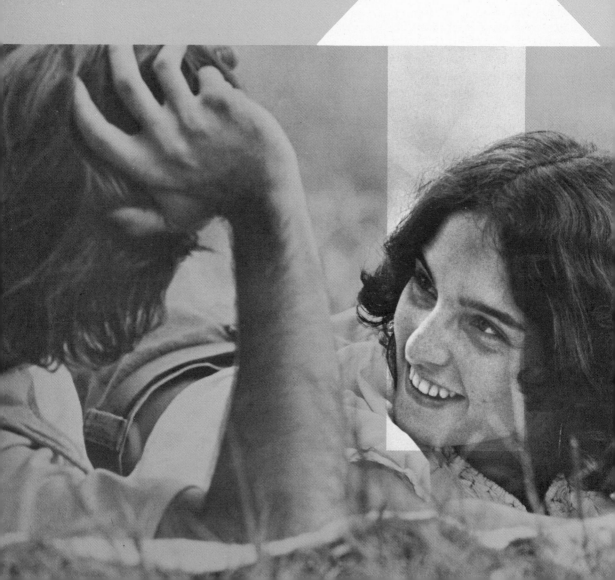

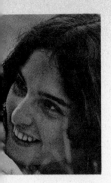

Young adults become increasingly aware of their masculinity and femininity as they grow toward maturity. Masculinity and femininity are not static conditions. They change with age and are determined by biological, emotional, and social factors.

An understanding of masculinity and femininity helps one to define and to fulfill more successfully the male or female role in the process of human life. The successful fulfillment of the male or female role directly reflects the degree to which a person achieves physical, mental, emotional, and social maturity. This chapter discusses important aspects of growing toward maturity.

Growing up means more than merely growing taller and heavier. It is important to recognize that **human development includes physical growth, intellectual advancement, emotional maturity, and social responsibility.** The process is somewhat long and may be different for each individual. It does not necessarily take place in an even, orderly fashion. One individual may have a physical growth spurt, but the other aspects of development may not keep pace with the physical. Another individual may grow in ability to acquire knowledge, but physical growth may be slow.

The word *adult* is often used to indicate a fully "grown" person. This emphasis on size often causes a person to overlook a number of other important factors that are involved in being an adult. As people grow and mature, the different systems in the body become more refined. People develop a greater ability to reason and to solve problems. They learn and acquire socially desirable attitudes and values. Throughout life, this maturation process is reflected in behavior. Each society tends to determine which behavior is appropriate at a particular age level. One of your tasks is to learn what behavior is acceptable where you live.

The youth of today are the parents of tomorrow. You should, therefore, understand the importance of prenatal care, what takes place during the birth process, and the physical and emotional changes that occur during infancy and childhood. In addition, it is important for you to understand the physical and emotional changes that take place during puberty, changes that signal the beginning of adolescence.

Prenatal Development

The growth toward maturity begins prior to birth. Human life starts with the fertilization of an ovum (egg) by a single sperm. The human ovum is so small as to be barely visible to the naked eye. This tiny cell, which measures approximately 1/1000 of an inch, is about 90,000 times larger than a sperm. Yet the ovum and the sperm contribute equal portions to the hereditary blueprint which will govern to a great degree the "growth toward maturity" pattern.

Fertilization

Fertilization of the ovum normally takes place in one of the Fallopian tubes of the female. Once a month, a mature ovum leaves one of the nearby ovaries and starts to travel down the Fallopian tube. If sperm are deposited in the vagina (the passage leading from the uterus to the external surface of the female reproductive system), they will move toward the site at which they are likely to encounter the ovum. When a single sperm enters the ovum, conception takes place and growth and development begin. On the average, a full-term human pregnancy takes approximately 280 days.

Cell Division and Implantation

The fertilized ovum immediately begins a process of cell division. As the dividing cells slowly travel down the Fallopian tube, a membrane forms around these cells. Tiny projections begin to grow. These projections attach the developing ovum to the wall of the uterus. The placenta (the uniting structure between mother and embryo, through which food and waste products are exchanged) will begin to form here. Other membranes also develop around the rapidly multiplying cells. One of the membranes, the amnion, will enclose the cells (the em-

bryo) in a fluid that keeps them moist and helps protect them from injury. Some membranes contribute to the formation of the umbilical cord. The umbilical cord contains blood vessels that connect the embryo with the placenta. There is no direct connection between the mother's blood and the blood of the developing baby. Each circulatory system is separate to itself. The blood vessels of the umbilical cord end in the placenta. They provide the means by which nutrients and oxygen from the mother's blood are made available to the baby. Waste products from the baby are transmitted to the mother's blood in the same way. This exchange is the result of diffusion through a semipermeable membrane. The scientific name for this process is osmosis.

Hereditary Blueprint

Each person grows and matures within the potential of what has been inherited from both parents. All the inherited characteristics are carried in a chain of molecules known as DNA (deoxyribonucleic acid). Thousands of these molecules make up a chromosome. Chromosomes are found in each body cell. The mature germ cell (ovum or sperm) has fewer chromosomes. In the germ cell there are only 23 chromosomes. When the germ cells unite during fertilization, the newly created cell will contain 46 chromosomes. Genes are found within the chromosomal structure along the DNA chain and are the actual carriers of hereditary instruction. One gene may affect many characteristics, and most characteristics may be affected by many genes. The combination of genes determines what a person inherits.

When genes for opposing characteristics are inherited from the two parents,

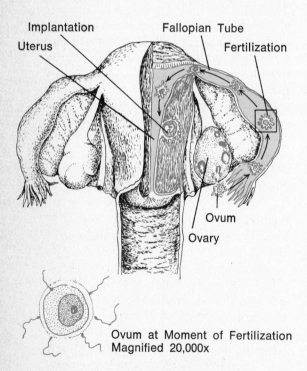

Implantation
Uterus
Fallopian Tube
Fertilization
Ovum
Ovary

Ovum at Moment of Fertilization
Magnified 20,000x

Figure 3-1 • Ovulation, fertilization, and implantation precede the formation of the embryo.

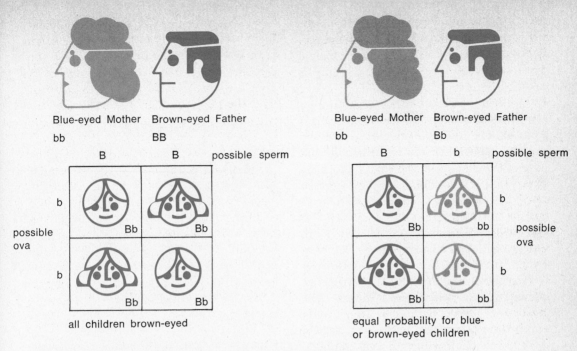

Blue-eyed Mother Brown-eyed Father
bb   BB

B   B   possible sperm

b   Bb   Bb

possible
ova

b   Bb   Bb

all children brown-eyed

Blue-eyed Mother Brown-eyed Father
bb   Bb

B   b   possible sperm

b   Bb   bb

possible
ova

b   Bb   bb

equal probability for blue-
or brown-eyed children

Figure 3-2 ● Results of dominant and recessive gene combinations in producing eye color. Can you explain how you inherited the color of your eyes?

some characteristics are more likely to be present than are others. Genes for these characteristics are known as dominant genes, those for characteristics that are hidden are called recessive genes. For example, in eye color, brown is dominant, blue recessive. If both parents have genes for brown eyes only, all their children will be brown-eyed. If one parent has a recessive gene for blue eyes, all the children will be brown-eyed. If one parent has a recessive gene for blue eyes and the other parent is blue-eyed, there is an equal chance that their children will be blue-eyed or brown-eyed.

Transmission of Characteristics

A basic knowledge of the natural laws which govern a person's hereditary blueprint is helpful in understanding the growth toward maturity.

Of the 23 pairs of chromosomes that form each fertilized egg, one pair is identified as the sex chromosomes. It is this pair that determines the sex of the new individual. There are two types of sex chromosomes, X and Y. Females have only X chromosomes, while males have an X and a Y chromosome. Before fertilization every ovum contains one X chromosome. Every sperm cell has either one X chromosome or one Y chromosome. It is the combination of the X and Y chromosomes that determines whether the fertilized ovum will develop into a boy or a girl.

If the ovum is fertilized by a sperm with the X chromosome, the child will be a female with two X chromosomes in each cell. If the ovum is fertilized by a sperm with the Y chromosome, the child will be a male with an X and a Y chromosome in each cell. From Figure 3–3 it can be seen that the possible fertilization combinations result in a 50 percent probability of the child's being a boy (or a girl). However, for various reasons, this mathematical law does not hold true. The number of male births is usually greater than that of females.

The X-Y chromosomes are also important in determining characteristics such as color blindness. This is referred to as a sex-linked characteristic. It is estimated that approximately 7 to 8 percent of the male population is color-blind for the red-green range of colors. This condition seldom occurs in females.

Sickle cell anemia is an inherited disorder for which no cure has as yet been found. The disease is found primarily among blacks and, to a much lesser degree, among Cubans and Puerto Ricans. The most severe form of the disease occurs when both parents transmit sickle cell anemia genes. Individuals with this gene combination often die in infancy or before reaching adulthood.

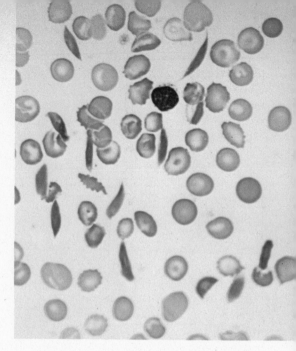

Figure 3-4 ● Sickle cell anemia is characterized by the quarter-moon or sickle-shaped red blood cells.

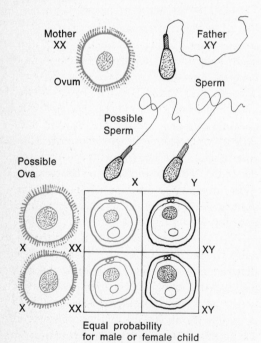

Equal probability
for male or female child

Figure 3-3 ● Results of X and Y chromosome combinations in determining the sex of a baby.

Most persons with only one gene for sickle cell anemia live normal lives. It is estimated that about one in 10 blacks in the United States carries one gene for this disease. If both parents have one gene for this trait, there is a 25 percent chance that their children will be born with a severe form of sickle cell anemia.

Symptoms of this disease include bone, joint, or abdominal pain which may or may not be accompanied by fever. The disease begins to manifest itself when the red blood cells begin to change their shape. The abnormal cells resemble quarter-moons, crescents, or sickles. A mutation in the hemoglobin molecules of the red blood cells is responsible for the change in the shape of the red blood cells. The elongated blood cells clog blood vessels, causing destruction of nearby tissues.

Medical science believes that the immediate solution to this problem depends on early detection by testing, and also on genetic counseling. The testing program requires a sample of blood for a screening procedure that is simple, fast, and painless. Those identified as having characteristics of the disease can be treated and counseled regarding their potential to transmit sickle cell anemia to their children.

Effect of Environment

It is important to realize that **the environment will influence the degree to which some potential characteristics will develop in the individual.** Intelligence is inherited, but the extent to which it grows is influenced by environment and by the manner in which an individual uses or abuses the original potential. Knowledge is acquired. The amount of knowledge a person can acquire is in part related to intelligence. If, however, some people do not use their opportunities to acquire knowledge, then their intelligence is not put to use. If, for example, they do not study, their intelligence will not be used and they will usually get a lower grade. The inheritance of musical ability may be viewed in a similar fashion. If the potential musical ability is not developed, it will lie dormant, despite the fact that it is a part of an individual's hereditary blueprint.

Prenatal Care

It is very important for a pregnant woman to be under the care of a physician during the entire term of pregnancy. The physician will perform a complete physical examination and take her health history, including information about other members of her family. The physician will also be concerned about smoking and excessive eating,

since both may be hazardous during pregnancy. Various tests will help the physician learn whether the pregnancy is proceeding normally or not.

One particular type of blood test is used to determine the Rh factor. The designation *Rh* represents the first two letters in the name of the animal used in early experimental work, the rhesus monkey. Certain Rh combinations may result in health complications that involve the destruction of red blood cells in the baby. It is estimated that about 85 percent of the population is Rh-positive, the remainder being Rh-negative. Since males and females are found in both groups, the following combinations may be observed in marriage partners:

Female		Male
Rh+	$\times$	Rh+
Rh+	$\times$	Rh—
Rh—	$\times$	Rh+
Rh—	$\times$	Rh—

The only combination that is potentially hazardous is the Rh-negative female married to the Rh-positive male. If their child inherits the Rh-positive blood of the father, a sequence of events may be set in motion that could cause damage to the future embryo. What can occur is this: The Rh substance in the child may pass across the placenta into the blood of the mother. This causes the production of antibodies to destroy the substance. Usually not enough antibodies are produced to harm the first child, but when the mother has children at a later date, the antibodies may cross the placenta into the embryo and begin destroying its red blood cells. This can occur only if the baby is Rh-positive. Each successive pregnancy with an Rh-positive baby, where the antibodies have developed, increases the possibility of damage to the developing child.

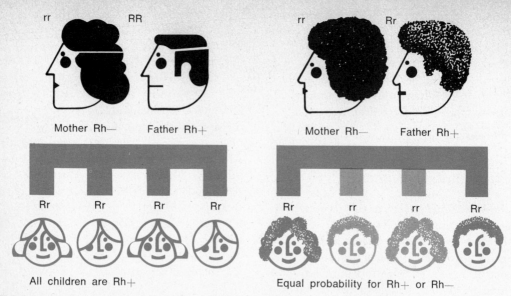

rr   RR   rr   Rr

Mother Rh—   Father Rh+   Mother Rh—   Father Rh+

Rr   Rr   Rr   Rr   Rr   rr   rr   Rr

All children are Rh+   Equal probability for Rh+ or Rh—

Figure 3-5 • The probability of an Rh+ father producing an Rh+ child when the mother is Rh— depends on the gene combination of the father. (a) All children are Rh+. (b) Equal probability for Rh+ or Rh—.

During pregnancy physicians carefully analyze and watch the antibody production level of the mother's blood if she is Rh-negative and her husband is Rh-positive. If a child is born with this condition, a correction can be made in most cases by transfusions of Rh-negative blood, replacing the entire original blood supply of the infant. In recent years, medical science has even been successful in transfusing the blood of the baby while it is still developing in the uterus. Research on vaccines may provide a way of immunizing the mother so that her system will not attack the red blood cells of her children.

The Birth Process

Human reproduction is a normal physiological process. While gestation (pregnancy) takes approximately 280 days, there is no way in which the date of birth can be exactly predicted.

Labor

The birth process begins with contractions of muscles in the uterine walls. These "labor pains" are relatively infrequent at first, but recur at closer and closer intervals as the birth process continues. At some point during labor, the membrane holding the embryo in fluid ruptures and releases the fluid (amniotic fluid). This now serves as a lubricant to aid in the birth process.

Delivery

Continued contractions of the uterus gradually force the baby out of the uterus and through the birth canal. The baby is usually born head first. It is still attached to the mother by means of the umbilical cord. This, in turn, is attached to the placenta, which is clinging to the uterine wall.

Under certain circumstances, when the baby is too large to go through the birth

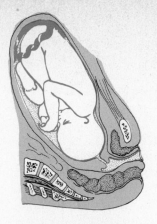

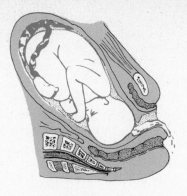

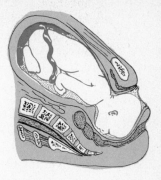

A. Contraction of uterine walls during labor

B. Breaking of the "bag of waters"

C. Dilation of the cervix

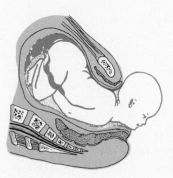

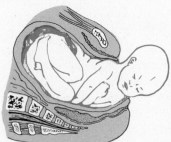

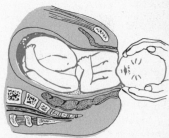

D. Head emerges through birth canal

E. Rotation of body begins

F. Rotation of body continues and baby completes the birth process

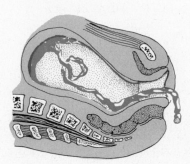

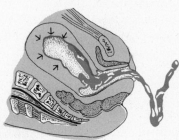

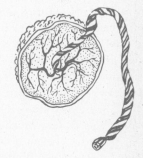

G. Continued uterine contractions start to expel placenta (afterbirth)

H. Afterbirth continues to be expelled

I. Expelled placenta

Figure 3-6

canal, a surgical procedure (Caesarean section) may be used to remove the baby through the abdominal wall. Most births, however, proceed in an orderly way.

When the baby reaches the outside world, its lungs become functional and the umbilical cord is no longer needed to supply oxygen. The cord is carefully tied off and cut, thus separating the baby from the placenta and the maternal tissues. Thus a new life is brought into the world and the cycle of human reproduction continues.

After the birth of the baby, the mother continues to have uterine contractions to expel the placenta (now called the afterbirth).

Multiple Births

Most pregnancies result in the birth of a single baby. However, there are occasions when two or more babies are born at approximately the same time or within a very few hours of each other. The single birth is the result of the fertilization of a single ovum by one sperm, and the development of that ovum into an individual. Identical twins also originate from one ovum fertilized by one sperm. In this case, the process of cell division results in two separate and distinct groups of cells. Both groups of cells continue to develop in the same embryonic sac and utilize the same placenta. Why this type of cell division occurs is not fully understood. Since these twins originate from one ovum fertilized by one sperm, the babies will be either both boys or both girls and will look very much alike.

On extremely rare occasions, the complete process of cell division in the development of identical twins is interrupted. The partially separated groups of cells continue to develop, but are joined together by certain tissues. One of the first reported instances of this type of multiple birth was of Siamese children. For this reason, the term *Siamese twins* is used to describe this rare phenomenon.

On occasion, two ova are fertilized by two different sperm at or about the same time. Each of these twins develops in a separate embryo sac attached to the uterine wall by its own placenta. The twins in this instance can be both of the same sex, or one of each sex. The sex determination of each twin depends entirely upon the individual sperm which functioned in the fertilization process. For this reason, these twins are no more alike and no more different from each other than are other siblings (brothers and sisters). Babies that are the result of this process are called fraternal twins.

Triplets, quadruplets, and quintuplets are the result of various possible combinations of ova fertilization and/or separation of cells during the cleavage process. Instances of multiple birth seem to follow a "rule of thumb" pattern called the "law of 86." Twins are born once in approximately 86 births. Triplets occur once in 86^2 (7,396) births. Quadruplets occur once in approximately 86^3 and quintuplets once in approximately 86^4 births. In recent years, the use of fertility drugs has increased the possibility of multiple births for some women.

Usually multiple births occur more regularly in certain families. When such is the case, we say there is a predisposition toward multiple births in that particular family.

Infancy and Early Childhood

The newborn child enters a period of development referred to as infancy. This period is characterized by complete dependence upon parents to provide those necessities that would best promote the child's total development. In addition to food, warmth, cleanliness, and protection from disease and injury, total development is strongly influenced by love, understanding, and security. Many parents become overly concerned at this time if their child appears to be growing more slowly than their friends' children. It is important to understand that growth is continuous and orderly, but each child has its own individual rate.

The average newborn baby is about 21 inches long and weighs about 7 pounds. Actually, throughout the period of infancy (the first year of life), growth is very rapid. It is not unusual for a child to triple its birth weight during this period.

Infancy is followed by the period of childhood. In addition to growth, a great deal of maturation takes place during this time. There is a constant refinement in the functions of all body systems. This refinement, at times, seems to be relatively slow. However, the child's hereditary blueprint has determined its rate of growth and maturation. There is no "right" or "wrong" time for various abilities to develop. Each child must be considered as an individual. Sooner or later each will learn and improve upon the ability to talk, run, jump, swim, make decisions, and assume responsibility.

Parents have an important responsibility. They must help their child make the social and emotional adjustments necessary for the development of a well-balanced personality.

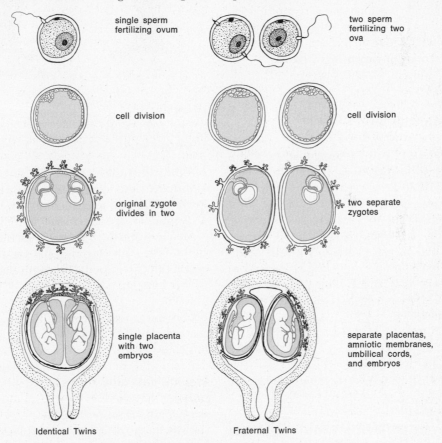

single sperm fertilizing ovum

two sperm fertilizing two ova

cell division

cell division

original zygote divides in two

two separate zygotes

single placenta with two embryos

separate placentas, amniotic membranes, umbilical cords, and embryos

Identical Twins

Fraternal Twins

Figure 3-7 ● Development of twins. (Left) Identical twins. (Right) Fraternal twins.

Puberty

During the later childhood period, an individual experiences a very important change in development. This change (puberty) occurs for most individuals when they are 12 to 14 years old, and is the beginning of adolescence or early adulthood.

Puberty starts when certain hormones are released by the pituitary gland. While this gland is involved with growth, it also affects the so-called sex glands, which are part of the reproductive system. The hormones from the pituitary gland act as chemical stimulators which cause the gonads to start functioning. The gonads (the ovaries in girls and the testes in boys) in turn produce hormones which cause many changes in the body. The most important change, perhaps, is that **at puberty each person has the potential of becoming a parent.**

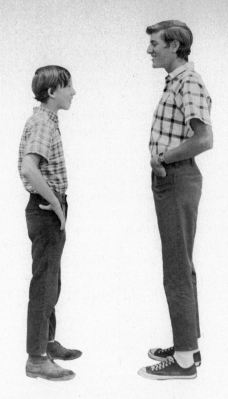

Figure 3-8 • Hormones control the rate of development of physical adult characteristics. Note the difference in size of these two 16-year-old boys.

Physical Changes in Boys

Hormones released by the gonads and circulated through the body by the blood cause hair to grow on the face, under the arms, and in the pubic region. A boy's shoulders begin to broaden, his physique develops, his larynx (Adam's apple) grows larger, and his voice starts to lower in pitch.

It is at this time that the boy can potentially become a parent. This is because the reproductive system has matured and is now functional.

The Male Reproductive System

Several weeks before birth, the testes descend from the pelvic cavity through a special opening (inguinal canal) and come to rest outside the body cavity in a pouch of skin called the scrotum. These testes, in addition to producing hormones which influence the characteristics of masculinity, also produce sperm. Sperm are the male reproductive cells. The testes produce millions of these microscopic cells, yet only one sperm cell is required to perform the fertilization function.

The matured sperm are passed into the epididymis, a tightly coiled tube adjacent to the testicles. The sperm leave the epididymis by way of larger tubes known as the vas deferens. From this point they enter the urethra (the tube that carries sperm and urine to the exterior) to be discharged from the male body by way of the penis. Before the discharge of sperm takes place, fluids from the seminal vesicles and the prostate gland are added. This provides the sperm

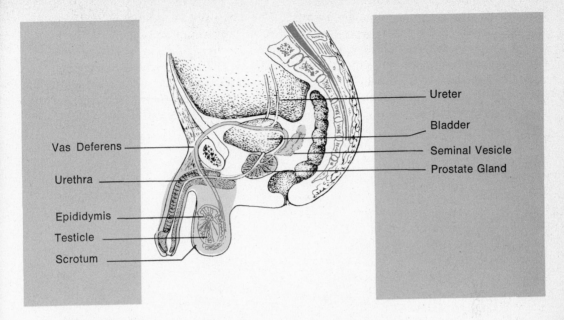

Ureter

Bladder

Seminal Vesicle

Prostate Gland

Vas Deferens

Urethra

Epididymis

Testicle

Scrotum

Figure 3-9 • Male reproductive system.

with a liquid medium in which they can then propel themselves by lashing their whiplike tails (flagella). The sperm in its fluid medium is called semen. At this point the sperm, with its ability to travel, is ready to perform its function—the fertilization of an ovum.

Physical Changes in Girls

On the average, girls reach puberty at a somewhat earlier age than boys do. As with boys, hormones from the pituitary gland stimulate certain changes in the girl's body. The ovaries, activated by hormones from the pituitary gland, now produce hormones of their own. These in turn cause hair to grow under the arms and in the pubic region. In addition, the mammary glands (the breasts) begin to develop and the more femininely proportioned figure begins to

take form. It is at this time that the girl acquires the potential of parenthood.

The Female Reproductive System

In addition to producing hormones which influence characteristics of femininity, the ovaries also contain sex cells called ova or eggs. Ova are the female reproductive cells. At birth, the two ovaries contain all the ova the girl is to have for her entire life.

At the time of puberty the ova, which have been present in the ovaries since birth, start to mature. As it matures, an ovum rises to the surface of the ovary, where it is contained in a blisterlike capsule called a follicle. Rupture of the follicle releases the ovum, which then enters the fallopian tube and begins its passage toward the uterus. This process occurs in alternating ovaries. It takes place about every 28 days.

If sperm are present in the fallopian tube, the ovum exerts a biochemical attraction which results in attempts by many sperm to penetrate the female reproductive cell. By some unknown selective process, one sperm eventually penetrates the egg cell and fertilization is accomplished. The process of cell division begins almost immediately after fertilization.

Ovulation

The entire process dealing with the release of an ovum from an ovary is called ovulation. It does not occur as an independent activity. While the ovum is nearing maturation in the ovary, hormones from the ovaries transmit a biochemical message to the uterus. The chemical message alerts the

Figure 3-10 ● Female reproductive system.

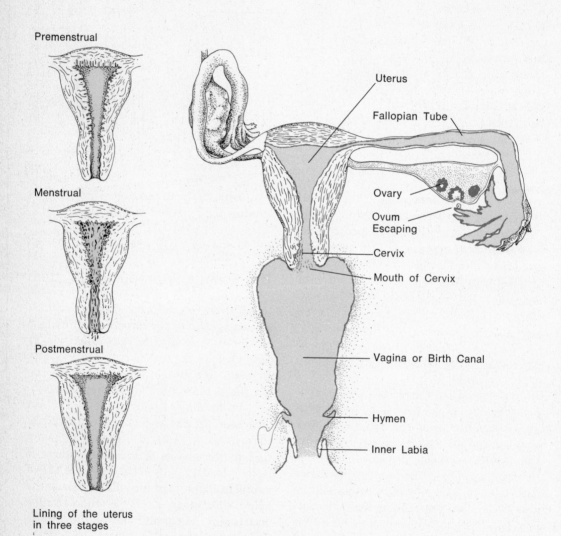

Premenstrual

Menstrual

Postmenstrual

Lining of the uterus in three stages

Uterus

Fallopian Tube

Ovary

Ovum Escaping

Cervix

Mouth of Cervix

Vagina or Birth Canal

Hymen

Inner Labia

uterus to the possible arrival of a fertilized ovum. The chemically alerted tissues of the uterus begin to store the nutrient-rich blood. The walls of the uterus continue to store the nutrient-rich blood in anticipation of the fertilized ovum's arrival. Should this anticipation be fulfilled, the ovum nestles into the tissues of the uterine wall, which contains ample nutrients until a more permanent system of nourishment can be established.

If, on the other hand, the ovum is not fertilized, other biochemical messages from the ovaries announce the forthcoming maturation of another egg cell. The walls of the uterus then begin to release the stored blood, which leaves the body through the vagina. This normal flow of blood from the female body is called menstruation.

Menstruation

One of the most important changes in girls at puberty is the beginning of the menstruation process. This change is an announcement that the girl now has the priceless gift of being able to bring a new life into existence. For this reason, the process of menstruation should be understood and regarded with respect and dignity.

The menstruation process begins at different ages for different girls. For some, it may begin as early as 10 or 11 years of age. For others, it may not begin until they are 15 or 16 years old. For most girls, it starts around the age of 12. The age at which the menstruation process begins happens to be right for that particular person.

The menstrual cycle is usually about 28 days for most girls and women. There is nothing wrong, however, if the menstrual cycle takes 24 days or even 30. Again, these differences happen to be right for these individuals.

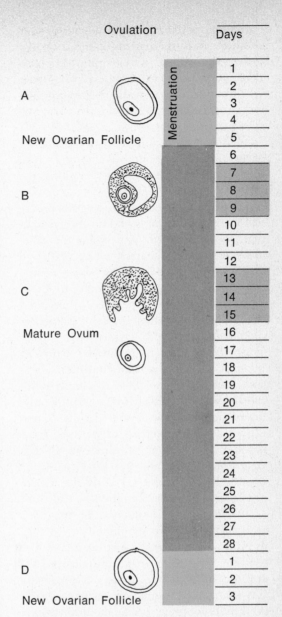

Figure 3-11 ● Ovulation and menstrual cycle. (a) During the menstrual flow (which may last from three to seven days) the new ovum begins to mature in the ovary. (b) The ovum continues to mature and the lining of uterus is being prepared to receive a fertilized egg. (c) On approximately the 14th day after the beginning of the menstrual period the mature ovum is expelled (ovulation). The lining of the uterus continues to be enriched with blood. (d) If the ovum is not fertilized, the uterine lining and blood are discharged (menstruation), and a new follicle begins to mature.

Some girls experience a considerable variation in menstruation before a regular cycle is established. The length of the menstrual period also varies among individuals. The average length is about five days. For some individuals three, four, six, or seven days is normal.

There is also a difference in the amount of flow, but in any case the amount is relatively small and is soon replaced by the body.

Even in our scientific age, there are still many superstitions and misunderstandings about menstruation. Many of these misunderstandings started many years ago and have continued because some people have lacked the proper information. Medical science is generally agreed that good total physical and mental health influences good menstrual health. Dysmenorrhea, commonly referred to as menstrual pains or "cramps," is not a normal condition. Freedom from dysmenorrhea is closely associated with desirable attitudes and the practice of simple but important habits. These include adequate exercise, proper diet, good posture, and regular elimination. If dysmenorrhea occurs and persists in spite of sensible health habits, certainly the family physician should be consulted.

Menstruation should not be regarded as a sickness. There should be no reason, therefore, for a normally healthy girl to discontinue most of her usual physical activities. On infrequent occasions, a physician may recommend limited or restricted physical activity for some specific medical reason. For the great majority of individuals, continuance of the normal pattern of physical and social activities helps to promote better total health.

It is also safe to bathe during the menstrual period. Good judgment should be exercised in avoiding drastic temperature changes which might influence the menstrual flow. While cleanliness is important at all times, it is especially important at this time, since the body tends to perspire more during the menstrual period.

When the ovaries no longer produce ova, the menstruation process stops. This occurs about the age of 46 to 48 for most women. For others, it may be somewhat earlier or later. The cessation of the menstruation process announces the end of the childbearing age. This change in the body is called the menopause.

Hormonal secretions are altered and may lead to a change in feelings. For some women, menopause creates an emotional problem. They feel that they are growing old. As a result, they become depressed (the same feeling may be brought about by hormonal changes). The fact that they can no longer have children may also contribute to feelings of depression. For those who experience physical and emotional problems related to menopause, hormonal therapy may be required along with psychological assistance.

Figure 3-12 • Menstruation should not interfere with a girl's daily activities or recreation.

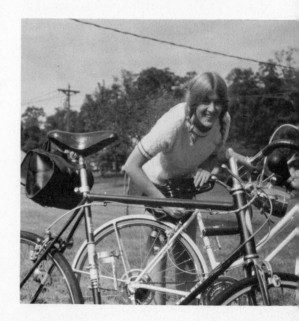

Most women accept the menopausal transition without any difficulty. They understand that motherhood is merely one function of womanhood. Their interests are broadly based, so that when their children grow up and leave home, they do not feel alone and useless.

Adolescence

Adolescence is the period beginning adulthood. At this time most individuals, especially girls, have reached over 95 percent of their adult height. A great deal of physical growth has taken place. Maturation has also occurred in varying degrees.

Some of the results of the "growing toward maturity" process are easily identified. This is particularly true of the changes which have taken place in the various systems of the body. The young adult now has almost all the permanent teeth; his or her skeleton has enlarged and the bones have hardened; the nervous system has matured so that there is better coordination of brain, nerves, and muscles; the maturation of the endocrine (hormone-secreting) system has further refined all the body systems.

The period of adolescence is sometimes characterized by the appearance of skin problems. It is perfectly understandable that the occurrence and recurrence of blackheads, pimples, and other skin blemishes is a major annoyance to young adults.

Although much maturation has taken place by the time adolescence is reached, additional maturation processes are still in progress and will continue for years to come. These processes will affect judgment, responsibility, the acquisition and use of knowledge, personal and social values, personal and social attitudes, and emotions.

Adolescence is the time of preparation for more mature adulthood. Many young people become confused about dating, courtship, love, and marriage. They also may have difficulty in understanding and coping with feelings of infatuation, affection, and love. It is important to realize that everyone has these feelings. Each person grows in ability to handle them.

Skin Problems

All the underlying causes of skin problems are not entirely understood, and there does not seem to be general agreement as to precise methods of preventing them.

Various possible contributing factors have been suggested from time to time. These include the possible influence of hormones at the beginning of puberty and the resultant glandular activity; the rapid growth process experienced during adolescence; and foods containing high levels of starches and sugars, as well as fried foods. Some of these factors may cause or contribute to the problem of skin eruptions. There seems to be no consensus on this point, however, among members of the medical profession.

All authorities agree, on the other hand, that skin cleanliness, exercise, rest, and a nutritionally balanced diet contribute to total health and, therefore, also contribute to skin health.

Pimples. Bacteria become lodged in skin pores and trapped by deposits of dirt and oil or by constriction of the pore as the result of very rapid cell division during an adolescent's accelerated growth period. In some instances the bacteria cause localized infections which occur inside the skin pore and involve the immediate adjoining tissue. This results in inflammation and swelling.

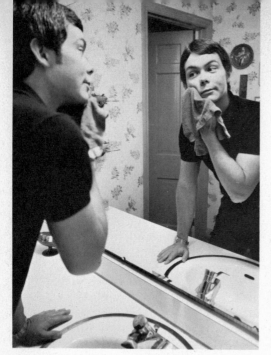
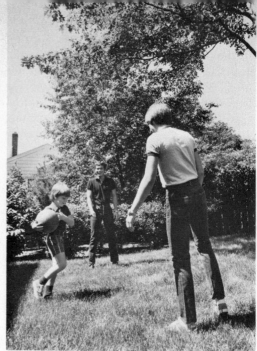
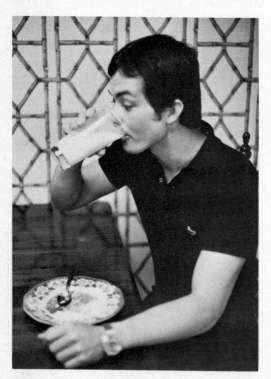
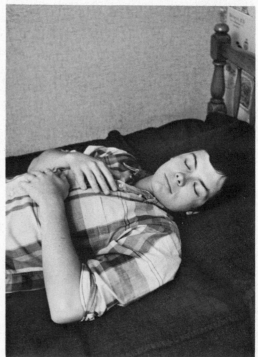

Figure 3-13 • You can reduce the risk of skin problems by using proper health practices such as those illustrated.

Pimple squeezing should be avoided. Instead, resort to regular but gentle use of a soft washcloth, mild soap, and warm water. Extreme or stubborn cases should be brought to the attention of a physician.

Blackheads. Blackheads also result from dirt-clogged skin pores. Bacteria trapped within the pore cause white blood cells to concentrate along the walls of the pore. The white blood cells, which are destroyed by bacteria along with impacted dirt and oil, constitute the core of the blackhead within the pore. As in the case of pimples, squeezing should be avoided in favor of regularly established and performed procedures for skin cleanliness.

Acne. Some adolescents may have a rather large area of skin affected by pimples, blackheads, and other skin blemishes. This condition is called acne. In some cases, improper care of this condition can result in further spread of the infections or in the formation of undesirable scar tissue.

Regular habits of skin cleanliness, along with adequate rest, exercise, and wholesome food can do much to improve the acne condition. Squeezing and picking at skin blemishes should be completely avoided. Acne which does not clear up as the result of practical and regular personal efforts should receive medical attention.

Emotions and Feelings

The development of your emotions and feelings is a very important part of your total maturation. Even during infancy you made your feelings quite clear when you felt the need for food, comfort, and love.

During early childhood, your feelings and emotions continued to develop in an introverted pattern, focusing on your own needs and wants. As you entered the period of later childhood, fairly definable patterns of affection and love became evident. Your friends were usually of your own sex. You merely tolerated peer group members of the opposite sex. On occasion, you permitted them to become a part of the "group," but did not usually accept them too well on an emotional basis.

In varying degrees and at different times, these basic emotions are channeled toward members of the opposite sex. For some, this may occur prior to puberty. It is not unusual for the individual at this stage of development to have a "crush" on a member of the opposite sex. The unknowing object of this emotional involvement might be a member of a peer group, or perhaps a TV or movie star, or even a teacher.

During young adulthood, some complications arise because of the striving for personal independence and for decreased parental control. Wanting to be grown-up and independent is perfectly normal and desirable. The basic problem is that most parents think young people do not yet have the judgment and mature sense of responsibility to run their own lives completely. Even young people themselves have some concern about taking on more responsibility. Their quick changes of mood at this time are particularly puzzling to parents and other adults. Both adults and adolescents need to understand that erratic behavior of this type is transitional.

As you move toward greater independence, infatuation, affection, and love play an increasingly important role in your life. This seems to complicate things even more when you begin to realize that these emotions are also being influenced by feelings of physical and biological attraction for members of the opposite sex.

There is no simple solution to the development of emotional maturation during the period of adolescence. However, the primary responsibility for resolving problems or conflict must rest with you. The key factor is how you use and control your personal attitudes and values. Young adults are well along toward maturity when they understand and can cope with feelings of infatuation, affection, and love.

Dating, Courtship, and Marriage

As young people reach puberty, they begin to develop an increasing interest in the opposite sex. This represents a change in their feelings and attitudes, because for a period of time they had little or no interest in the opposite sex. These changes and the reasons for the changes are discussed in some detail in the next chapter.

For many young people, dating begins as a part of group activity. Later, as individuals get to know one another, they begin to pair off. Gradually, they move toward that time when they will settle on one particular person for dating and enter the period of courtship. Of course, dating practices vary from one part of the country to another, from one country to another, and from one age to another. Part of growing to maturity is knowing what is acceptable for your age and for where you live.

Dating provides you with the opportunity to see how some members of the opposite sex react to various situations. You are able to learn something about the way these friends feel about life in general, and more specifically about how they feel about other people, their home, and school.

Courtship allows people to develop a genuine knowledge and understanding of others—their likes and dislikes, their habits (both pleasing and annoying), their beliefs, and their deep inner feelings. It is the time when people can realistically evaluate whether they can live on a day-to-day basis with the potential marriage partner.

When a couple have honestly faced the realities of marriage, such as responsibility for each other, and feel sure they have the capacity to adjust to each other, they have arrived at the time for marriage. Their chance for a successful marriage is great, because their decision to marry has been maturely made.

Of course, some people choose to live their adult lives without marrying. For them, dating provides opportunities to establish friendships which will enrich their lives.

Adulthood and the Future

Adulthood is that state of physical, mental, emotional, and social maturity which most nearly reaches the potential with which each individual is endowed by nature. It is the time during which the individual makes a contribution to the never-ending bridge from the past to the present and into the future. You can make no greater contribution to civilization and to humanity than to use your abilities to their greatest extent, with pride and dignity.

Each person differs in thousands of ways from all others. People are also alike in many ways. Basically, they experience much the same hopes, fears, dreams, failures, and successes. No matter what they do—whether it be driving a truck, practicing medicine, farming, or orbiting the earth—there is for most adults a common ground called parenthood. This is the beautiful and priceless gift of being able to reach into the future with a part of what they are today. It is a form of immortality. Since this contribution to the future will reflect what people do with life today, parenthood should be based on total ability to assume responsibility for one's own maturity.

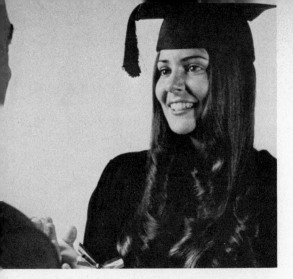

Figure 3-14 • How does the young adult gain independence?

Some of your roles as an adult may include:

■ Selecting a mate
■ Learning to live with a marriage partner
■ Starting a family
■ Raising children
■ Establishing a home

■ Managing a home
■ Getting started in an occupation
■ Assuming civic responsibility
■ Finding a congenial social group

The future is yours. You and your peers are the parents of tomorrow. You represent the hope of the future. The responsibility is a serious one, perhaps even a frightening one.

In spite of temporary differences of opinion between parents and their children, most adults have a great deal of confidence in the ability and integrity of today's young people. This is right and proper, because you deserve this confidence. You are faced with difficult problems in growing up; you are acquiring more difficult and technical knowledge; you are growing larger and healthier than any of your ancestors. You are fortunate people, and many adults envy you. They would give a great deal to be in your shoes, to be a part of the wonderful, almost unbelievable world to which you will contribute when you are fully mature.

Summary

Human development involves physical growth, intellectual progress, emotional maturity, and social responsibility. The process of development is somewhat long and may proceed at a different rate for each individual. Growing toward maturity begins prior to birth and follows fertilization, cell division, and implantation. Each person grows and matures within the potential of what is inherited from both parents. That potential is carried in the genes. The combination of genes determines what a person inherits. The environment, however, will influence the degree to which some potential characteristics will develop.
Prenatal care is important. The physician conducts a number of tests to determine whether the pregnancy is proceeding normally. Approximately 280 days are required for the completion of a pregnancy. Multiple births are not uncommon.
Infancy is characterized by complete dependence on parents. Infancy is followed by childhood. During this time a child develops many skills and learns to make decisions and to assume responsibility. During the period of later childhood, puberty occurs. This is the beginning of adolescence and usually takes place when the individual is 12 to 14 years old.

Adolescence or young adulthood is the period in which people face varying problems, from skin blemishes to handling feelings of infatuation and love. Dating, with its attendant emotions and feelings, is also part of adolescence. Courtship and marriage may occur during this time. Young adults can avoid many problems by developing judgment and a mature sense of responsibility, as well as the ability to handle their emotions.

Adulthood is that state of physical, mental, emotional, and social maturity which most nearly reaches the potential with which a person is endowed by nature. For most people, it is the time of homemaking and parenthood.

in making health decisions . . .

Understand These Terms:

adolescence
embryo
hormones
identical twins
maturity

menopause
ovulation
placenta
puberty
sickle cell anemia

Solve This Problem:

A family with twins has just moved into your neighborhood. For each set of observable characteristics listed below, indicate the reasons that the children might be identical or fraternal twins:

1. One child is a boy and the other a girl. Their facial features are very much alike.

2. Both children are girls. One has blue eyes and the other brown eyes. Otherwise, they look very much alike.

3. Both children are boys, and all observable characteristics look very much alike.

4. Both children are girls. One has dark hair and the other blonde hair. Otherwise, all observable characteristics look very much alike.

Try These Activities:

1. Mr. and Mrs. Hyfield have two brown-eyed children and two blue-eyed children. Can you determine the possible eye-color determining gene combination for each parent? What color eyes does each parent have?

2. Compile separate lists of personal characteristics that you associate with either your mother or your father. Identify those items on each list that are inherited characteristics and those that are acquired traits. With which parent do you seem to share more acquired characteristics? How can you account for this?

3. As you think about your future role of masculinity or femininity as an adult, how would you arrange the following items in a priority sequence?

   - Selecting a mate
   - Learning to live with a marriage partner
   - Starting a family
   - Raising children
   - Establishing a home
   - Managing a home
   - Getting started in an occupation
   - Assuming civic responsibility
   - Finding a congenial social group

   Write a one-page rationale for your choice of sequence priorities.

Interpret These Concepts:

1. Each person grows and matures within the potential of what has been inherited from both parents.
2. There is no simple solution to the development of emotional maturation during the period of adolescence.

Explore These Readings:

Bauer, William W., M.D., *Moving into Manhood.* New York: Doubleday & Company, Inc., 1963.

———— and Florence Marvyne Bauer, *Way to Womanhood.* New York: Doubleday & Company, Inc., 1965.

Beadle, George W. and Muriel Beadle, *The Language of Life: An Introduction to the Science of Genetics.* New York: Doubleday & Company, Inc., 1966.

de Schweinitz, Karl, *Growing Up,* 4th Edition. New York: The Macmillan Company, 1968.

Landis, Judson T. and Mary C., *Building a Succesful Marriage,* 6th Edition. Englewood Cliffs, N. J.: Prentice-Hall, Inc., 1973.

————, *Building Your Life,* 3rd Edition. Englewood Cliffs, N. J.: Prentice-Hall, Inc., 1964.

————, *Personal Adjustment, Marriage, and Family Living,* 5th Edition. Englewood Cliffs, N. J.: Prentice-Hall, Inc., 1970.

Landis, Paul H., *Coming of Age: Problems of Teen-Agers,* Public Affairs Pamphlet No. 234. New York: Public Affairs Committee, Inc., 1966.

Scheinfeld, Amram, *Twins and Supertwins.* Philadelphia: J. B. Lippincott Co., 1967.

Tanner, J. M. and G. R. Taylor, and the Editors of Life, *Growth.* New York: Life Science Library, Time-Life Books, a Division of Time, Inc., 1965.

————, *A Baby Is Born.* New York: Maternity Center Association/Grosset & Dunlap, Inc., 1964.

Four | Developing an Understanding of Sexuality

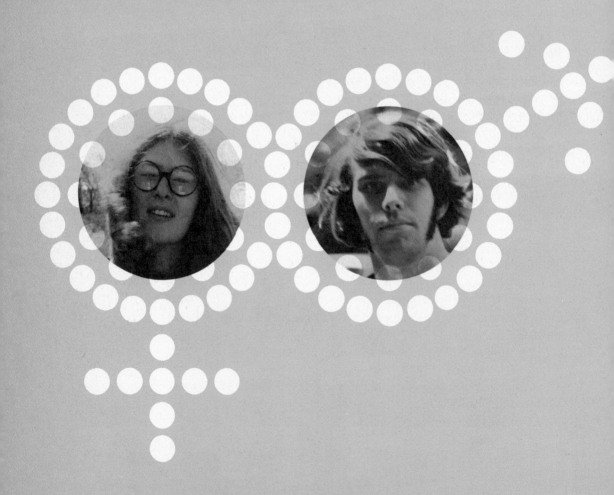

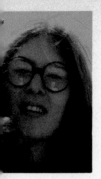

The way you feel about yourself as a male, if you are a young man, or as a female, if you are a young woman, and about your male or female traits is called your masculinity or femininity. The way you feel about the opposite sex also is an integral part of your masculinity or femininity.

These masculine and feminine traits are also called your sexuality. Such traits do not appear suddenly. They began when you were born and will continue to develop throughout your life. As you evolve from birth through adulthood, what you will become and what you will achieve within your inherited potential, what kind of man or woman you become, depends on the social, psychological, and moral environment in which you are raised. For example, how parents feel about the sex of the child (whether they wanted a child of the opposite sex or were pleased about the gender of their child) will affect the child's own feelings later on about being a man or a woman. In a similar fashion, the development of an individual's feelings about love, attitudes toward the sex relationship itself, and feelings about the opposite sex also develop within that particular individual's social and psychological environment.

The Development of Sexual Attitudes

Your masculinity and femininity, or your sexual feelings, develop continuously throughout life. This development of sexuality is a never-ending process that begins quite early.

Early Sex Interest

Early in life, the child learns that touching the sex organs with the fingers produces a pleasant sensation. When adults see a child touch his or her sex organs, they often attribute to the child the impulses and emotions an adult might have. It is not uncommon for adults to push the child's hand away. They fail to realize that the child's interest is purely physical and just as natural as any other physical activity.

About the same time, the child becomes curious about other people's sex organs and begins to notice sex differences. This also is normal and natural. Gradually, the child develops an interest in the opposite sex.

Preadolescence

During preadolescence, hormones begin to increase the rate of sexual maturing. At this time, the girl is usually ahead of the boy in physical development. She is often taller, stronger, and more mature physically. As a result, boys may feel inferior to girls at this stage.

Some researchers have suggested that boys stick together and show little interest in girls because of this difference in their development. By so doing, they can minimize their embarrassment. At the same time, probably because of their advanced physical maturity, girls are much more interested in boys. There is sexual curiosity, but no great amount of emotion is involved.

Early Adolescence

Between the ages of 12 and 14, physical maturing is accelerated. Secondary sex char-

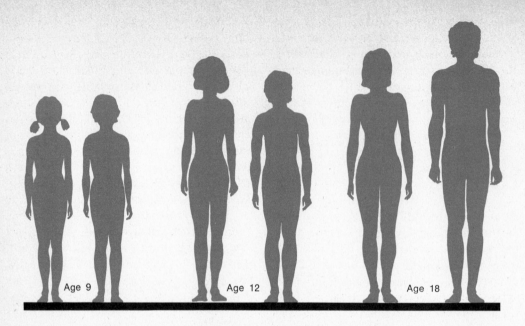

Age 9   Age 12   Age 18

Figure 4-1 ● As individuals mature through adolescence they change in both size and body shape. Can you explain how males and females may vary in growth rate and development of secondary sex charactertistics?

acteristics begin to develop. The girl starts to menstruate, her breasts develop, she acquires pubic hair, and her body begins to have an overall womanly look. The boy's voice deepens, his larynx enlarges, and he begins to develop hair on his face. The penis and testes become larger and heavier and he may start to experience sexual dreams which result in ejaculation (discharge of semen).

Unfortunately, psychological or emotional growth does not keep pace with this rapid physical maturing. This produces conflict within the individual and with adults with whom he comes in contact. It is probably the heart of the "growing-up" problem for many young people.

Whereas earlier only the girl was interested in the opposite sex, the boy now begins to share this interest. The interest of both is still of a general nature. A boy is interested in almost any girl and a girl in almost any boy. Dating begins and each individual tries to find out what the opposite sex is like. Group dating or double dating may be quite prominent in their activities.

In this attempt to discover what the opposite sex is like, adolescents look around them for models of behavior. They observe the way their parents treat each other. They see how other young persons and adults conduct themselves with members of the opposite sex. They examine behavior exhibited on television, in the movies, and in articles and pictures in newspapers and magazines.

Sexual curiosity, desires, and anxieties become more intense at this time. This is due in part to the increased activity of the hormones. It is also due to a strong psychological drive to grow up quickly and become independent. It is difficult for the sexual tension to be released. As a result, masturbation is often practiced by both males and females.

Aroused sexual feelings, apprehension about masturbation and menstruation, the developing personality of the individual, the striving for freedom and independence from the family all combine to create anxiety in young people during early adolescence.

Late Adolescence

As maturing continues, the sex drive becomes stronger. Both sexes experience sexual dreams, with the boys' culminating in nocturnal emissions (discharge of semen during sleep). As the end of adolescence approaches, young people begin to adjust to the physical and emotional changes taking place within them, and learn to cope with them. They develop attitudes about sexual dreams, masturbation, petting, and intercourse.

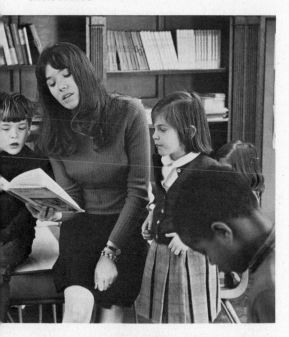

Figure 4-2 • Young children look up to young adults as models of behavior. Do you set a good example?

Almost all adolescents go through the same phases of sexual development. However, the rate at which the development takes place is highly individual. **Each young person's needs and expectations of love and sex are unique to that individual.** They develop from experiences during psychological and sexual growth. There are as many different kinds and degrees of needs in love and sex as there are different kinds of people. Every young person should have some standard of behavior as a guide in attaining goals and meeting needs within the framework of society.

Adjusting to Your Sex Drive

The sex drive is a normal component of growth and development. It is a natural part of life that needs to be understood and properly channeled. The goal of the sex drive is biological sexual maturity, which includes the capacity to live, mate, reproduce, and care for the young. It is a sharing of interests and ideas, mutual acceptance of responsibilities, self-realization and fulfillment, and love.

If the sex drive is to become a positive force in the development of the total personality, it should be controlled and used within the rules set down by the particular society in which we live.

Dating

Part of the process of learning how to adjust to your sex drive involves dating. As mentioned earlier, when young people reach puberty and enter the period of adolescence, they undergo a subtle but definite change in feelings toward the opposite sex. This change occurs at a somewhat earlier age for girls than for boys. In either case, a developing attraction toward and interest in the opposite sex is a normal and healthy result of the maturation process. For most people, it is this attraction that eventually leads to marriage.

About this time, young adults begin to date those individuals whom they like and enjoy being with. It is the beginning of a friendship relationship that includes having mutual interests, respect for each other, and mutual trust. In addition, it encompasses the biological boy-girl differences which influence people's attitudes and help them understand and control their emotions and behavior. Dating helps young people acquire the experience to understand and adjust to the opposite sex.

Because of this, the attitudes and values that boys and girls bring into their dating activity are very important. These attitudes reflect whether the persons respect themselves as human being and bear themselves with fitting dignity. They also reflect whether they respect the friend they are dating.

Since dating is an exploration period, it is to an individual's advantage to date a number of people. This provides the individual with a greater opportunity to learn about the positive qualities in the opposite sex. In this way, **dating plays an important role in preparation for marriage.**

The assumption of responsibility on the part of the young adult extends also to recognizing and observing dating guidelines developed with parents. All families need to establish reasonable rules involving the frequency of dating, time to be in, use of the car, and handling of money, to mention a few of the aspects of dating behavior to be settled by parents and youth. While many young persons feel that this type of decision should be made by them alone, they must remember that parents cannot abdicate their responsibility to guide their children and help them develop into responsible adults. This is part of their moral and legal adult role.

Some young people find it more difficult than others to get dates. Part of the difficulty is usually within the individuals themselves. This is often reflected by their feelings about themselves (feelings of inferiority), their attitudes about the opposite sex, how well they make friends, and how well they function in mixed groups. Fortunately, many difficulties and handicaps can be overcome by learning important social attitudes and skills.

A great asset in overcoming these difficulties is developing the ability to put oneself in another's place and gain insight into how that person feels. By so doing, an individual finds it somewhat easier to communicate wtih the other person. One of the best ways a person can acquire social skills is by participating in social functions. This type of experience is probably the best teacher. Take advantage of contacts at school, at religious functions, and in other group situations to gain social experience. These skills cannot be learned by sitting home.

A common problem you may face is the question of going steady. The term "going steady" has different meanings for different people. Many adults associate the practice with courtship that has marriage as its objective. Many young people look upon the practice as simply an indication of friendship and fondness. To reduce the possibility of misunderstanding, you need to help your parents understand the kind of dating behavior you are practicing.

You should also be aware of the advantages and disadvantages of going steady. Some of the advantages include the personal security of being assured of a date, the opportunity to get to know each other well, and the natural transition to becoming engaged and then married. Some of the disadvantages are that going steady may reduce the possibility of wider social contacts for both individuals, may limit their choice of a marriage partner, and may cause them emotional anguish because of worries about breaking up.

Petting

Whenever dating is discussed, questions about petting usually come up. This is another term that has different meanings for different people. Some consider hugging, kissing, and other physical contacts that are simple expressions of affection as petting. Others feel that petting is the deliberate stimulation of various parts of the male and female bodies. It is important for you to help your parents understand what you mean by petting.

Boys often believe that it is up to the girl to decide how far petting should go. Many girls believe this, as well. Actually, both have a responsibility for establishing the right relationship for the couple.

Petting emphasizes the physical aspects of a relationship. There are couples who gradually drift into a petting relationship because they can no longer relate to their partner in any other way. To some extent, this may be a reflection of their need for affection. It may also reveal their inability or unwillingness to explore and develop other aspects of their personalities.

The problem of petting is keeping it within bounds. Without self-control on the part of both individuals, it may lead to sexual intercourse. Various parts of the human body are sensitive and stimulated by touch. This is particularly true for the male since his sex organs are external. He can be sexually aroused much more quickly than the female. Strong sexual excitement can occur in the male in a few seconds, very often simply as the result of thinking about things of a sexual nature.

No specific rules for petting can be put forward. However, it is important to understand the factors involved in this form of sexual behavior. Many couples who engage frequently in heavy petting find themselves becoming irritable with each other; they quarrel often; they lose their enjoyment in associating together; they lose respect for each other; and their friendship eventually breaks up. This kind of petting keeps a couple upset emotionally, builds up desires, and creates serious problems of self-control.

Premarital Intercourse

The question of sex before marriage has always faced the maturing individual. Arguments in favor of premarital intercourse stress physical satisfaction and pleasure. Those who favor these arguments overlook the emotional, mental, and social aspects of life and try to consider the sexual act in isolation. They often ignore the fact that intercourse is the closest relationship that two people can have with each other. In marriage, it is a merging of two unique persons who are expressing their deepest affection.

The attitudes that are developed about sex are extremely important. Does the boy think of girls as good companions, good fun, and persons he can enjoy in a social setting? Or does he think of them only as a means of satisfying his physical desires? What about the girl? Does she build friendship on the basis of companionship, shared interests, and fun, or does she encourage boys to think of her only in a physical way?

A girl who participates in premarital intercourse often finds her conduct more severely criticized by people than that of the boy who participates with her. This "double standard" is obviously unreasonable. Sexual activity should be judged as appropriate or inappropriate for the boy or girl equally.

People who can attract desirable companions on a basis other than the purely sexual will be more likely to achieve an enduring and satisfying love relationship when the proper time comes.

Many research studies also have demonstrated that premarital intercourse does not provide the proper setting for this important part of the deep experience of love. The feelings of worry, guilt, and fear often affect the emotional well-being of both parties, particularly the female. These worries and fears may result in an attitude about intercourse that prevents the individual from establishing normal sexual relationships in marriage.

A number of questions should be considered when the decision regarding premarital intercourse is made: What value do you place on yourself? What value do you set on the other person? How able are you to exercise common sense and self-control, to sacrifice a pleasurable moment now for lasting later benefit?

Satisfactory adjustment in marriage is not determined by previous sexual experience. It is dependent upon the partners' having wholesome attitudes toward sex, upon a real understanding of each other, and upon their consideration and appreciation of each other as persons.

Masturbation

Obtaining sexual gratification by self-stimulation of the sex organs is called masturbation. It is estimated that more than 90 percent of the males in the United States over 15 years of age have engaged in some form of masturbation. Some males masturbate once or twice in their lives; others much more frequently. About 50 to 60 percent of all females are believed to masturbate. For young people, masturbation is the chief source of sexual outlet before marriage.

The great majority of modern medical opinion is agreed that masturbation does no physical harm. Some authorities caution against carrying it too far. They are concerned that it might become an obsessive habit and the excess they refer to is psychological. In this sense, masturbation is excessive when it is substituted for other outlets to relieve tensions and anxieties which are not sexually derived. These may be concern over one's schoolwork or job, rejection by friends, or uncertainties about self-worth.

Another symptom of psychological excess is worry caused by masturbating more than one might wish. A person who masturbates a great deal sometimes develops guilt feelings and begins to worry about losing self-control.

Part of the worry is caused by misconceptions. Throughout the years, there have been those who believed that masturbation "drives one crazy." More common is the association of masturbation with pimples, feeble-mindedness, loss of weight, fatigue, or weak eyes. No relationship between masturbation and any physical disorder has ever been found.

Parents sometimes contribute to worry about the act. They believe it will do their child harm, and try to discourage the child with threats of physical punishment.

Another worry of those who masturbate is that they are being betrayed by physical symptoms—moist palms, pimples, and certain expressions of the eyes. There is no scientific basis for these beliefs. Common sense should help us understand that no one can tell by looking whether a person has been masturbating recently, or excessively, or at all.

Even when people know a great deal about masturbation, they may still be troubled by it as a habit. Most problems which develop from masturbation are not due to lack of knowledge but to deep feelings that masturbation is wrong or harmful. But the feelings do not prevent the act; they simply make the individual worry about it all the more. Sometimes, even though people have assured themselves that masturbation is all right, they unconsciously worry about it. They develop feelings of guilt, inferiority, and fear of social disgrace. Even though such fears are unwarranted, they still exist.

Nocturnal Emission

Nocturnal emissions are the result of sexual stimulation during sleep. An individual dreams he is engaging in a sexual experience and at some time during it has an orgasm. In the male, there is an ejaculation and thus the common name "wet dream." (The female experiences no ejaculation, but she is also subject to sexual stimulation during sleep.)

Sexual dreams are common; almost everybody has them. Their frequency varies with the individual and seems to be related to the amount of sexual tension, need, or stimulation that that person is experiencing. Sometimes the dreams are fostered by conditions that irritate the sex organs, such as a full bladder or constricting clothing.

Some young men tend to worry about nocturnal emissions. They should realize that emissions simply take place, and that they are considered by all authorities to be quite normal.

Homosexuality

Homosexual behavior involves sexual relations or emotional attachments arising from sexual attraction between individuals of the same sex.

During childhood it is normal for boys to look down on girls, have male heroes, and enjoy the company of other boys. It is also normal during this early development period for girls to hate boys, have crushes on girls, and love some best girl friend intensely. This kind of behavior is not considered homosexuality, because it is transitional and temporary. It is more proper to apply the term "homosexual" to those individuals, both male and female, who chronically feel an urgent sexual desire toward members of their own sex. They then seek to gratify these desires with members of their own sex.

It is not easy to identify a homosexual. You cannot tell by physical appearance. There is a common misconception that men who appear to be physically feminine, with extra fat deposits, small sex organs, wide hips, and feminine hair distribution are more likely than others to be homosexuals. Similarly, there is a misconception that women who have a mannish physical build are homosexual. This has not been proved by research. In other words, homosexuals are no different physically from individuals with heterosexual tendencies (attracted to the opposite sex).

There is little agreement in scientific circles as to what causes homosexuality, beyond the widely accepted belief that psychological, social, and cultural factors do play key roles. The causative factors are probably multiple. One outstanding researcher suggests the following as possible contributing factors: inappropriate identification with a parent of the opposite sex; fear of, or hostility to either parent; reversal of masculine and feminine roles in parents; and feelings of inadequacy where "masculinity" is emphasized.

Can a homosexual change his behavior and drives? Studies have shown that long-term psychotherapy has helped some homosexuals become heterosexual. However, the prospect for change in an adult with a long-established pattern of exclusive homosexual behavior is not too encouraging at this time. The greatest chance for success in treating homosexuality still lies in reaching young persons who exhibit such tendencies at an early age. A still better approach lies in preventing homosexuality by helping boys and girls learn their appropriate sex roles in a way that is more satisfying.

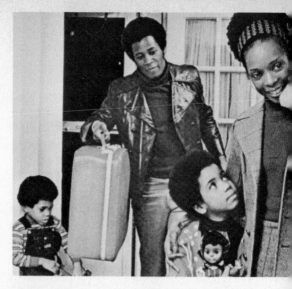

Figure 4-3 ● For most people the culmination of developing sexuality is marriage and a family. Success in marriage is partly dependent on your present attitudes and practices.

Preparing for Marriage

A basic prerequisite for a happy marriage is love. Yet the question might well be asked: What is love?

Some authorities try to distinguish between romantic love and mature love. Romantic love is usually characterized by thrills and excitement. It is the type of love described in the lyrics of many modern songs. These lyrics proclaim that love is the mysterious attraction that two people have for each other; that there is a one-and-only mate whom you will recognize as soon as you meet; that nothing can or should stand in the way of love. Mature love contains many of the concepts of romantic love, but is built on firmer ground, since it also includes understanding, mutual respect, shared interests and goals, and mutual consideration. It is love based on the realities of everyday family living. Mature love is not fleeting. It persists despite difficulties and arguments or disagreements.

How does a person learn about love? First, by observing the marriage relationship of parents. If this is sound and based on mutual respect and consideration, it provides a model for the children to follow. If it is an unhappy relationship, it may suggest pitfalls that children should avoid in seeking marriage partners. Then the young couple can also gain understanding of love by experience, through dating and courtship. **Careful preparation enhances success in marriage.**

Courtship

Courtship is the period during which partners find out a great deal about each other. They have an opportunity to take an honest look at themselves and each other to determine whether or not their marriage would have a chance for success.

If the courtship process is to be conducted within the guidelines of maturity, the following questions must be considered by both parties:

- Am I sure that I love this person and that he or she loves me?

- Is this the person with whom I wish to spend the rest of my life?

- Am I prepared educationally to earn a living which will permit me to provide or help provide at least the basic necessities and comforts of a home?

- Am I prepared to bring a new life into the world, for whom I can provide love, a sense of being wanted, security, understanding, and at least the basic essentials necessary to health and happiness?

Truthful answers to these questions can help you better evaluate your feelings. Avoid mistaking infatuation and affection

Figure 4-4 ● What is love?

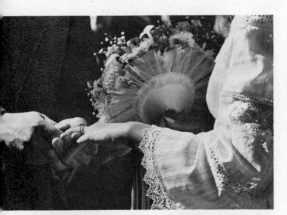

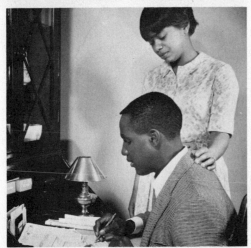

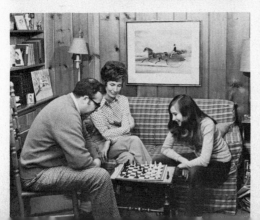

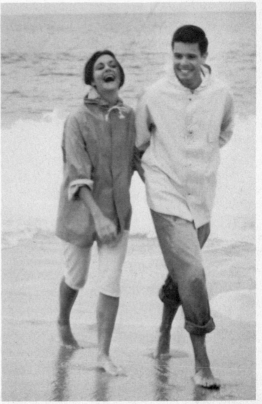

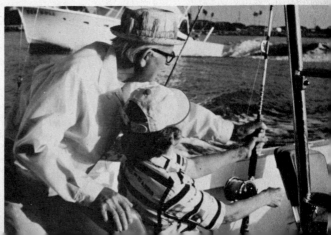

for love, or thinking that love will outweigh all the other considerations that go into making a happy marriage.

Choosing a Marriage Partner

Most persons marry because they are in love and want to establish a happy home and have children. They want to enjoy life and raise children who will be a credit to their community. The ability to reach the goals of marriage and responsible parenthood is dependent to a great extent on the individual's maturity.

Unfortunately, a number of young people marry merely on the basis of biological and physical attractions. One of the regrettable facts concerning early marriages is that these marriages result in the highest divorce rate in the nation. Certainly some early marriages are successful, but it is generally agreed that lack of maturity in one or both partners is a contributing factor to the failure of many such marriages.

A successful marriage depends upon the selection of the right person as a marriage partner. This implies consideration of psychological and biological suitability, economic security, and a readiness for and commitment to marriage. An equally important consideration is the ability of each marriage partner to look at situations through the eyes of the other and make adjustments for the benefit of the entire family. **Effective preparation, the ability** **to adjust, and respect for and understanding of one's marriage partner tend to produce successful marriages.**

Summary

The development of human sexuality is a continuous, never-ending process that has its beginnings quite early in life. The development takes place within your genetic inheritance and is shaped by your social and psychological environment.

Sex interest also begins early in life and increases during preadolescence, early adolescence, and late adolescence.

Around the age of puberty, as physical maturing speeds up, there is an increase in interest in the opposite sex. Since physical maturing occurs earlier in girls, it seems logical that girls are interested in the opposite sex somewhat earlier.

The sex drive is an important force in the development of your personality when it is properly used and controlled. It is important that you understand the many factors that can influence or be influenced by your sex drive.

This involves developing sound attitudes and values about dating, learning acceptable standards of behavior in respect to petting, making sound decisions about premarital intercourse, and developing a thorough understanding of masturbation, nocturnal emission, and homosexuality.

The ability to establish a happy and stable marriage is dependent on much more than physical attraction. Psychological and biological maturity in each of the marriage partners who are suited to each other, economic security, and readiness for and commitment to marriage are most important for a successful marriage.

in making health decisions...

Understand These Terms:

courtship   masculinity   semen
ejaculation   nocturnal emission   sex drive
femininity   obsessive habit   sexuality
homosexuality   physical desires   social maturity

Solve This Problem:

A couple has been going out steadily for approximately one year. Both the young man and young woman are beginning to take each other for granted and their relationship is becoming more and more physical. Do you feel that this relationship will benefit the couple? In which ways might this relationship be harmful to both?

Try These Activities:

1. Survey several young men to determine what characteristics they like most in a young woman they would like to date. Now question several young women as to the characteristics they like most in young men. Compare the answers given by both sexes and discuss your findings.

2. Interview a marriage counselor, a minister, a priest, or a rabbi to determine what basic adjustment problems married couples have who ask his help. Ask several couples who have been married for five years or more how important they feel are the adjustment problems identified by the marriage counselor. Be prepared to discuss your findings in class.

3. Make a list of people you could go to for advice if you were worried about your developing sexuality or relations with the opposite sex. Who might help you compile a list of basic adjustment problems in marriage?

Interpret These Concepts:

1. Your masculinity and femininity, or your sexual feelings, develop continuously throughout life.

2. The sex drive is a normal component of growth and development.

3. Dating plays an important role in preparation for mariage.

Explore These Readings:

Brenton, Myron and Oscar Rabinowitz, "How to Talk to Your Parents About Sex," *Seventeen,* 30:152–153 (March, 1971).

Carr, Gwen B., ed., *Marriage and Family in a Decade of Change.* Menlo Park, Calif.: Addison-Wesley Publishing Co., Inc., 1972.

Jermann, T. C., "Can the Young Make Good Marriages?" *America,* 128: 329–330 (Apr. 14, 1973).

"Male and Female: Differences Between Them," *Time,* 99:43–44 (Mar. 20, 1972).

"Understanding Sexual Attraction," *Story of Life,* Part I. London, England: Marshall Cavendish, Ltd., 1970, pp. 6–10.

Five | Developing Sound Nutritional Practices

workbook p. 32
33
34
35
36
45

See if Scarsdale diet compares with chart on p. 70-71

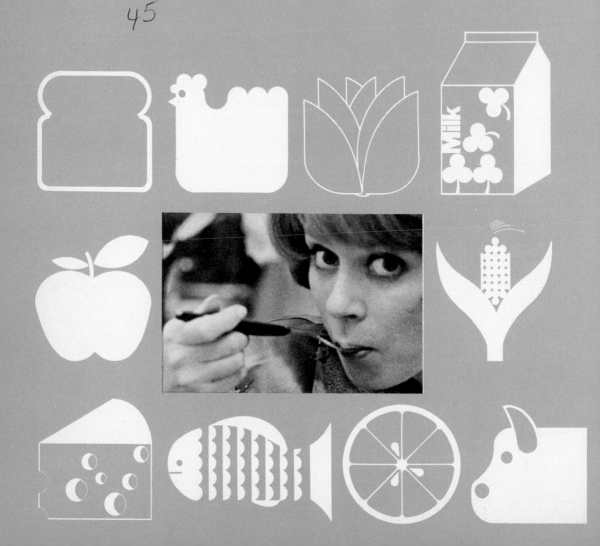

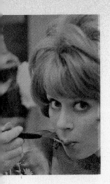

Good nutrition is basic to your health and well-being. The foods you eat can have an effect on how long you live and how well you live. But there is no magic formula or special preparation that will provide you with a shortcut to good health. Don't be fooled by those who stress the need for special "health foods" and "food supplements" (vitamin pills). With a basic understanding of the principles of sound nutrition and some common sense, you can have a well-balanced diet with all the nutrients you need from the foods you find in the grocery store.

Eating Practices

Eating practices are complex and depend on many factors. How and what you eat may depend on the food that is available to you at any given time. Your eating practices may also be related to emotional problems. Some persons will cut down on their eating or will not eat at all because of certain emotional problems. Others will try to meet emotional needs by overeating. Some persons base their eating habits on food fads and fallacies.

Family traditions and cultural patterns also have a great deal to do with how and what you eat. While most of these traditions and patterns are in keeping with sound nutritional practices, some are not. Certain families consume too many rich foods; others eat too much of everything. Some prepare most of their foods by frying while others boil or broil most of their foods. Still others eat their foods raw.

Your eating habits develop early in life. They result from a combination of many factors. Because of this, changing poor eating habits may be extremely difficult. Understanding the reasons for poor eating habits and recognizing the benefits of good nutrition may help you change poor habits for better ones. As you study this chapter on nutrition, try to decide which of your eating practices are beneficial and which are not. Determine the reasons for poor habits, if there are any, and try to change them. In later years you may be responsible for developing sound nutritional practices for your own children. Your application of the information presented in this chapter can be of benefit to you now and to your children in the future.

The Basic Four

One of the simplest yet surest ways of receiving the nutrients you need is to include in your diet foods from the four basic food groups. These groups are: (1) milk and milk products, (2) meat and meat substitutes, (3) vegetables and fruits, and (4) breads and cereals. The role in your diet that each food group plays is found in the chart on page 66.

To give you the full advantage of these foods, your daily diet should include four or more glasses of milk or equivalent amounts of milk products, two or more servings of meat or meat substitutes, four or more servings of vegetables and fruits (including dark green or yellow vegetables and citrus fruits or tomatoes), and four or more servings of breads and cereals. This constitutes a properly balanced diet.

Your body requires so much energy that your nutritive needs are high. One of the values of using the basic four food groups as a guide of good nutrition is that a variety of inexpensive foods can be found in each group. This variety makes it possible for you to obtain a well-balanced diet without too much difficulty or expense, thereby meeting your nutritioanl needs with ease.

better understanding of why you should eat foods from each of these groups, examine the importance of the various nutrients found in these foods.

Essential Nutrients

Individuals throughout life require the same nutrients but in varying amounts. One way to get essential nutrients is through the basic four food groups. These nutrients include proteins, carbohydrates, vitamins, minerals, and fats. To give you a

Proteins

Meats are an excellent source of proteins. Other sources include cheese, nuts, eggs, cereals, and beans. The percentage of protein found in various foods is illustrated in Figure 5–1.

The Role of Basic Food Groups *

Group	Role in Diet
Milk Group Milk, cheese, ice cream	Valuable sources of protein, calcium, other minerals, and vitamins
Meat Group Meats, poultry, fish, shellfish, and eggs. Dried beans, peas, and nuts as alternates	Valuable sources of protein; also furnish certain minerals (e.g., iron) and B vitamins
Vegetable-Fruit Group All fruits and vegetables, including potatoes Leafy, green, and yellow vegetables Citrus fruits, tomatoes, raw cabbage, etc.	Chiefly important as carriers of minerals, vitamins, and fiber (cellulose) High in iron and vitamin A Rich in vitamin C
Grain Group Bread, flour, cereals, baked goods (whole-grain or enriched preferred)	Inexpensive sources of energy and protein. Whole-grain or enriched products carry more iron and B vitamins.

* Adapted from L. Jean Bogert, George M. Briggs, and Doris Howes Calloway, *Nutrition and Physical Fitness,* 8th ed. Philadelphia: W. B. Saunders Company, 1966.

Proteins should be included in your diet because they are essential in building and maintaining body tissues and because they provide fuel which produces energy. Another reason for eating protein-rich foods is that they contain necessary minerals and vitamins.

Because of their importance in building tissue, proteins are most needed during periods of rapid growth. However, there is still a need for protein when you have stopped growing. The repair and replacement of cells and tissues that are worn out require that protein be constantly included in the diet.

You are in a period of rapid growth right now. You should be sure that your diet contains an adequate amount of meat or meat substitutes. However, do not make the mistake of thinking that protein-rich foods alone will provide all of your dietary needs. It is essential that you eat other foods as well.

Carbohydrates

Foods containing carbohydrates are the most abundant and economical today. The percentage of carbohydrates found in various foods is illustrated in Figure 5–2.

Carbohydrates are important because they serve as a source of energy. One of the difficulties you face is selecting foods which provide the right amounts of carbohydrates. Candy, soft drinks, and pastry have a high level of this nutrient. However, these foods may have a detrimental effect on your teeth and, in addition, contribute to obesity (overweight). They are also lacking in other nutrients that are essential to you.

You can meet your carbohydrate needs and at the same time supply yourself with certain vitamins and minerals, by eating fruits, vegetables, and whole-grain products.

Practice moderation in your choice of sweets and extras. Although they add enjoyment to your meals, they are not essential.

Care also must be taken not to reduce your intake of carbohydrates drastically, as is called for in some weight-reducing diets. Your health can be adversely affected if carbohydrates are eliminated or reduced to fewer than 60 grams per day over a period of time. The hazard of engaging in such a practice is that you eliminate an important source of energy as well as needed vitamins and minerals.

Vitamins

Each food group contains certain types and amounts of vitamins. A balanced diet, including foods from each basic food group, will provide all the essential vitamins you need.

Although vitamins are required in extremely small amounts, they are essential to your normal growth and the regulation of your body activities. They usually act as catalysts in allowing certain processes to be carried out.

Major vitamin deficiencies will result in disease. Some of the more common deficiency diseases are scurvy, caused by a lack of vitamin C; beriberi, caused by a lack of thiamine, one of the B vitamins; and rickets, caused by a lack of vitamin D. Because of the abundance and variety of food available here, vitamin deficiency is only a minor problem in the United States.

Vitamins may be categorized as fat-soluble or water-soluble. Fat-soluble vitamins A, D, E, and K can be stored in your body until needed. Water-soluble vitamins C and the B complex are not stored. What is not utilized by the body in a given day is excreted through the urine.

It is not necessary to know the names of all vitamins and their food sources to maintain your health and vigor and avoid deficiency diseases. Since only small amounts of the various vitamins are needed, a daily intake that includes food from the four basic groups will provide all that you require.

Figure 5-4 contains a list of the more common vitamins, their food sources, and their functions in maintaining and promoting health.

Minerals

Minerals, like vitamins, are found in each of the basic food groups, with certain minerals more abundant in some foods than in others. By having a well-balanced diet, you will receive all the minerals you need. You need many different kinds of minerals, but some of the more important minerals you require are iron, calcium, phosphorous, potassium, sodium, and iodine.

The amount of each mineral needed by your body is extremely small. In spite of this, minerals are extremely important because they help regulate the body and serve as building materials. The chart on page 72 describes the major minerals and how they are utilized by the body.

One important body-regulating function of minerals is maintaining the acid-base balance, that is, ensuring that your blood composition is neither too acid nor too alkaline. This balance is necessary to sustain life. Changes in the balance can become a problem if certain minerals are not supplied on a regular basis. This lack might be the result of "crash" reducing diets or the loss of excessive amounts of water. The loss of water may reduce the dissolving of minerals so that they are not as readily available for use by your body.

Fats

Fats or fatty acids are found in both plant and animal sources of food. Many persons believe that fats serve no useful purpose and should be eliminated as much as possible from the diet. This is indeed a misconception. Your fat intake should be no less than 20 to 25 percent of your daily caloric requirement. More will be said of this caloric requirement in the section on "Weight Control" in this chapter.

Fats are necessary in your diet for several reasons. They provide energy because they are concentrated sources of body fuel. In addition, they add flavor to various foods, act as carriers of fat-soluble vitamins, and provide the body with fatty acids necessary for certain body functions. Eating food with some fat content keeps you from getting hungry for a longer period of time. Eliminating fat from the diet may cause you to feel hungry more often. In addition, this practice removes an important source of energy and vitamins.

Figure 5-3 shows the percentage of fat found in various foods.

Elimination of Wastes

The basic function of the digestive system is to break down foods so that nutrients within the foods can be absorbed into the bloodstream and put to use by the body. This is accomplished by mechanical and chemical means. The mechanical part of the digestive process includes the chewing of food in the mouth and the churning of food in the stomach and intestines. The chemical part of the digestive process is the action of the digestive juices on the food particles. Not all of the food eaten is utilized by the body. The "leftover" food, or residue not digested, and the other waste products must be removed from the body.

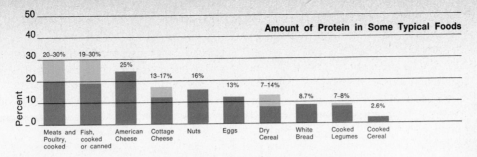

Figure 5-1 • Adequate protein is particularly important for your growth and development now. Does your diet include regular amounts of enough protein?

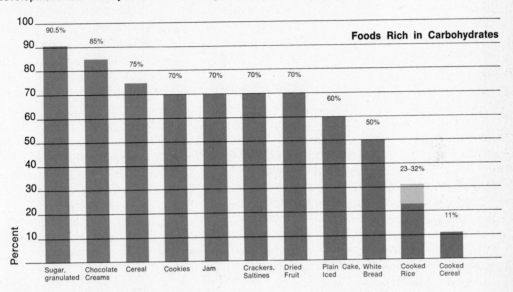

Figure 5-2 • Carbohydrates are energy foods. Does your diet provide you with enough energy to function at your peak?

Figure 5-3 • Fats are essential but should not constitute more than one-fourth of your caloric intake. Are you exceeding that amount?

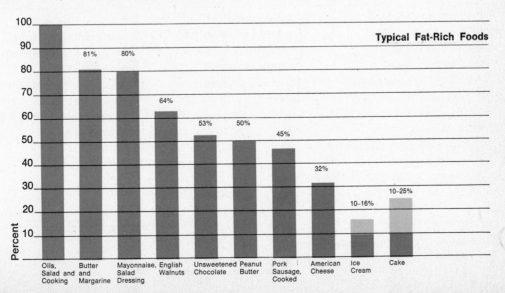

Vitamins
Their Functions
and Important Sources

	Vitamin A	Thiamine (B₁)	Riboflavin
Best Sources	Liver Sweet Potato Spinach Carrots Cantaloupe Squash, Winter Dark Green, Leafy Vegetables	Pork Pork Link Sausage Dried Beans and Peas Liver Lamb, Veal Luncheon Meat Nuts, Peas	Liver Poultry Milk Beef, Veal, Lamb, Pork Luncheon Meat Oysters Tongue Fish Cheese, Cottage
Functions	Promote growth and repair of body tissues Build general good health Help maintain normal vision and healthy eyes Help keep soft, smooth skin Help maintain healthy mucous membranes of mouth, nose, etc.	Help convert carbohydrates to energy Help maintain good appetite Aid in digestion and assimilation of food Help the heart, nerves, and muscles function properly	Help maintain good vision and clear, healthy eyes Build healthy skin and mouth tissue Help use carbohydrates efficiently promote well-being and vitality
Deficiency Symptoms	Retarded growth "Night blindness" Dry eyelids and reddened eyes Weakened respiratory system Increased susceptibility to infection Defective tooth formation	Poor appetite Retarded growth Nervousness and irritability Poor digestion Abnormal fatigue **Beriberi** (deficiency disease)	Reddened eyes oversensitive to light Cataract-like symptoms in eyes Cracks in corners of mouth Dimness of vision Inflamed and painful tongue Premature aging

 Developing Sound Nutritional Practices

Figure 5–4 ● If you select your foods properly, you will meet your daily vitamin requirements. Vitamin supplements are then unnecessary.

Niacin	Ascorbic Acid	Vitamin D
Liver Fish Poultry Lamb, Veal, Beef, Pork Peanut Butter Pork Link Sausage Luncheon Meat	Grapefruit, Orange Broccoli Strawberries Tomato Melon Dark Green, Leafy Vegetables Cabbage Liver Potato	Fish-Liver Oil Liver Milk (fortified) Eggs
Build and maintain healthy skin and tongue Help use carbohydrates efficiently Aid digestion Help the nervous system function	Help maintain firm, healthy gums Help build and maintain bones, tissues, and blood Utilize iron properly Help build resistance to infection Help heal wounds and fractures	Needed for calcium and phosphorous metabolism Promotes normal growth
Rough, inflamed skin Mental depression and nervousness Digestive disorders Pellagra (deficiency disease)	Possible bleeding in any part of body Weakened bones which may become deformed Tendency to bruise easily Swollen, painful joints Scurvy (deficiency disease)	Soft bones Poor tooth development

Your Mineral Needs [2]

Use	Elements Especially Needed	Results of Lack of These Elements
As Building Materials:		
To develop sound bones and teeth	Calcium and phosphorus	Stunted growth Weakened or soft bones Malformed or decaying teeth Rickets
Hair, nails, and skin Soft tissues, chiefly muscles	Sulphur All salts, especially potassium, phosphorus, sulphur, chlorine	Malfunction or improper development of specific tissues
Nervous tissue	All salts, especially phosphorus	
Blood	All salts, especially iron, calcium, sodium, phosphorus, copper	Lack of iron or copper results in less than normal amounts of hemoglobin in blood, a condition called nutritional anemia.
Glandular secretions	Stomach secretions— chlorine Intestinal secretions— sodium Thyroid secretion—iodine	Lack of iodine results in enlargement of thyroid gland—simple goiter.
As Body Regulators: To maintain normal Exchange of body fluids	All salts	
Contractility of muscles Irritability of nerves	All salts, especially balance of calcium with sodium and potassium	
Clotting of blood	Calcium	Improper regulation of body processes involved
Oxidation processes	Iron and iodine	
Neutrality of body	Balance between: Basic elements—sodium, potassium, calcium, magnesium, and iron Acidic elements—phosphorus, sulphur, and chlorine	

[2] Bogert, Briggs, and Calloway, *Nutrition and Physical Fitness.*

Undigested food residue is eliminated through the large intestines. Excessive amounts of water and salts are eliminated through the skin and kidneys. Carbon dioxide and water vapors are expelled from the body by the lungs. Keeping these processes functioning in a normal manner is essential to your health and well-being. Some of the steps that you can take to insure proper elimination of waste products are:

- Include recommended amounts of fruits and vegetables in your diet.
- Drink sufficient amounts of water daily.
- Exercise regularly.
- Maintain body cleanliness.
- Establish a regular time for evacuation of your bowels.
- Avoid the habitual use of laxatives.

If you are having problems with elimination of waste products (excessive bowel movements or constipation) see your physician. The use of laxatives, self-diagnosis, and self-medication can be extremely dangerous and can result in unnecessary pain and discomfort. Be especially careful not to take laxatives if constipation is accompanied by abdominal pain. If the pain is due to appendicitis (inflammation of the appendix), taking a laxative could result in a ruptured appendix. This in turn could lead to peritonitis (inflammation of the entire digestive tract).

Weight Control

A brief discussion of energy needs may give you some insight into the problems of weight control. You can estimate your own energy needs and determine whether or not you are meeting these needs through your daily intake of food.

Energy balance determines an individual's weight. There are three basic ways in which you expend energy: basal metabolism (internal work), muscular work (external work), and eating and digesting food (food cost).

Basal Metabolism

Basal metabolism is the minimum amount of energy required to maintain life processes. It is the energy needed for the internal work of the body.

Although basal metabolism varies from individual to individual, you can make a rough estimate of your own basal metabolism. For boys, basal metabolism equals one calorie per hour for each kilogram of body weight. For girls, it equals 0.9 calories per hour for each kilogram of body weight. One kilogram equals 2.2 lbs. A calorie is a unit of heat used for measuring energy that the body utilizes or takes in by means of food. Technically, this calorie is defined as the amount of energy required to raise the temperature of one kilogram of water one degree centigrade. To maintain your body weight, you must have a balance between the number of calories coming into your body and the number of calories used by your body. If your intake is greater than the amount used, the result is a gain in weight. If the intake is less than the amount used, the result is a weight loss.

A rough estimate of basal metabolism for a girl who weighs 150 lbs. would be computed as follows:

Basal metabolism = calories per day × kilograms of body weight

Calories per day = $0.9 \times 24 = 21.6$

Kilograms of body weight = $\frac{150}{2.2} = 68$

Basal metabolism = $21.6 \times 68 =$ 1469 calories

Basal + Effect of Food + Physical Work

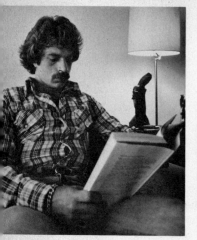 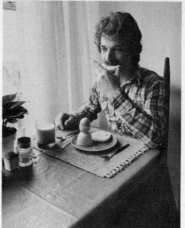 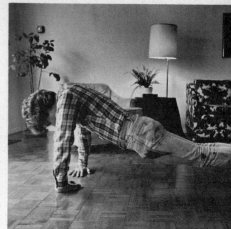

1632	326	1632	3590
Calories +	Calories +	Calories =	Calories

Figure 5-5 ● The total daily energy requirement for a male teen-ager who weighs 150 pounds and is very active in athletics.

Muscular Work

Energy requirements beyond one's basal metabolism are mainly to allow for muscular activity. A rough estimate of the amount of energy expended in muscular activity can be quickly calculated by taking a percentage of the basal metabolism (determined by the kind and amount of activity in which you are engaged) and adding it to your base figure. A general guide for calculating your energy requirements follows.

Very light activity . . . Increase the basal metabolism requirement by 30 percent.
A combination of sitting a greater part of the day, studying, talking, and walking or standing approximately two hours

Light exercise . . . Increase the basal metabolism requirement by 50 percent.
A combination of some sitting, typing, standing, laboratory work, and some walking.

Moderate exercise . . . Increase the basal metabolism requirement by 75 percent.
A combination of standing, walking, housework, gardening, carpentry work, etc., and a little sitting

Strenuous and service exercise . . . Increase the basal metabolism requirement by 100 percent.
Skating, outdoor games, sports

Thus, if a young man had a basal metabolism requirement of 1632 calories and he estimated that he engaged in moderate activity, his energy requirement would be 1632 + (75% of 1632) or 2856 calories.

Eating and Digesting Food

The food you eat provides you with energy. On the other hand, you use energy in eating and digesting this food. It is estimated that if you have a balanced diet the energy cost of eating and digesting your food will be approximately 10 percent of your total intake of food. Thus, if your basal metabolism and muscular activity energy needs come to 2856 calories, you will need to consume about 286 calories more if you are to maintain your weight.

It must be remembered that the above estimates of energy consumption are approximations. The figures and the discussion should indicate to you the need for a balance between caloric intake and energy output. You can readily see that the active person uses more energy than the inactive person. Therefore, physical activity can affect weight maintenance. If two persons were the same in regard to basal metabolism, amount of food eaten, and sleep, but differed in regard to activity, their weights would differ. If one of these persons sat for one hour daily for one year while the other person walked for that hour, at the end of the year the person who sat would be approximately 12 pounds heavier than the person who walked.

It also should be noted that it takes relatively few calories beyond one's requirements to cause a significant increase in weight. If you were to eat as few as 200 calories a day more than you need (200 calories = approximately 1½ doughnuts or 3 pieces of chocolate candy), at the end of one year you would have gained about 15 to 17 pounds.

Overweight

The problem of being overweight affects children, teen-agers, and adults. In the teen-age group, it is estimated that 10 million are overweight. Are you one of these? If not, good. Keeping the excess weight off is important. If you are overweight, you should do something about it.

Why You Should Be Concerned

The major cause of obesity is overeating. The individual simply takes in more calories than he can use, and the excess is stored as body fat. Most persons know by looking in the mirror when they are overweight. If you are in doubt, check with your doctor. You might also try the simple pinch test. Pinch a fold of skin at your midsection between your thumb and forefinger. If you can pinch an inch or more, it is usually an indication that you are overweight. If you find that you are overweight, do not make any hasty decisions about what to do. Again, consult your physician.

The obese person is generally not a very healthy person. **As excess weight increases, health hazards increase.** The health hazards become more severe if the gain in weight takes place after the age of 30. In general, studies indicate that individuals who are overweight do not live as long as those who do not have this problem. Overweight persons seem to have greater risk from kidney, heart, and circulatory disorders. The obese person also has a poorer chance of recovery after an operation or serious illness than does the nonobese one.

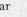

As you grow older, you may find that you gain weight rather easily. This happens quite often because your eating habits that were established at a young age have remained the same while your energy requirements have become less. To keep from gaining weight as you grow older, it is a good idea to reduce your caloric intake while maintaining a program of regular physical activity.

Dieting To Lose Weight

It is generally agreed that if an individual wants to lose 10 pounds or less, it can be done without necessarily calling for the advice of a physician. If, however, a greater weight loss is desired, it is wise to consult the family doctor. Losing too much weight or losing weight too quickly can be hazardous to one's health.

The best rule for reducing is to maintain a balanced diet while cutting down on the amount of food consumed. It is also wise to reduce slowly, one to two pounds per week. This can be accomplished by decreasing the daily food intake by 500 to 1000 calories and maintaining a good level of physical activity.

Some individuals have a more difficult time losing weight than others do. For example, a number of persons overeat (and are therefore overweight) because of emotional insecurity or frustration. Food for them is a means of satisfying a need. They cannot or will not reduce the amount they eat. For these individuals, the problem of obesity can be resolved only when the underlying causes for their overeating are uncovered and treated.

Losing weight and maintaining this loss is dependent upon an individual's changing his eating habits. If an individual reaches a desired weight and then goes back to his old eating habits, his weight will increase once more. Some people do this over and over again. In a sense, they are playing "Ping-Pong with pounds." You should remember that it is easier to keep pounds off than to take pounds off.

Underweight

In recent years the concept of what constitutes desirable weight has been revised downward. Consequently, many individuals who at one time might have been called thin are now considered normal. Life insurance statistics generally suggest that those who are slightly or moderately underweight live longer than those who are overweight. Some persons, in trying to attain what they consider an ideal weight, go too far below normal and become markedly underweight. If you are underweight, be sure you are not too far below the weight considered normal for good health.

Why You Should Be Concerned

If you are more than 10 percent below your ideal weight, you may be operating at a level somewhat below that which you should maintain. You may have reduced vitality and stamina, conditions which may be dangerous to your health. These conditions, in turn, may contribute to such factors as irritability, lowered resistance to disease germs, a tendency to tire easily, and a tendency to chill easily. This latter condition is frequently caused by inadequate subcutaneous fat.

Sometimes underweight is caused by an underlying disease or organic problem. The underweight individual needs the advice of a physician to determine the cause. If disease is involved, this must first be taken care of before the problem of weight can be resolved.

Dieting To Gain Weight

If you are underweight simply because you have an insufficient supply of nutrients, you can correct this merely by adding to your daily intake. One approach is to consume more high-calorie foods. However, it is also important to remember that increased amounts of protein, minerals, and vitamins are also necessary.

The best approach is to eat slightly larger portions than usual at all meals. This will help set a pattern which can be easily maintained. Along with the increase in food consumption, it might be necessary to decrease physical activity slightly. Too much activity can burn up the added calories. Be cautious. In dieting to gain weight, do not develop eating habits that may lead to the other extreme, obesity. Both extremes are dangerous to your health.

It is still important to select foods from the basic four food groups. A well-balanced diet is also important when you are trying to gain weight. Just getting heavier is not necessarily healthy. Merely adding rich foods to gain weight establishes bad eating habits that will be difficult for you to break later on.

Food Fads and Fallacies

Dietary fads and misconceptions can be detrimental to health. There are a number of fads and fallacies associated with nutrition and eating. Some of these are the outgrowth of social customs and traditions. Others are the result of a lack of adequate knowledge. Still others are based on the recommendations of food faddists who are trying to get rich by taking advantage of people's weight problems and worries. If you follow these fads or believe in these fallacies, there is a potential hazard to your health. In addition, you may be spending a great deal of money unnecessarily. Read carefully the following pages and determine if you are operating under some misconceptions about food and nutrition. Also determine to what extent you might be wasting your money or jeopardizing your health.

Vitamin Pills

Some food faddists would have you believe that everyone needs vitamin supplements. The fact of the matter is that if you have a well-balanced diet you will be getting all the nutrients you need for good health and attractive appearance.

Self-treatment with vitamins may be both hazardous and costly. For instance, water-soluble vitamins cannot be stored for later use by your body. Therefore, if you take more of these vitamins than your body can use in a given day, the excess will be eliminated through the urine. Vitamin C is an example of this. Because the body can use only the amount of vitamin C found in one orange, any extra vitamin C that might be taken is a waste. The fad of taking massive doses of vitamin C to ward off a cold or modify its severity is not backed by any reliable research.

Fat-soluble vitamins, on the other hand, can be stored by the body for future use when needed. However, care must be taken not to overdose the body with these vitamins. The accumulated effects of certain fat-soluble vitamins such as A and D can be toxic (poisonous) to the body. The American Medical Association and the United States Food and Drug Administration have issued warnings against taking, without the consent of a physician, one-a-day multipurpose vitamins containing more than half of the minimum daily requirement. This amount will safely supplement the vitamins in your food.

Vitamin E has received a great deal of attention in recent years. Claims for it include increased sexual virility, protection against heart attack, and clearing of skin blemishes. To date, however, there are no studies that can substantiate these claims. One researcher indicated that the folklore about vitamin E is 90 percent wishful thinking.

Special Foods

Many food faddists advocate the use of special foods or combinations of foods to promote good health. Common fallacies in this category include the following:

Fish is a brain food.

Tomatoes clear the brain.

Lemons aid digestion.

Oranges cause an acid stomach.

Brown sugar or honey is better for you than white, refined sugar.

Vegetable or fruit juices are better for you than the whole fruit or vegetable.

NONE OF THESE STATEMENTS CAN BE SUBSTANTIATED. In fact, most of them can be labeled as out-and-out falsehoods.

It is true that the nerve tissue does require phosphorus for proper functioning. However, food such as meat, poultry, eggs, and milk provides adequate amounts. Fish does contain phosphorus, but not in any unusual amounts that would require it to be eaten as a special aid to the brain.

Acid is necessary for proper digestion of foods. The stomach secretes HCl (hydrochloric acid) for this purpose. Eating lemons has no effect upon the process.

Oranges cannot cause an acid stomach. Your stomach already produces an acid to aid the digestive process.

There is nothing wrong with eating honey or brown sugar. Indeed, many persons do so because they enjoy the taste. These foods, however, offer no special health benefits. The difference between the nutrients found in honey or brown sugar and those found in white, refined sugar is too small to have any effect on health.

Vegetable juices and fruit juices are tasty and enjoyable, as well as being good for you. However, when the juices are made, there are left in the fibers some mineral salts and some pigment from which vitamin A is synthesized for use by the body. Therefore, drinking fruit and vegetable juices may not be so nutritious as eating the whole fruit or vegetable. Certainly these juices are not the cure-alls that some health faddists claim them to be.

"Organically Fertilized" Foods

A claim made by some "health food" faddists is that the foods grown in their "special soil" with organic fertilizers are more nutritious and better for you than other types of food. These faddists say that much of the food sold in the grocery store is grown in depleted soil, or soil that does not contain rich nutrients. The claim is that food produced under such conditions is lacking in important nutrients. They say also that chemical or inorganic fertilizers reduce the food's nutritive value. THESE CLAIMS ARE COMPLETELY UNFOUNDED.

The nutritional quality of foods is determined by the genetic structure of the seed and not by the soil or fertilizer used. Even if foods were grown in depleted soils, it is the size and the yield, not the nutritional value of the food, that would be affected.

"Enriched" Foods

A common cry from many food faddists is that we are eating overprocessed foods. These faddists claim their product is superior to other foods because no important nutrients have been lost through processing. What they neglect to say is that most food processing either conserves nutrients or restores what might have been lost. Restoring nutrients is called enrichment. White bread is a good example of enrichment. During processing, some nutrients are lost when kernels of wheat are husked. The producers of "enriched" bread replace some of these lost nutrients. In some instances, they add even more than the amount lost. As a result, there is no significant nutritional difference between whole wheat and white enriched bread.

Diet Fads

You cannot go into a drugstore or supermarket today without seeing claims for many preparations to help you control weight. These preparations are expensive and using them may not be the most effective way to solve your problem. **If you need to control weight, you should follow the advice of your physician.** If he decides to prescribe special medications for you or put you on a special diet, well and good. Do not make such a decision on your own; you may not need to change your weight. Then, too, taking certain preparations or changing weight too rapidly could cause serious health problems. For example, special canned liquid diets have been shown to have an irritating effect on the digestive system of some persons, resulting in chronic colitis (inflammation of the colon). In addition, these diets might be supplying more vitamins than you need to meet your daily requirements. It is a good idea to consult with your physician before substituting these special canned diets for other forms of food.

Diets which alter the balance of certain nutrients also come into vogue from time to time. In the long run, they are no more effective for controlling weight than eating proper amounts of a well-balanced diet is. Eliminating carbohydrates or eating only proteins might lead to certain deficiencies.

Unbalanced diets can cause an abnormal acid-base balance (acidosis) as well as abnormal fatigue.

Many people use low-calorie sweeteners, carbonated drinks, and specially prepared foods in an attempt to lose weight. Such foods and beverages, if substituted for sugar and regular beverages and foods, can reduce the intake of calories. They are, however, expensive and are not necessary if the individual merely reduces the total intake of food. If a person is attempting to gain weight, the best approach is to try to eat larger portions of a balanced diet at each regular meal.

For many years, special devices such as vibrating machines, baths, and massages have been used by individuals in an attempt to lose weight. There is no evidence that such devices or techniques work. Fatty tissue cannot be broken down by massage or vibrators. Systematic exercise may tone certain muscles. If there is also a reduction in calories taken in, extra fat can be eliminated. Steam and water baths cause little weight reduction other than the water lost through sweating. You should be suspicious of establishments that promise quick reducing, spot reducing, or easy reducing. The only thing that will be reduced will be the size of your bankroll.

Cholesterol and Animal Fats

In recent years there has been a great deal of emphasis on reducing the intake of animal fats which supposedly increase blood-cholesterol levels. Some researchers believe that there is a relationship between high levels of blood cholesterol and atherosclerosis (closing and hardening of the inner artery walls). However, there is a wide variation in blood-cholesterol levels among individuals regardless of their diet. Other researchers have called attention to a variety of factors that might influence this level. These factors include the number of cigarettes one smokes, the amount and kind of activity one engages in, and the kind of emotional stress one undergoes. The way one handles stressful situations also seems to be important.

You should remember that reducing the intake of animal fat is not a cure-all for heart disease nor does it completely eliminate the risk of this disease. Reducing animal fat consumption may benefit some persons but not others. In reducing the risk of heart disease, there are many other factors that must be considered.

Summary

Good nutrition is important to your everyday functioning. Your vigor and vitality, your degree of susceptibility to certain disorders, and your general emotional and physical efficiency are dependent, to some extent, on adequate intake of essential nutrients. There are no shortcuts, no special foods or pills that can take the place of a well-balanced diet.

Once the food is digested, it is important that the waste products be properly eliminated. Good eating practices plus regular exercise and rest help to ensure proper elimination.

Some of you are from families that have certain special cultural patterns of eating. After studying this chapter, you should be in a better position to evaluate these patterns.

If you have a problem of weight control, you should do something about it. You should first understand the potential dangers of being overweight or underweight. You should try to evaluate your reasons for improper eating, then you should take steps to regulate your weight. You may be able to handle the problem on your own, but in most cases you should seek the advice of a physician.

You and most of your friends will always have available all the food you need. No one can force you to have a well-balanced diet. No one can prevent your following the advice of a food faddist, and no one can make you disbelieve certain fallacies about eating. You must make your own decisions. The decisions you make now about the kinds and amount of food you eat can affect the quality and length of your life.

in making health decisions . . .

Understand These Terms:

atherosclerosis	calorie	food enrichment
balanced diet	digestion	food fads
basal metabolism	fat-soluble vitamins	water-soluble vitamins

Solve This Problem:

Manuel is a high-school student interested in pursuing a career in the nutrition field. His girlfriend tells him he would be wasting his time because nutrition careers are primarily for girls.

1. What careers are available in the nutrition field?
2. Can both males and females gain employment in such fields?
3. Would Manuel need training beyond high school in order to be qualified in some of these fields?
4. Are there any jobs in the nutrition field available for a person who does not have training beyond high school?

Try These Activities:

1. In class, select and invite a home economist to come to your class to discuss various career opportunities in the nutrition field that might be available to both males and females.
2. Have selected students prepare dinner menus containing foods from different countries (i.e., China, Italy, Mexico, Germany, etc.). As a class, discuss the similarities and differences among the menus and determine which of the menus contain adequate amounts of the basic four food groups.
3. Before making a hasty decision about dieting, estimate your energy needs and determine whether or not you are meeting these needs through your daily food intake.
   a. Check pages 73–75 for steps to follow in estimating your energy needs (basal metabolism, eating and digestion, and muscular work).
   b. Use of calorie counter to determine your caloric intake. (You must account for all food consumed, including snacks.) What is your caloric intake? Discuss what adjustments are necessary to enable you to meet your energy requirements. Analyze whether or not you are eating a balanced diet (check the basic four food groups).

Interpret These Concepts:

1. Individuals throughout life require the same nutrients but in varying amounts.
2. Energy balance determines an individual's weight.
3. As excess weight increases, health hazards increase.
4. Self-treatment with vitamins may be both hazardous and costly.

Explore These Readings:

Ahrens, Richard A., *Nutrition and Health.* Belmont, Calif.: Wadsworth Publishing Co., Inc., 1970.

"Are You Digging a Grave with Your Teeth?" *Story of Life,* Part I. London, England: Marshall Cavendish, Ltd., 1970, pp. 24–28.

Singer, Steve, "When They Start Telling You It's Easy to Lose Weight," *Today's Health,* 50:46–49 (November, 1972).

Stare, Frederick J. and Mary McSherry, "Right Diet for You," *Reader's Digest,* 102:89–92 (February, 1973).

"What's So Great About Health Foods?" *Life,* 73:45–47 (Sept. 29, 1972).

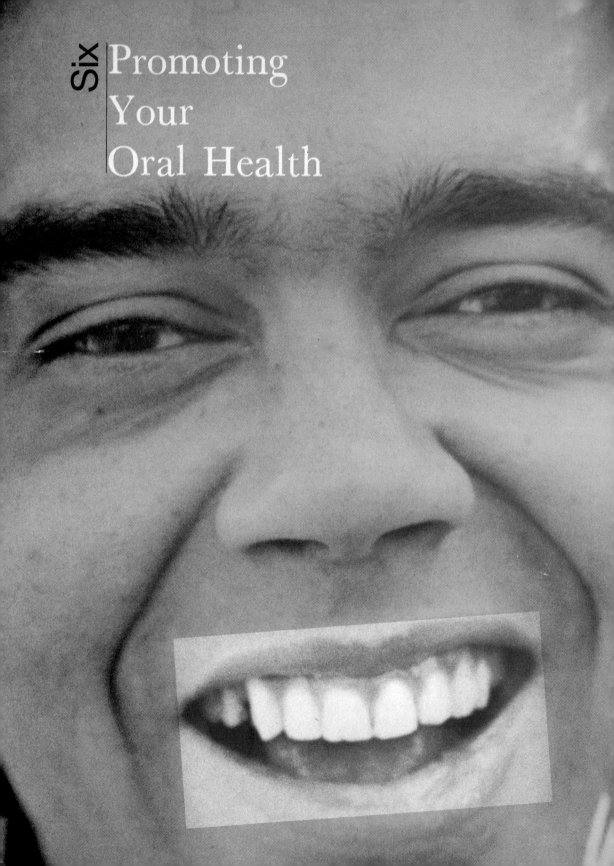

Six

Promoting Your Oral Health

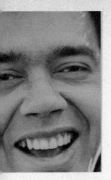

Neglect of oral health affects individuals of all ages. Your oral health not only affects your teeth and gums; it can affect your total health. Whether or not you have good oral health depends on the decisions you make. For tooth decay and gum diseases can be prevented by applying sound health practices.

As you read this chapter you will learn more about dental problems and how they affect your teeth and gums and your total well-being. You will learn what research scientists now know about tooth decay, its causes, and how it can best be prevented. Diseases of the supporting structures of the teeth (periodontal diseases) will be discussed. In addition, you will learn how these diseases can be prevented. Information about the causes of and problems related to malocclusion (poor alignment of teeth) will be presented. Finally, you will study about fluoridation and why it is beneficial to your oral health.

Why Be Concerned?

Dental neglect can result in serious infections of the teeth, gums, jawbone, and major organs of the body.

In addition, this type of neglect can have an effect upon behavior in a social setting, since a person's appearance and personality are often involved. One of the first things you notice about a person's smile is the teeth. When you see unsightly teeth, you become bothered and feel rather uncomfortable. As a result, you tend to avoid people whose teeth seem neglected.

In a similar fashion, you feel more comfortable when you know that your teeth are clean and your breath is pleasant. You feel more like mixing or talking with people.

Dental neglect and the results of neglect are unnecessary. For **most oral disorders can be prevented.** With a little effort, you can attain good dental health and avoid unsightly teeth.

The Tooth Decay Process

Dental caries (tooth decay) is one of the most common problems in the United States in that it attacks approximately 95 percent of our total population. Furthermore, your age group has more tooth decay than any other age group.

Study Figure 6–1, which shows the process of tooth decay. In this illustration you can see that once decay passes the enamel, it spreads very rapidly through the dentin. This is because the dentin is not so hard nor so compact as the enamel. The dentin is composed of tubules that enable bacteria and acids to spread more rapidly throughout the tooth. It should be noted that the bacteria present spread out farther than does the decay itself. If allowed to continue, the decay process penetrates the pulp. When the infection reaches this stage, an abscess may form. From this point on, your general health may be affected. Each tooth is supplied with nutrients from blood vessels that are contained within the root canal and are a part of the main circulatory system. The bacteria may invade the circulatory system and then be deposited in other parts of the body.

Factors Contributing to Tooth Decay

Many factors contribute to tooth decay. Knowing these factors will enable you to take preventive measures that will help reduce tooth decay and related problems.

Figure 6-1 • Note the progression of tooth decay and how microorganisms can invade the bloodstream, enabling the infection to reach other parts of the body.

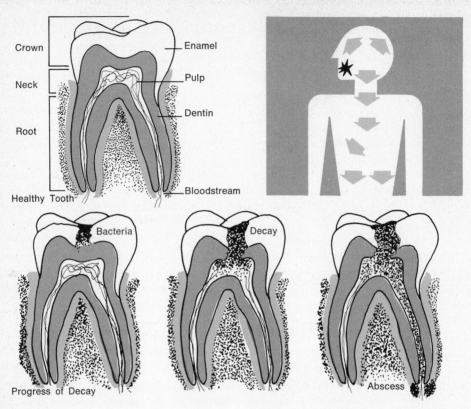

Some of these factors include structure of teeth, sweets, bacteria, saliva, and heredity. **Tooth Structure.** The quality of your teeth is determined in part by the foods eaten by your mother and the nutrients you consequently received when you were developing as an embryo. In addition, heredity plays a vital role.

During the first half of pregnancy the primary teeth (baby teeth) of the embryo begin to develop their protein base. Insufficient amounts of protein, vitamin C, and vitamin A at this time can result in faulty or poorly structured teeth. During the last half of pregnancy, as the primary teeth begin to calcify, a lack of or improper portions of calcium, phosphorus, and vitamin D might result in inferior enamel and dentin structure. If this occurs, the teeth become more susceptible to decay. The balance between phosphorus and calcium is important. If there is too little phosphorus and too much calcium in the mother's diet, the fetus will develop an inferior enamel structure of the primary teeth.

The secondary teeth (permanent teeth) of the fetus begin to develop during the second half of pregnancy. During this period, the protein base is being formed and adequate amounts of protein, vitamin C, and vitamin A are again needed. After birth, these secondary teeth begin to calcify and it is essential once more to supply proper amounts of calcium, phosphorus, and vitamin D for healthy growth.

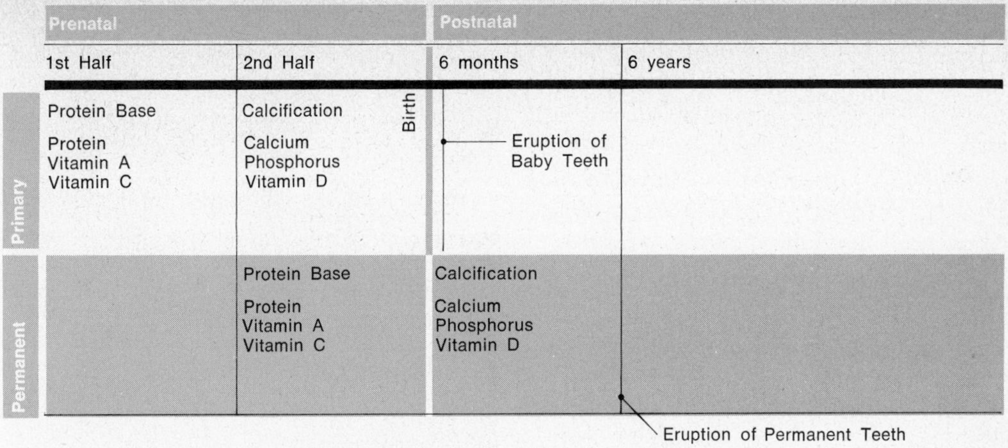

Prenatal		Postnatal	
1st Half	2nd Half	6 months	6 years
Primary Protein Base Protein Vitamin A Vitamin C	Calcification Calcium Phosphorus Vitamin D	Birth • — Eruption of Baby Teeth	
Permanent	Protein Base Protein Vitamin A Vitamin C	Calcification Calcium Phosphorus Vitamin D	

Eruption of Permanent Teeth

Figure 6-2 ● Developing primary and permanent teeth and their required nutrients. What foods should the expectant mother eat to ensure proper development of the embryo's teeth?

You can see that the structure of teeth can be altered by nutrients taken in during the development of the teeth. For the most effective structure, a well-balanced diet is necessary from early embryonic stages through birth until all the permanent teeth have fully developed. Once the enamel of the teeth has been formed, food taken in will not improve their structure. While you have little or no control over this part of your development, this information is still important to you. In a few years, you and many of your peers will probably be parents. You will have the responsibility of planning proper diets so that your children will have the best possible start in life.

While the development of your teeth can no longer be affected by what you eat, your diet can still be beneficial or detrimental to your teeth and gums. The lack of certain nutrients can, for example, make you more susceptible to gum disease. In addition, excessive sweets can contribute to the development of tooth decay.

Sweets. Studies have shown that before teeth can decay, sweets or refined carbohydrates must be present in the mouth. In animal experiments, where carbohydrates

were fed directly into the stomach through a tube, no decay developed. However, if carbohydrates were fed into the mouth, tooth decay developed in all of the animals. As a result of these studies, it was determined that sugars, or refined carbohydrates, must be present in the mouth before decay will develop.

Another important point brought out in these studies was that the longer the sugars or refined carbohydrates remained in the mouth, the greater were the chances that decay would develop. As a result, the consistency of sweets or the kind of sweets eaten becomes an important factor. Sweets that tend to stick to the teeth pose a much greater problem than those that do not. **Bacteria.** Tooth decay will not develop without the presence of bacteria in the mouth. There is some evidence to suggest that certain bacteria involved in the decay process can be transmitted from individual to individual. If these observations are correct, tooth decay may be considered a communicable disease.

Experiments at a number of universities have shown that animals without bacteria in the mouth did not develop tooth decay. When these animals were fed a diet containing highly concentrated amounts of refined carbohydrates, they still did not develop decay. A second step involved placing animals with decay in the same germ-free environment as the animals without decay. When this occurred, all animals became infected and developed decay. The bacterium isolated in these experiments was a streptococcal organism.

The possibility that tooth decay is a communicable disease has led many investigators to study new measures of control. Some investigators have developed antibiotic toothpastes as a possible means of control. These toothpastes have been tested in laboratory experiments, but so far have been ineffectual for the following reasons:

■ The antibiotic used could destroy essential or needed bacteria in the body.
■ The bacteria responsible for the development of tooth decay could adapt to the antibiotics used and thus render them ineffectual.
■ Using antibiotics continuously and without control in large groups of the population could result in many severe reactions or side effects that might be more serious than tooth decay.

Another area of investigation for control measures has to do with the development of a vaccine. Such a vaccine could increase the resistance of human beings against the bacteria that are involved in the tooth decay process.

While evidence that tooth decay may be communicable has led to the consideration of new preventive measures, it has also made us realize that the results of decay are not necessarily limited or restricted to the mouth. We are more aware that neglected teeth can result in disease or disorders in various parts of the body. If, for instance,

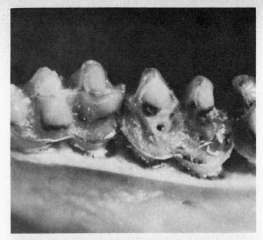
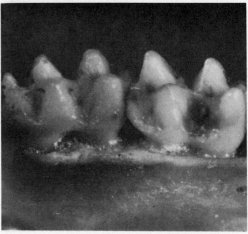

Figure 6-3 ● Microorganisms must be present in order for tooth decay to occur. (Top) The molars of hamsters raised in a normal environment are heavily decayed. (Bottom) The molars of hamsters raised in a germ-free environment are entirely free from decay.

a tooth abscesses (infection penetrates the pulp of the tooth and causes pus to form at the tip of the root), the bacteria can enter the bloodstream and travel to other parts of the body. Acute infections could thus spread to the throat and head area or to more distant organs, such as the heart, kidneys, or liver. Disorders resulting from these infections are referred to as systemic effects of tooth decay.

Saliva. Saliva is absolutely essential in the maintenance of healthy tooth structure. It helps prevent tooth decay in three ways:

- By diluting acids that may develop from the action of certain bacteria on refined carbohydrates, saliva helps neutralize the essential decay-producing material.

- By acting as a lubricant to reduce the friction produced when teeth rub against one another. Without this protection, the enamel of the teeth would be quickly destroyed.

- By serving as a medium that permits the exchange of minerals from itself to the enamel. This exchange is thought to be quite important in establishing the quality of tooth enamel. Once the enamel has developed, a well-balanced chemical exchange prevents the enamel from breaking down and in this way inhibits decay.

Some individuals are able to produce more saliva than others and as a result have a more effective mechanism for preventing decay. While the exact role of saliva is not yet clear, several types of investigation are being conducted. Some researchers are exploring the possibility that the saliva contains a hormone that increases the chances for transmission of minerals to the enamel. Other researchers are looking at the possible inhibiting effect hormones may have upon bacterial growth. Still others are concerned with a relationship among all these factors. If a specific hormone can be shown to be implicated in the prevention of tooth decay, it might be possible to stimulate its production as a means of decay prevention.

The diluting action of saliva is an important consideration in the prevention of decay. Decay is related to the time of day you eat sweets and the frequency with which you eat them. Normally it takes approximately two hours for saliva to dilute all the acid that has developed after you have eaten a candy bar or some other sweet. Obviously, if you eat sweets continuously (with less than a two-hour interval between each serving) you are providing a continuous acid bath for your teeth. This, of course, increases your chances of developing tooth decay. If you eat sweets before going to bed and fail to brush your teeth, the acids produced will stay in your mouth all night. At night, the diluting action is not so efficient because the salivary glands do not secrete sufficient amounts of saliva to dilute any acids present.

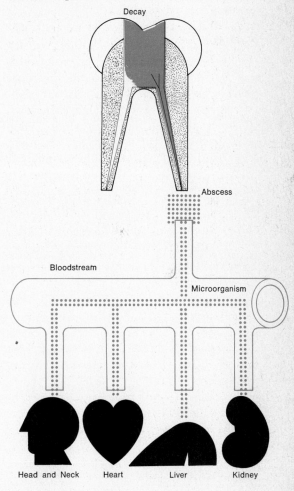

Figure 6-4 • Possible sites in the body where infection, beginning with tooth decay, can spread.

Heredity. The relationship between heredity and tooth decay is under investigation. By controlling breeding, it has been possible to produce animals that were either extremely susceptible to tooth decay or virtually free from decay. In one experiment, rats were inbred until decay was present as early as 25 days after birth. Another group of rats was inbred until no decay was detected before 550 days after birth. These studies are important because they may help to identify other factors causing tooth decay.

You have learned that the development of tooth decay is dependent on many factors. Some factors are determined by your biological makeup (heredity). Others are affected by poor practices or environmental conditions (eating habits, tooth brushing, and the presence of bacteria). In addition, you have learned that decay is not merely a problem affecting the teeth alone. Your total well-being can be affected. As more research is completed, new information will become available that will help you prevent this disease. If you apply what is already known, however, **you can effectively prevent or control tooth decay.**

Periodontal Disease

Another major dental health problem is gum disorder or periodontal disease. This is a disease that affects the gums and other supporting structures of the teeth. The most common periodontal disorder develops in two stages. The first stage is referred to as gingivitis and the second stage is called periodontitis.

Gingivitis

Look into a mirror and examine your gums. If they are healthy and free of disease, they will be firm or tight near the teeth. In addition, they will appear to be slightly stippled (a little rougher in texture than the inside of your cheek). If the gums change color, look shiny and swollen, and are loose near the teeth, and if they bleed easily when you

Figure 6-5 ● Progression of periodontal disease. (1) Beginning stage is gingivitis with red, swollen gums. (2) and (3) Gingivitis progressing to advanced stage of periodontitis. Bone tissue is actually being destroyed. (4) Final stages of periodontitis where structure is lost due to complete destruction of bone tissue.

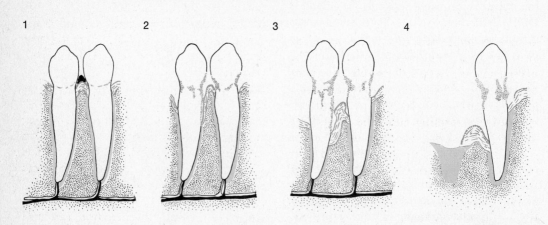

1 2 3 4

eat or brush your teeth, you may have the initial stages of gingivitis. This condition is commonly called inflamed gums. When gum inflammation is neglected, it usually advances to the second and more serious stage, periodontitis.

Periodontitis

This type of disorder (also known as pyorrhea) is much more serious and involves not only the gums but also other supporting structures of the teeth. These supporting structures include periodontal fibers (the tissues that attach the teeth to the jaws), cementum (a bonelike substance that covers the roots of the teeth), and the jawbone itself (where the teeth are embedded). If this stage of gum disease is neglected, it ultimately results in loss of teeth. When the disease is allowed to run its course, there simply is no bone left to hold the teeth in place. Furthermore, the bacteria may invade the bloodstream and cause damage in another part of the body.

Factors Contributing to Periodontal Disease

Gingivitis and its advanced stage, periodontitis, can be prevented and controlled. The primary cause of these disorders is poor oral hygiene. If you clean your teeth and gums properly, you will prevent tartar (calculus) from forming near the gum line. When the tartar does accumulate and is not removed, an irritation is established that causes the gums to swell. The swelling and inflammation constitute what is called gingivitis. If this condition is not corrected, the gums continue to swell and the space between the gum line and the tooth deepens.

Food particles, tartar, and bacteria can then penetrate deeper into the space, causing more irritation and deeper pockets. Finally, the bone itself is infected and begins to deteriorate.

Once tartar has developed, it must be removed by a dentist. The prevention of this condition depends on proper oral hygiene.

Diet. Insufficient amounts of vitamin C may destroy gum tissues and add to the development of periodontal disease. A contributing factor may be a general nutritional deficiency which can also be reflected in poor response to treatment. Nutritional factors that may be involved in the development of periodontal disease are:

- Inadequate or unbalanced diet
- Inability of the body to utilize foods properly
- Texture of food eaten

All these factors may lower resistance to gum disease, and the vicious cycle is started. The insufficient diet can contribute to gum disease and the subsequent gum condition may in turn cause poor selection of foods, with the nutritional habits and gum condition becoming progressively worse.

Breathing Habits. Breathing through the mouth tends to dry the gums and lower resistance to injury and infection. As a result, the susceptibility to gingivitis is increased.

Malocclusion. Poor alignment of the teeth so that they do not mesh together is called malocclusion. This improper impact, occurring thousands of times a day, may set up bone and gum irritation which results in periodontal disease. In addition, if the teeth are not straight, food may be diverted into the space between the teeth and into the gums. As a result, an irritation can take place that may lead to periodontal disease.

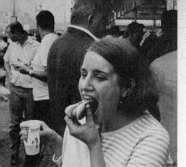
Diet Lack of Vitamin C

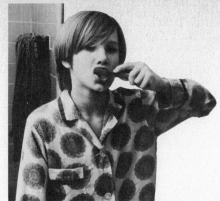
Oral Hygiene Poor brushing habits

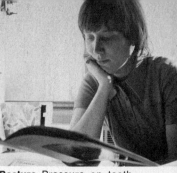
Posture Pressure on teeth

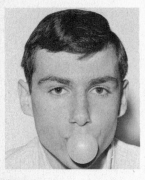
Gumchewing
Pounding teeth together

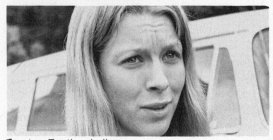
Tension Tooth-grinding

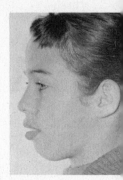
Malocclusion
Bone and gum irritatio

Figure 6-6 ● Many factors influence the development of periodontal disease. Are you a candidate for this disease? Evaluate your own practices.

Emotional Tension. People who are tense or worried have a tendency to grind or clench their teeth. The continuous practice of this habit results in unusual pressure on the bones that support the teeth. This is especially true of the bones supporting the large molars. The continued pressure can result in bone destruction and irritation of the gums. It is not unusual to discover that many people suffering from periodontal disease are also under a great deal of emotional tension.

Gumchewing. Chronic gumchewing is similar to toothgrinding. It causes unusual pressure on the bones supporting the large molars. The resulting periodontal conditions usually take a number of years to develop. As a result, the deterioration may not be detected until much of the bone structure surrounding the molars has been destroyed.

You and your dentist should both be concerned about periodontal disease and its related problems. Usually, your dentist is able to detect early signs of this disease by visual examination or by X ray. Upon diagnosis, the dentist can stop the progress of the disease. However, a dentist can correct only an existing condition. No dentist can prevent the disease from developing unless you cooperate. You are the only one who can maintain a clean and healthy environment for your teeth by means of proper cleaning procedures and good nutritional practices.

Periodontal disease usually affects those over 25 years of age. In fact, after this age, it is the chief cause for the loss of teeth. However, the disease begins to develop much earlier than this. Oral neglect, if continued through the teens, can result in permanent damage to the teeth and gums that may not be noticeable until age 25. Thus the prevention of periodontal disease should begin early in life.

If the disease is neglected and the symptoms persist, you may require the services of a periodontist, a dentist who specializes in the treatment of periodontal disorders.

Malocclusion: An Orthodontic Problem

Malocclusion, the poor alignment of teeth, has been discussed as a contributing factor to the development of periodontal disease. Whether you consider your teeth or the teeth of the children you may someday have, you should be aware of the problems related to this disorder. **Malocclusion can be controlled.**

Most people have the misconception that malocclusion simply means crooked teeth. This is not true. When the condition exists, the teeth are misplaced or out of alignment. Furthermore, the disorder involves not only the positioning of the teeth but also the growth of the jaw. Correcting malocclusion does not involve merely moving the teeth. It requires the services of a specialist, an orthodontist, who must alter the growth of the jawbone. In some cases, extractions must be made if there are too

Figure 6-7 • Malocclusion has a definite effect on one's appearance. (1) Before orthodontic treatment. (2) After treatment.

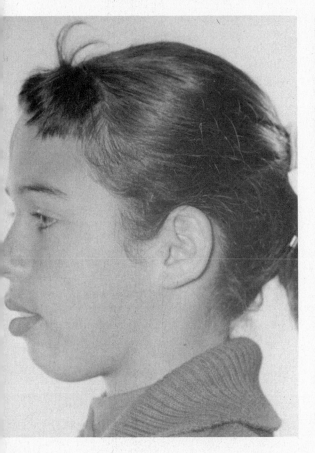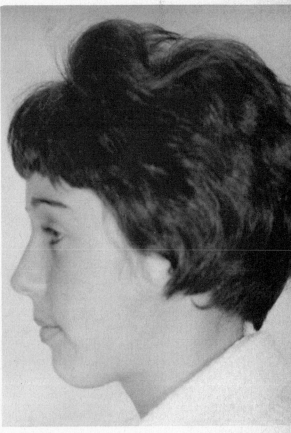

many teeth for the size of the jawbone. The age at which corrections should be made varies greatly and depends on the kind of malocclusion, the severity of the disorder, and the growth and development of the jawbone. Thus, an orthodontist may recommend that one child start corrective treatment around the age of seven or eight. For another child, it might be better to wait until he is 10 or 11 before treatment starts.

Causes of Malocclusion

Although orthodontists report that heredity is the primary factor contributing to malocclusion, there are a number of circumstances that can aggravate this condition.

Missing Teeth. If a tooth is lost prematurely and the space that is left is not properly filled, the teeth can become malaligned. The adjacent teeth tend to drift toward the space and the opposite tooth tends to leave its socket because there is no opposing force to hold it in place.

Tongue-Thrusting. Some children have the habit of pushing the tongue forward against the top front teeth as they talk or swallow. Since a person swallows approximately 2,000 times a day, it is possible to exert a great deal of pressure on the upper front teeth. Over a period of time, this pressure will cause a malalignment of the upper arch. Before the orthodontist can effectively correct this malocclusion, the habit of tongue-thrusting must first be broken. The aid of speech therapists is often needed to correct this habit either before or during treatment by the orthodontist.

Thumb-Sucking. Pressure on the upper front teeth is also produced by thumb-sucking. If the habit is continued over a period of years, it can cause malocclusion. A child usually stops thumb-sucking by school age or shortly thereafter. Unless there is a heredity factor, any malocclusion that might have resulted from sucking the thumb will correct itself. If continued, however, thumb-sucking may lead to serious orthodontic problems. In addition, this practice may be a symptom of emotional disturbance. In this case, the services of a psychologist or psychiatrist might be necessary to solve the emotional disturbance before the orthodontic problem can be corrected.

Poor Resting Habits. When a person develops the habit of cradling the jaw in the hands, pressure is exerted on the jaw. When this habit persists, it may result in problems related to malocclusion.

Fluoridation

One of the greatest discoveries of our time in the prevention of tooth decay is the fluoridation of water. **Flouridation reduces tooth decay.** By adding approximately one part of sodium fluoride to one million parts of water (1 ppm.), communities have been able to lower the average amount of tooth decay by at least 60 to 75 percent. (See Figure 6–8.) This relationship between fluoridation and the reduction of tooth decay was first noticed in communities where fluorides occurred naturally in the water supply. We now know that the fluoride reacts with certain chemicals and forms a denser and harder enamel that is resistant to decay. This process is beneficial when the developing teeth are becoming calcified.

Fluoridation of the water has undergone extensive tests and research and the results have been conclusive. It is a sound public-health measure for the reduction of tooth decay. During the past 40 years no adverse effects on health have been attributed to fluoridated water. Major health organizations in the United States have endorsed fluoridation. They include such

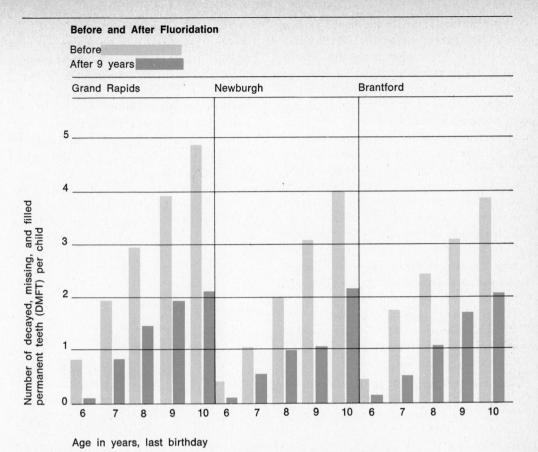

Before and After Fluoridation

Before

After 9 years

Grand Rapids   Newburgh   Brantford

Number of decayed, missing, and filled permanent teeth (DMFT) per child

Age in years, last birthday

Figure 6-8 • Before and after fluoridation. A comparison of the dental condition of children living continuously in Grand Rapids, Michigan; Newburgh, New York; and Brantford, Ontario, Canada, before fluoridation and after approximately nine years of fluoridation. Does your community need to add fluoride to the water supply?

groups as the American Dental Association, the American Medical Association, and the American Public Health Association.

In spite of the knowledge we have of the benefits of fluoridation, a number of communities still refuse to add fluoride to their water supply. One reason is that a small number of persons have made unwarranted statements concerning fluoridation. Antifluoridationists have stated that almost any disease that affects human beings can be caused by fluoride or made worse by this chemical. Extensive research has been conducted regarding these and other claims.

None have proved to be valid. However, the antifluoridationists have been successful in preventing many communities, and millions of people, from receiving the benefit of fluoridated water. Their most effective weapon has been the lack of knowledge on the part of the public. They have used emotionally charged half-truths and have raised unwarranted suspicions about fluoridation. They have been most successful where the issue is put on the ballot for public vote. The highly emotional charges tend to raise doubt and fear in the minds of voters, with the end result of defeating the issue.

It seems unfortunate that some proven public-health measures such as fluoridation are put to a vote of the public. If a vote were taken on every proposed health measure, it is conceivable that important health programs such as sewage disposal, chlorination of water, pasteurization of milk, and immunizations against smallpox, measles, and polio might not be available today.

Some of the individuals who are against fluoridation are quite sincere and simply do not have the knowledge or will not accept the scientific evidence produced by public-health officials. Others are either extremists or food faddists and are out to promote their cause. If you are ever required to vote on this issue, you should remember that:

■ Studies by our federal government and by university research authorities have shown that fluoridation has absolutely no harmful effect on health.

■ Communities using the optimum amount of fluoridation in their water supply have had a 60 to 70 percent reduction of tooth decay.

■ Fluoridation is endorsed by major health organizations as being a safe and effective public-health measure in the reduction of decay.

■ Fluoridating the water supply is the most economical means of preventing tooth decay. It costs approximately 10 cents per person per year, much less than the cost per person of one filling.

Other Means of Receiving Fluorides

Until such time as your community does have fluoridated water, there are other ways of receiving the benefits of fluoride. For example, fluoride tablets equal to one part per

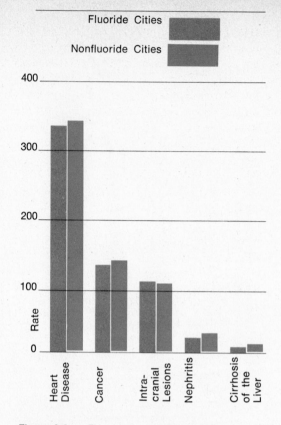

Figure 6-9 ● Fluoridation does not cause disease. This chart shows deaths per 100,000 population from five causes in fluoride and nonfluoride cities in the United States.

million (ppm.) can be mixed in your own drinking water or taken by mouth. These tablets are quite expensive compared to the fluoridation of a community's entire water supply. Another limiting factor of these tablets is that people tend to forget to use them.

Dentists can apply fluorides directly to the enamel of the teeth of patients at certain ages. This is called topical application of fluoride. Studies show that groups receiving topical application have 40 percent less tooth decay than do groups using no fluoride. Topical application is much more expensive and more inconvenient than utilizing fluoridated water.

Proper Oral Hygiene

You may brush your teeth 20 times a day and still not be cleaning your teeth properly. Proper oral hygiene means more than counting the times you brush your teeth. Toothbrushing techniques vary with individuals. Your best source for proper toothbrushing information is your family dentist. Most dentists now recommend a soft-bristled brush to clean the teeth and gums. Some dentists stress cleaning the area just above or beneath the gum line adjacent to the teeth. They recommend using a slight circular motion at the gum line and then brushing away from the gum. This strengthens the gums while cleaning the teeth. Most dentists recommend using dental floss to remove food and plaque deposits between the teeth.

Two other oral hygiene devices are the electric toothbrush and the Water Pik. Some dentists feel that the electric toothbrush offers advantages, such as easier and better cleaning of the teeth and more effective massaging of the gums. A possible disadvantage is that excessive use of the electric toothbrush could lead to receding gums.

The Water Pik provides a pressurized stream of water for cleaning between the teeth and near the gum line without causing irritation. It is often prescribed for those who have periodontal disease, but it can also benefit others. As with the electric toothbrush, its excessive use might be harmful to the supporting tissues of the teeth. It is best to use these two devices, or any new device, only after consulting your dentist.

Dental Checkups

It is not always possible for you to detect tooth decay or periodontal disease. Waiting can be potentially dangerous to your health and eventually expensive. Regular dental checkups are needed so that the dentist can spot what you cannot observe. These checkups keep the cost of dental care at a minimum because problems are detected when they are easier to correct. In addition, disorders are prevented from growing progressively worse.

The cost to repair teeth increases as damage progresses. In addition, your chances of losing a tooth or developing more serious dental problems increase if this work is neglected. It is for these reasons that you should visit your dentist for a checkup at least every six months.

Summary

Your oral health is closely related to your total health. Dental neglect can not only cause problems in your mouth, but can also create serious disorders in other parts of your body.

Three major dental health problems are tooth decay, periodontal disease, and orthodontic defects. Factors that contribute to the development of tooth decay include poor tooth structure, excessive amounts of sweets, bacteria, saliva, and heredity. Periodontal disease affects the supporting structure of the teeth. Diet, breathing habits, malocclusion, emotional tension, and gumchewing contribute to this problem. Orthodontic defects (poorly aligned teeth) are caused by missing teeth, tongue-thrusting, thumb-sucking, and poor resting habits.

No one can provide you with good oral health. It is your responsibility. You can reduce oral health problems only by putting into practice current procedures regarding their prevention and treatment.

in making health decisions...

Understand These Terms:

abscess
caries
fluoridation
gingivitis

malocclusion
orthodontics
periodontitis
systemic effect

Solve This Problem:

A young man complained to his doctor that he always seemed to have a sore throat and an earache. After examining the young man, the doctor advised him to consult with a dentist.

1. Give possible explanations of how the young man's sore throat and earache could be related to dental neglect.

2. What other systemic effects might result from dental neglect?

Try These Activities:

1. Assume that you had to teach a lesson on good dental-health practices to children in the primary grades. Summarize the major points you would stress.

2. In class discussion select a dentist, a dental hygienist, and a dental assistant and delegate someone to invite them to your class to discuss their role in helping you prevent oral disorders. Ask each to review the education required for their specialty.

3. Survey your community to find out their views on fluoridation. Be prepared to report the results of the survey in class. As a class, decide whether an educational program on fluoridation is in order.

Interpret These Concepts:

1. Neglect of oral health affects individuals of all ages.

2. Most oral disorders can be prevented.

3. Many factors contribute to tooth decay.

4. Gingivitis and its advanced stage, periodontitis, can be prevented and controlled.

5. Malocclusion can be controlled.

Explore These Readings:

Alban, A. A., "What Do You Want to Know About Your Teeth?" *Consumer Bulletin,* 56:14–17 (February, 1973).

"Ecology of the Tooth," *Scientific American,* 226:42 (February, 1972).

"Effects of Acids on Teeth," *Consumer Bulletin,* 55:22–24 (February, 1972).

Schrep, H. W., "Dental Caries: Prospects for Prevention," *Science,* 173:1199–1205 (Sept. 24, 1971).

"Tooth Coating Stops Decay," *Science Digest,* 69:59 (June, 1971).

Seven

Achieving Vitality for Living

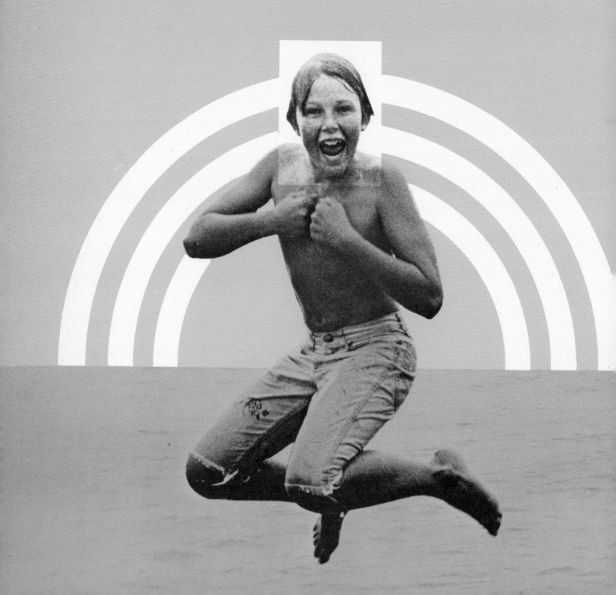

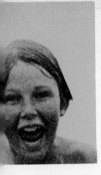

Modern conveniences and inventions have changed people's habits and produced a life-style that emphasizes passive and sedentary pursuits. Instead of the vigorous labor that strengthened earlier generations, today's workers have machines to perform many of their tasks. Many become spectators instead of participants in active sports. Overreliance on modern transportation has resulted in a reduction in walking, a much needed physical activity. Television viewing has usurped precious hours that could be put to better use. These changes in people's activities have had a widespread effect on people's health, both physically and mentally.

Factors Affecting Vitality

Your vitality level is dependent on a number of factors. What and how much you eat and your degree of freedom from disease greatly affect this level. Of equal importance are the amount and quality of your physical activity, your rest practices, and your posture. **The types of practices in which you engage can affect your level of vitality today and in the future.**

President John F. Kennedy commented on the need for physical fitness in his article "The Soft American," published in *Sports Illustrated,* December 26, 1960:

. . . physical fitness is not only one of the most important keys to a healthy body; it is the basis of dynamic and creative intellectual activity. The relationship between the soundness of the body and the activity of the mind is subtle and complex. Much is not yet understood. But we do know what the Greeks knew: that intelligence and skill can only function at the peak of their capacity when the body is healthy and strong; that hardy spirits and tough minds usually inhabit sound bodies. In this sense, physical fitness is the basis of all activities of our society. And if our bodies grow soft and inactive, if we fail to encourage physical development and prowess, we will undermine our capacity for thought, for work, and for the use of those skills vital to an expanding complex America.

The President's Council on Physical Fitness * reports that regular physical activity benefits the body by:

- Increasing strength, endurance, and coordination
- Increasing joint flexibility
- Reducing minor aches, pains, stiffness, and soreness
- Correcting remediable postural defects
- Improving general appearance
- Increasing efficiency with a reduction in expenditure of energy in performing both physical and mental tasks
- Reducing chronic fatigue.

Medical evidence shows that those who lead an active life and keep physically fit live longer than do those who lead a sedentary existence. Fewer deaths from chronic and degenerative diseases occur among active people. But the activity cannot be a haphazard, irregular occurrence. To be beneficial, it must be reasonable and regular. Developing the proper attitudes toward exercise early in life is important.

*President's Council on Physical Fitness, *Adult Physical Fitness.* Washington: President's Council on Physical Fitness, 1963, p. 6.

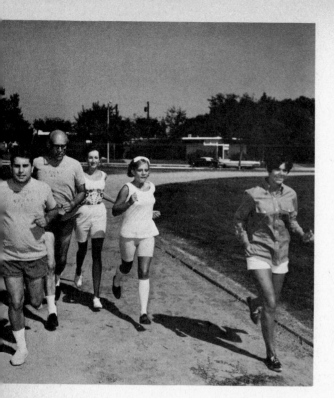

Figure 7-1 • Jogging, a popular activity.

Physical Activity and the Heart

Many heart specialists are interested in the relationship between coronary heart disease and lack of physical activity. They say American teenagers and young adults are underexercising and overeating themselves into future strokes and heart conditions that they will suffer by the time they reach middle age. The best preventive program for young adults is regular vigorous activity consistent with a balanced diet.

Physical activity does not harm the healthy heart. The heart is a muscle. Like all large muscles in the body, it must be properly used to maintain its appropriate function at optimum efficiency. In fact, when heart trouble does occur, medically prescribed activity often hastens recovery and rehabilitation.

Physical Activity and Weight

An individual's ability to achieve physical fitness can be hampered by overweight or underweight. Too little physical activity can contribute to the development of fatty deposits in the body. Too much activity can prevent the individual from achieving a proper weight.

A balance between caloric intake and expenditure of energy must be maintained. This, together with a planned program of physical activity, can help develop and keep firm the large muscles of the body. Some people who need to lose weight omit exercise because they fear it will increase their appetite and interfere with their efforts to reduce. This is a basic fallacy about exercise as a means of weight control. Because overweight people have large stores of fat, moderate exercise does not stimulate their appetites.

Analysis should bring you to the conclusion that proper diet can help you lose or gain the required number of pounds, and that proper activity can assist you in taking off or putting on the desired number of inches.

Psychological Benefits of Activity

There is a close relationship between physical activity and mental health. Everyone, regardless of age, should have some pleasurable form of physical activity. It is usually when people grow up and fail to include enjoyable activity in their daily programs that they are confronted with mental-health problems.

Activity helps relieve the tensions brought about by the pace of modern living. The stress of studying and other pressures of school need to be modified by a change

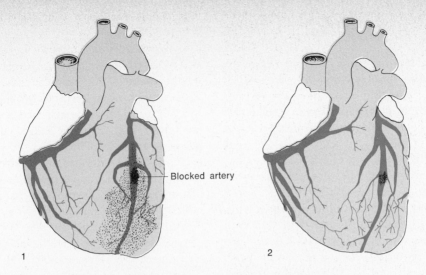

Figure 7-2 • How physical exercise can help protect the heart. (1) Heart of an individual who has suffered a heart attack and who has exercised little. Notice the extent of tissue damage as a result of the blocked artery. (2) Heart of an individual who has suffered a heart attack, but who has participated in regular physical exercise. Notice the lack of tissue damage due to the increased blood flow to the area. In what other ways does exercise help to prevent the risk of heart disease?

of pace. Studies have indicated that doctors, including psychiatrists, feel that moderate physical activity provides effective relief from tension. Most of these doctors actually prescribed an activity program for their patients with problems of tension and anxiety. It makes good sense for you to include active sports or exercise in your daily schedule to help maintain emotional balance.

Because of the fast pace of your activities, it is necessary for you to take time out for fun. For most individuals, fun involves other people. Participating in activity programs promotes the possibility of making friends and having fun.

Everyone usually needs to find a means of self-expression. Some individuals express themselves by developing skills in art, music, or writing. Others develop skills in various physical activities. You are more apt to improve your mental health if you develop skills in both passive and physical activities and then balance them in your daily living.

Figure 7-3 • How do you relieve tension?

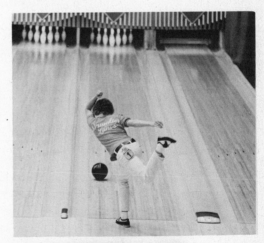

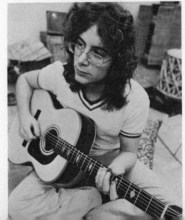

101

A Sensible Physical Activity Program

You can improve your physical fitness by adopting a sensible program of physical activity, following through with it, and modifying your activities as you grow older. You will feel better, look better, and enjoy life to the fullest.

Exercise is not necessarily a competitive sport, and you should not always try to "keep up with the group." You should slowly increase the amount of your activity until you reach the desired level for you. Then maintain that level by continuing the activity on a regular basis. Don't be a "weekend warrior." Plan your time in such a way that you have the opportunity to use your body in a vigorous fashion every day of the week. The desired level of activity depends on your general state of health. If you are in good health, you can increase your activity without concern. If you have a serious health problem such as heart disease, diabetes, or chronic fatigue, get your doctor's advice on the type and amount of physical activity in which you can safely engage. This applies to overweight and underweight as well. Your doctor will prescribe an activity program that takes into consideration the nature and seriousness of your problem.

Recommended Activities. There are many ways in which you can develop a sensible physical activity program. You need not engage in competitive sports or have special skills. Such activities as bicycling, hiking, or merely walking are very good for you. Many physicians prescribe walking for the relief of tension. Other activities that are often prescribed are swimming, golf, and bowling. Tennis and dancing are also frequently suggested. Most of these activities are inexpensive; thus a regular activity need not be a financial burden. The important thing to do is to select a variety of activities that you like. Then participate in these activities on a regular basis.

There is some interest today in isometric exercises as a means of developing physical fitness. An isometric exercise consists of pushing or pulling, for a short period of time (usually six seconds), against an object that does not move. An all-out effort is exerted during this brief period of time. Such exercises are designed primarily to develop or maintain muscular strength. An advantage of isometrics is that the muscles do the same amount of work in about one-third of the time needed for conventional exercise. Isometric exercises can also be valuable when equipment and facilities for other types of activity are not available. The main drawback is that this activity does not require the circulatory and respiratory systems to work harder. As a result, the entire body is not benefited. If you are interested in isometric exercises, you should try to combine them with other forms of physical activity so that you can obtain the full range of physical benefits.

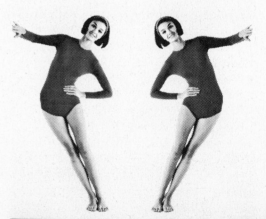

Figure 7-4 ● What are the advantages and limitations of isotonic exercise (bottom) and isometric exercise (top)? Is one preferable over the other?

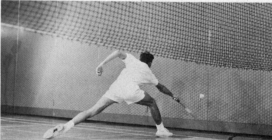

The following suggestions may help you get the greatest benefit and enjoyment from your personal physical activity program. They were developed by a joint committee of the American Medical Association and the American Association for Health, Physical Education, and Recreation.

- A program of exercise should be started at an early age and be continued throughout life with certain adjustments from time to time as life advances and needs, interests, and capabilities change.

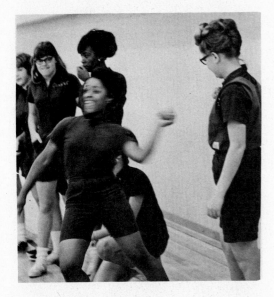

- The amount of vigorous exercise that is desirable each day is largely an individual matter. Recommendations range from 30 minutes to an hour daily as a minimum.

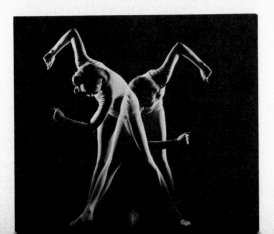

- Something of interest for every individual can be found to make exercise satisfying and enjoyable. In addition to numerous sports, the variety of choices includes daily habits such as walking, bicycling, and gardening.

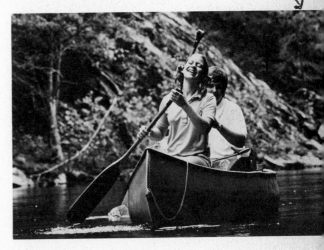

- Hard, fast, sustained, or highly competitive games and sports should not be played by persons of any age, unless these persons have attained an appropriate state of fitness through systematic training.

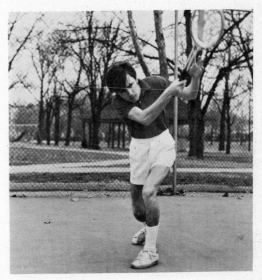

■ All persons should be shown by medical examination to be organically sound before training for competition or other strenuous exercise. The examination should be repeated periodically and whenever special indications appear.

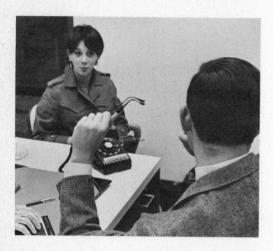

■ An individual in good physical condition may appropriately participate in an activity that might be harmful to another person of the same age who is not in a comparable state of fitness.

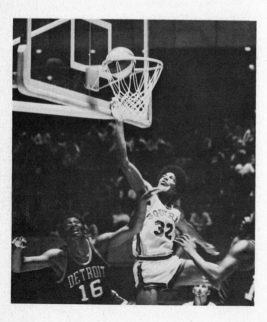

■ Persons who are out of training should not attempt to keep pace in any vigorous sport with persons who are properly conditioned and accustomed to regular participation in that sport. Being in condition for one sport does not always mean that a person will be in condition for another.

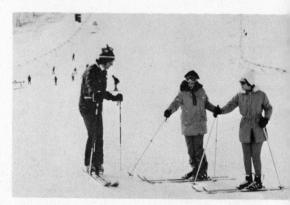

■ Persons long out of training, or "soft" (who have not practiced strenuous exercise regularly), will need an extended period of conditioning to facilitate gradual return to full activity.

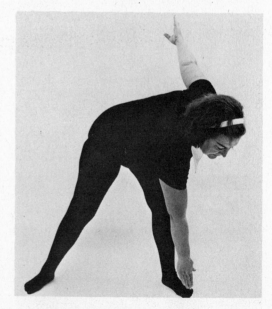

A person's ability to recover quickly after physical activity is a good indication as to whether or not the exercise is too strenuous. If breathlessness and pounding of the heart are still noticeable ten minutes after exercise, if marked weakness or fatigue persists after a two-hour period, if a broken night's sleep is attributable to exercise, or if there is a sense of definite and undue fatigue the following day, then the exercise has been too severe or too prolonged for that person in the present stage of training and physical strength.

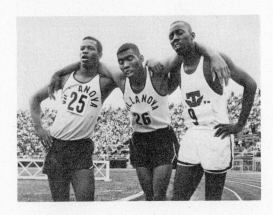

■ Medical supervision of the amount, type, and effect of exercise during convalescence is essential.

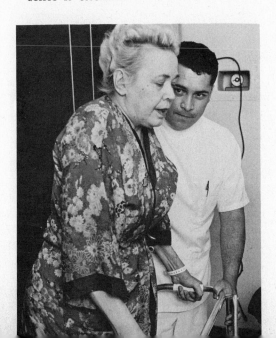

■ People should not compete in body-contact sports or activities requiring great endurance with others of disproportionate size, strength, or skill. If risk of injury can be controlled, carefully supervised practice periods against such odds may occasionally be warranted as a learning device for gaining experience or improving performance.

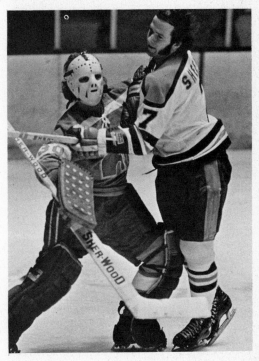

■ Sports involving body contact or traumatic hazards necessitate the provision of protective equipment. Such protection is especially important for the head, neck, eyes, and teeth. Other activities should be substituted when adequate protection cannot be provided.

■ Careful preparation and maintenance of playing fields and other arenas of sports are essential to reduction of injuries and full enjoyment of the activity. Competent supervision and proper equipment are necessary for the same reasons.

Fatigue and Rest

Fatigue is a natural warning system of the body. It goes into action when your body has reached the safe limit of activity for your health level. Different types of fatigue have different causes and, frequently, different methods of treatment.

Fatigue problems are common at your age. Sometimes they are due to the pressures of your academic, social, and home life. Sometimes they result from a particular disease or from poor health practices. You should know the different types of fatigue and how to recognize and overcome them.

Normal Fatigue

It is normal to become tired after studying, working, or engaging in sports or some other kind of physical activity. Healthy people awaken from a night's sleep refreshed and ready to meet the activity of a new day. As a result of daily living, they become tired or physically exhausted. Another night's sleep refreshes them once more. This illustrates the normal fatigue pattern.

It is also normal to become tired because of mental effort. The energy you spend in studying and in other forms of concentration can result in fatigue just as if you were engaged in physical activity.

Emotions can also play a role in producing fatigue. Worry and anxiety, as well as hatred, fright, anger, and other emotions can produce a feeling of tiredness.

If all of these factors are a part of a normal pattern of living and are producing normal fatigue, recovery should be relatively easy. Usually normal rest is all that is required. However, if you do not recover and your feeling of tiredness persists despite sleep or rest, you might require medical help.

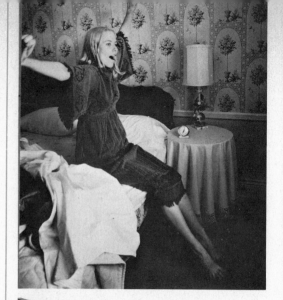

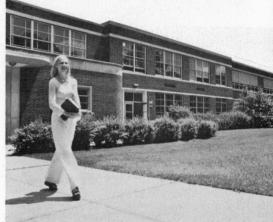

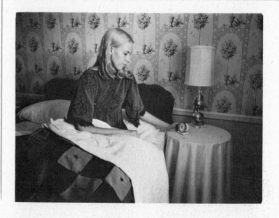

Figure 7-5 • Two extremes in fatigue patterns are illustrated. Where do you fit?

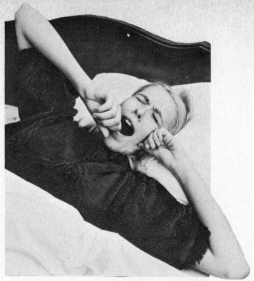

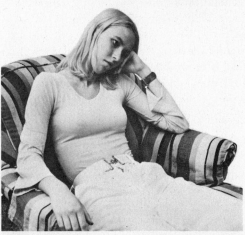

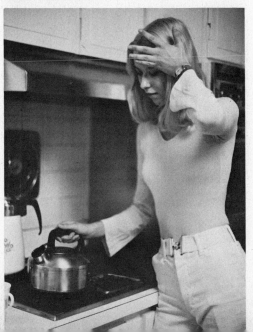

Chronic Fatigue

Fatigue is a normal part of everyday life. But if it persists and becomes a chronic condition, there may be some underlying factor which demands attention.

Unusual or excessive fatigue may be a symptom of disease. The ability of the body to restore itself is undermined by the disease. For example, fatigue is one of the most common symptoms of infectious mononucleosis. Until the disease is cured, the body will not be able to overcome the feeling of tiredness. Anemia is another possible cause of tiredness. Until the anemia is corrected, a person may continue to feel unduly tired.

People suffering from nutritional or glandular disturbances frequently experience undue fatigue. These underlying problems, too, must be corrected before it is possible to cope with the fatigue. The same applies to chronic fatigue that might be the result of undue worry or tension. The fatigue will probably persist until the worry or tension is removed.

Proper treatment of chronic or pathological fatigue consists of finding the cause and then eliminating it, if possible. A physician should make the diagnosis and treat chronic fatigue. If the fatigue is due to illness, the illness must be treated and cured. If the tiredness is due to emotional strain, the cause of that strain must be removed, if possible, or the individual must find a way to adjust to the emotional situation.

Prevention of Fatigue

One of the most important principles behind the concept of fatigue prevention is balance. **To prevent chronic fatigue, it is important to balance work with other types of activity and with adequate rest and sleep.**

The need for balance is illustrated in part by how the body works. When any muscle works hard, the body expends a great deal of fuel and oxygen. As the system burns more fuel it produces greater amounts of waste products such as carbon dioxide. Normally, the bloodstream carries away and disposes of the waste products. However, during periods of heavy work the waste products cannot be disposed of quickly enough.

Rest, relaxation, and recreation play an important part in maintaining a proper balance. They help provide the energy-saving periods that allow for the elimination of waste products.

Prevention of fatigue involves developing and maintaining balance and good personal health practices. To prevent undue fatigue:

- Avoid physical disease.
- Promote mental health.
- Maintain a varied, balanced diet.
- Allow time for adequate exercise or recreation.
- Plan for alternating periods of work and rest.
- Establish appropriate times for adequate relaxation and sleep.
- Maintain a balance of activity and rest.
- Maintain a balance of calories taken in and calories used.

Rest, Relaxation, and Sleep

Rest, relaxation, and sleep are important parts of your daily schedule. They are the restorers of energy and the amounts of each that you need will vary with the type and amount of your activity. **A balanced program of exercise and rest contributes to fitness.**

Rest

When physicians talk about rest, they usually imply inactivity. Many authorities recommend that everyone find one or two periods each day to sit or lie down, close the eyes, and rest for five or ten minutes. You might have some trouble finding an opportunity for this in your school schedule, but it is a worthwhile recommendation to keep in mind.

Relaxation

Relaxation is the process of changing the pace of your activity or "letting down" periodically. To relax, you need not be completely inactive. Select a form of relaxation that is enjoyable and fits conveniently into your daily schedule. Reading or engaging in some hobby after playing tennis are good examples of a change of activity.

Sleep

Getting the proper amount of sleep is one of the most important ways of overcoming normal fatigue. You must determine the proper amount for your needs. This varies for each person according to age, type of activity, and health status. Many people seem to get by with seven hours of sleep or less. Others seem to need nine hours. The important thing is that when you wake up at your usual time you should feel ready to go. If you are getting enough sleep, you will feel this way.

Insufficient sleep can result in health problems in addition to fatigue. When your body is run-down due to lack of sleep, you are more susceptible to infectious disease. Your emotions are also affected by this lack

Figure 7-6 ● Do you counteract your activities with relaxation, rest, and sleep to help you maintain optimal health?

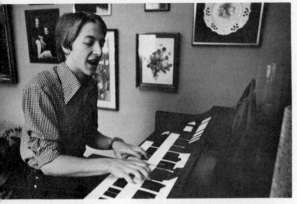
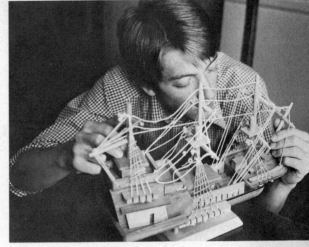
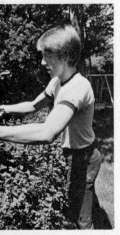
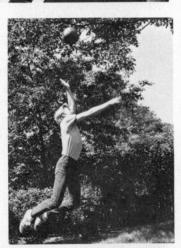
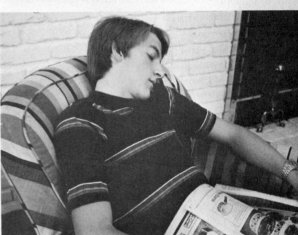
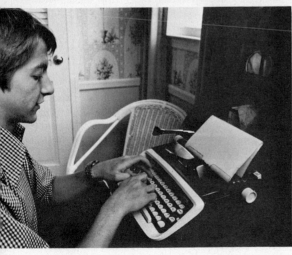
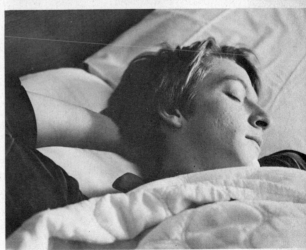

of sleep. Probably you become irritable and lose your temper more easily. This can certainly change your relationships with your friends and affect your mental health. Accidents are also related to insufficient sleep. Lack of sleep usually results in a loss of coordination, impaired vision, and retardation of the thought processes.

Insomnia, the inability to sleep, is a common complaint. It is not a disease, nor is it usually caused by a disease. Insomnia is usually brought about by tension, worry, pain, or nervousness. People with insomnia generally worry so much about not sleeping that they increase their inability to sleep.

For most individuals, a period of relaxation before bedtime might be the best solution for insomnia. This period might include moderate (but not heavy) exercise. A warm bath might be helpful, but a stiff rubdown with a towel should be avoided. A rubdown stimulates circulation and contributes to wakefulness. The bed should be comfortable and warm, and there should be an adequate supply of fresh air. The most vital aid is keeping the mind inactive once the individual is in bed. Counting sheep does not help because this requires concentration.

Avoid using drugs to help you sleep, unless they have been prescribed by your physician. Do not be misled by the advertisements that make all sorts of promises. If you constantly have trouble falling asleep, see your doctor. Never practice self-medication. It might be dangerous.

Posture

Good posture is proper body alignment in a variety of activities. These include sitting, standing, reclining, walking, working, or playing. While good posture contributes to a person's total well-being, no single posture is correct for everyone for all occasions. A general rule to remember is that good posture allows for freedom of movement, is most efficient for the task at hand, and utilizes the least energy.

Good posture improves an individual's appearance and body functions. It permits the proper positioning of his internal organs, such as the stomach, liver, kidneys, and intestines. Posture also appears to have some influence on blood circulation. Since the circulation of the blood is involved in the disposal of waste products, and thus affects fatigue, there is a relationship between poor posture and fatigue.

Poor posture results from a variety of poor health practices. Improper nutrition causes poorly developed muscles, nerves, and bones. Lack of activity inhibits the development of the muscles needed to support good posture. Overweight and underweight can also contribute to poor posture. To support his excess weight, an overweight person tends to throw his body out of alignment. The underweight person tends to slump because of weakness and fatigue.

Clothing that does not fit properly can also contribute to poor posture. Tight clothing does not allow for the proper movement of muscles. Poorly fitted shoes can cause a person to stand improperly to relieve foot discomfort.

If you need to improve your posture, you must start now. It is very difficult to do much about it after you are fully grown. In addition, the longer you persist in a habit, the more difficult it is to change. For young people like you, the desire to look attractive to others is enough incentive to do something about your posture. The impression that others have of you is greatly influenced by the way you stand, sit, or walk. Study Figure 7–7. Try to develop the proper techniques of good posture. Practice these techniques until they become a habit.

Some individuals have serious postural problems that require corrective exercises. They should consult with their physician and physical education instructor about their problem. With such guidance, they can start a corrective program. However, the real work and perseverance necessary for improvement are up to the individual.

Figure 7-7 ● Good posture is good body dynamics in a variety of situations. Does your posture improve your appearance and help your performance?

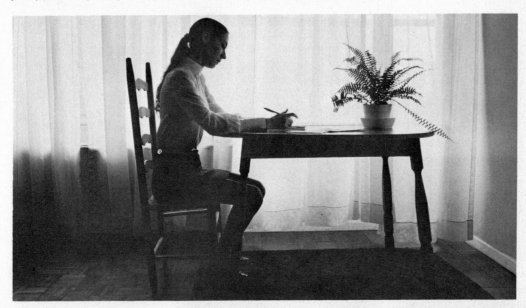

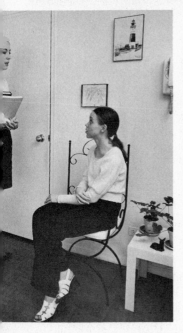

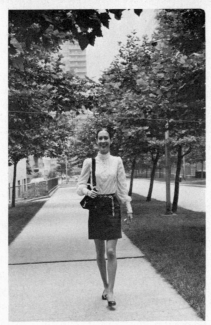

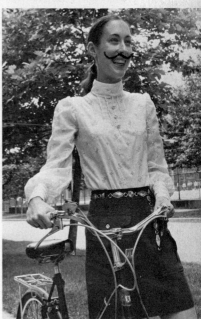

Summary

The state of your health, which includes your vitality, the way you feel, and the energy you spend conducting your daily activities is dependent upon many health practices. The amount and kind of physical activity you undertake are vital to your well-being. Physical activity is important to you physiologically, psychologically, and socially.

Medical authorities declare that lack of adequate activity can contribute to heart disorders and overweight. Psychiatrists affirm that tensions can be relieved by a sensible activity program. You should plan a program suitable to your own interests and needs and carry it out faithfully.

Alternating activity with rest or relaxation and sleep should help you recuperate from normal fatigue. If fatigue persists despite a proper balance, you should seek the aid of a physician.

Good posture contributes to both the prevention of fatigue and an attractive appearance. The habits you develop now are important because they tend to stay with you the rest of your life.

Take inventory today on your vitality level. Make the decision to develop the proper balance between physical activity, rest and relaxation, and sleep, to achieve vitality for living.

in making health decisions . . .

Understand These Terms:

correct posture
chronic fatigue
insomnia
isometric exercises

normal fatigue
physical fitness
relaxation
sedentary

Solve This Problem:

Susan is a high-school senior who is having a difficult time making up her mind about the kind of career she should prepare for. Susan is an above-average student and has special skills in modern dance and synchronized swimming. What type of careers might be challenging and enjoyable to her? What preparation would they require? What are the job-placement opportunities in these careers? How would you get information on these questions?

Try These Activities:

1. Make a list of common diseases. Carry out library research to identify those of which fatigue is a symptom.

2. List physical activities that you now participate in that will be more useful to you when you grow older. Then list the activities that you would like to learn now so that you could use them later in your life.

3. Select two friends, one who is athletically active and one who is not. Take their pulse rates and compare them. Now ask each one to hop up and down on one foot. Take the pulse rates again and compare them. How do you account for the difference?

Interpret These Concepts:

1. Your vitality for living is influenced by a balance between physical activity and rest.

2. Activity helps relieve the tensions brought about by the pace of modern living.

3. Good posture improves an individual's appearance and body functions.

Explore These Readings:

Cooper, Kenneth, *The New Aerobics.* New York: M. Evans & Co., Inc., 1970.

Galub, Jack, "What's So Bad About Exercise?" *Family Health,* Vol. V (May, 1973), pp. 32–33.

Johnson, Perry and Donald Stolberg, *Conditioning.* Englewood Cliffs, N. J.: Prentice-Hall, Inc., 1971.

Koch, J. and S. Petrillo, "What You'd Better Know Before Joining a Health Club," *Today's Health,* Vol. 50 (February, 1972), pp. 16–19.

Wallis, Earl L. and Gene A. Logan, *Figure Improvement Exercises for Women* (booklet). Englewood Cliffs, N. J.: Prentice-Hall, Inc., 1971.

Eight | Preventing Misuse of Alcohol

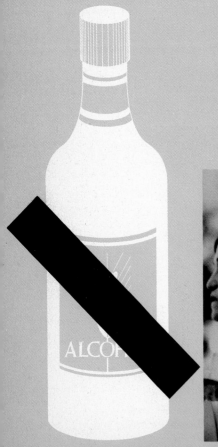
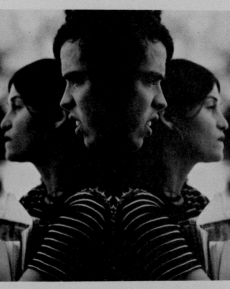
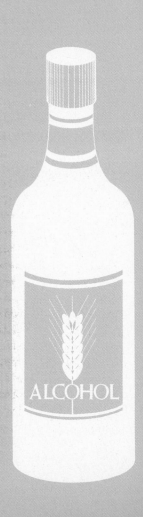

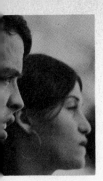

The use of alcoholic beverages, in one form or another, is very common in many parts of the world. In addition, drinking is a very old custom. Historically, alcohol was one of the first substances used by people to change moods. Over the years, alcohol has been used as a medicine to ease aches and pains and to produce general relaxation. Among certain groups, the use of alcohol continues to be important in religious and civil ceremonies.

In the United States today the number of persons who drink alcoholic beverages is estimated at about 100 million. For many of these, no difficulty arises from their use of alcohol. For a number of others, problems do arise. Throughout the centuries, problems related to alcohol have centered in improper and excessive use of these beverages. Because of the widespread use of alcohol, there has been—and continues to be—confusion as to how alcohol should be used in society.

Misuse of alcohol can have serious medical, economic, emotional, and social effects. It is one of society's most troublesome problems.

Although alcohol is usually considered to be a stimulant, in reality it is a depressant or sedative-like drug. It seems to be a stimulant because it takes the controls off emotional restraints. Thus you might engage in behavior you ordinarily would avoid. Alcohol works the same way in the bodies of children, adolescents, and adults. Of course, the same amount of alcohol in a smaller body has a stronger effect. But people are not the same emotionally and therefore react differently. Uncontrolled behavior because of intoxication is a major hazard for young people. This is particularly true when you consider the relationship between alcohol and accidents.

Influences on Drinking Practices

Research has indicated that an individual's drinking practices are closely related to those of the parents. When parents help their children understand the rules for drinking, and these rules are consistent with other values they observe, then problem drinking, including alcoholism, seems to be less prevalent. Apparently people in cultures where alcohol is used, but where there also is a low incidence of alcoholism, drink in a definite pattern. The alcohol is consumed slowly, usually taken along with food and generally in the company of other people. No rewards are given to the person who consumes a great deal of alcohol. Instead, qualities of alertness and control are admired.

Of course, there are many influences other than parents. Some young people drink in an attempt to prove that they are adults, and in so doing they consume large quantities of alcohol. They look forward to their legal drinking age as the beginning of a more sophisticated life. Some even attempt to begin drinking earlier as a form of rebellion against their parents or society itself. Still others drink because they think it will help them fit in with the crowd and be in on things. Having friends, being liked and accepted by the group, is important to everyone, particularly teen-agers. Yet those who drink because they feel it will make them more attractive, make friends, and fit in with the group are bound to be disappointed.

One can live a normal, full, and happy life without misusing alcohol. Those who choose not to drink at all should not feel any obligation to conform by yielding to the pressures of others. Those who choose to drink should be aware that there are dangers involved in the use of alcoholic beverages. These dangers should not be ignored.

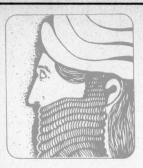

History shows that people tried to prevent intemperate use of alcohol. . . . In ancient Babylon (about 2225 B.C.) King Hammurabi set up the oldest known system of codified law, and several sections were devoted to problems created by the abuse of alcoholic beverages.

In China, laws that forbade making wine were enacted and repealed 41 times from 1100 B.C. to 1400 A.D.

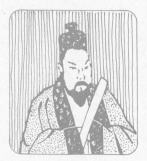

In the United States, prohibition during the 1920's was accompanied by good and bad results: a reduction in per capita consumption and alcoholism on one hand, a rise in lawlessness on the other.

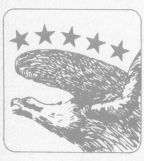

Figure 8-1 • The misuse of alcoholic beverages has been of concern to society throughout history.

The Extent of the Alcohol-Abuse Problem

The number of persons who misuse alcohol is extremely difficult to determine. There is a tendency to hide dependency on these beverages. Even so, it is estimated that there are approximately nine million men and women whose drinking is associated with serious problems. This includes persons who are alcohol abusers and alcoholics. Some of the sources of data for these estimates include the number of arrests for drunkenness, reports from industries, and admissions to mental hospitals for problems associated with the effects of alcohol.

Contrary to what you might think, problem drinking is not confined to "skid row" or to the "poorer sections of the community." About three-quarters of the problem drinkers are executives in large and small businesses, professional men and women, sales people, and skilled laborers. The frequency of the problem varies with sex and age. Excessive drinking is most common among males between 35 and 55 years of age. In recent years, however, a substantial increase in problem drinking has been noted among women and young persons under the age of 21.

Alcohol Abuse Is a Social Problem

The problem drinker is not the only person affected by the use of alcohol. Others who feel the effects are family members, friends, and co-workers. The dependency on alcohol interferes with the establishment of proper interpersonal relationships. The probability for a successful marriage is reduced, thus increasing the potential for divorce. In one large urban area of the United States, it is estimated that there are more than 450,000

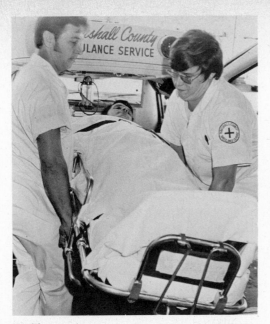

Health

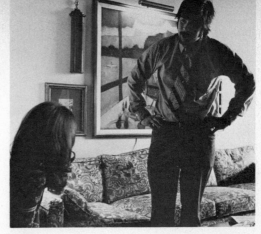

Family

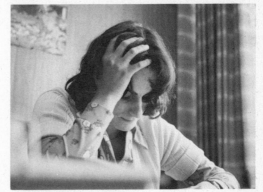

Personal Responsibility

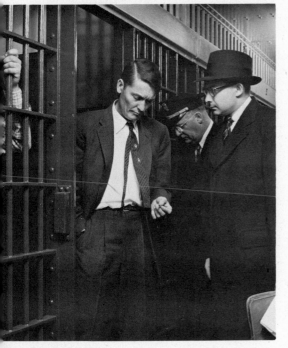

Legality

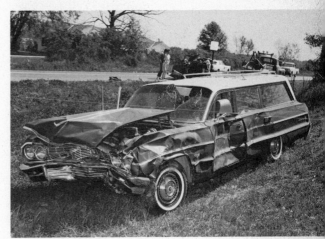

Injury and Liability

Figure 8-2 ● Alcohol abuse has an effect on many personal and interpersonal relationships. These problems can affect anyone who drinks.

alcoholics. These alcoholics, in turn, affect approximately 1½ million family members. There is a significant reduction in work efficiency and an increase in the number of accidents on the job. This cost to industry has caused great concern. Many industrial organizations have developed rehabilitation programs for their workers to reduce this economic problem. It is estimated that alcoholism costs industry more than 8 billion dollars a year. The cost of alcoholism for such items as care and treatment of alcoholics in hospitals and jails is great. This cost, together with money lost through crime, accidents, reduced wages and support of dependents comes to billions of dollars each year.

Alcohol Abuse Is a Law-Enforcement Problem

The abuse of alcohol is one of the chief causes for arrest in the United States. More than 50 percent of the fatal accidents that occur on highways involve persons who have had too much to drink. Police authorities in many parts of the United States report that a significant number of persons jailed for criminal acts or offenses have been found to have been drinking excessively. Approximately one-half of all homicides and one-third of all deaths reported as suicides are known to be alcohol-related. In addition, delinquency seems to be related to alcoholism. Approximately 30 to 40 percent of young people who are classified as delinquent come from homes where alcoholism exists. Some researchers feel that those who show a pattern of misusing alcohol will start misusing other drugs as well. They either discontinue the use of alcohol in favor of another drug or combine the misuse of alcohol with the misuse of another drug.

Alcohol Abuse Is a Psychological Problem

The most significant cause for the misuse of alcohol is the effort to cope with the problems and crises surrounding us. Wherever a person lives, there is stress from the physical and social environment. A person must adjust to changes within—maturing (physically, emotionally, and socially), getting old, and the effects of disease on the body and mind. A person must adjust to changes in living pattern—change of job, moving from one place to another, getting married, and finding new friends when the environment changes.

Most people learn to cope with these new situations. Some have so much difficulty, however, that they turn to alcohol for support. Psychologically, the individuals who misuse alcohol are considered immature. These persons have not developed the ability to cope successfully with their world. A dependency on alcohol has developed and it is used again and again to escape from uncomfortable situations. A great deal of psychological support is needed to help these individuals resolve their dependency on alcohol.

Alcohol Abuse Is a Medical Problem

The effects of excessive drinking can be devastating to the body. Most of the results are almost immediate but some develop slowly, not showing until the person has been a steady drinker over a period of several years.

Among the immediate and relatively minor physical effects are a feeling of warmth and a flushing of the skin. Glands that control important chemical processes in the body are affected by alcohol's action on the brain. This in turn affects the way other glands and organs work. Repeated occurrences of this type of mistreatment can cause serious and lasting injury to the body's tissues and organs.

Excessive drinking can lead to certain forms of vitamin deficiency, resulting in disease. When an adequate diet is not followed, for whatever reason and over a long period of time, nutritional diseases occur. Alcoholics receive a number of calories from the alcohol they consume, and this gives them a certain amount of energy to perform their daily tasks. These persons often skip meals and usually neglect to eat foods that would give them a proper balance of essential nutrients.

This lack of essential vitamins, minerals, and protein can adversely affect the body. Even those who have no deficiency diseases show signs of ill health. The general tone of their tissues often becomes poor. Their muscles tend to become flabby and their skin blotchy.

Those who drink excessively but continue to have a normal diet are likely to become overweight, because the alcohol adds many calories to their intake. Fatty deposits are formed, not only in the skin, but also in the internal organs. Cirrhosis of the liver, heart disease, and high blood pressure are among the conditions likely to result. Whenever a person is treated for problems related to excessive drinking, careful attention must be given to these and other medical difficulties that might be present.

Is Alcohol a Food or Medicine?

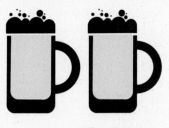 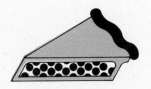 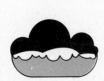 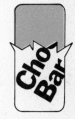

Two beers contain more calories than   a piece of pie,   **or**   a creampuff,   **or**   a candy bar.

Alcohol's medicinal value has been overrated in the past. Today it is sometimes used in small amounts as a sedative.

Nutritionally, alcohol resembles pure fat or starch in that it supplies only calories. If it replaces too much of a normal diet the resulting imbalance may lead to malnutrition.

Alcohol contains none of the essential vitamins, minerals or amino acids, so necessary in the daily diet, but it can make one fat!

Calorie Count

8 oz. beer	= 105 calories
1½ oz. gin	= 105 calories
1½ oz. rum	= 105 calories
1½ oz. whiskey	= 105 calories
2 oz. port	= 105 calories
2 oz. sherry	= 76 calories

Figure 8-3 ● Alcohol is an inefficient food or medicine.

Alcohol Abuse Is a Public-Health Problem

The misuse of alcohol is a major public-health problem because it is a serious threat to the individual, to public safety, and to general welfare. Programs to prevent, treat, and control misuse of alcoholic beverages are so complex that they require the co-operative efforts of many individuals and organizations. The success of these programs demands research, education of the public, and education of professional persons who must provide services to those who require such services. Additional services must be made available to those who have problems associated with the use of alcohol. More and more public funds will have to be spent on these types of programs. The development of preventive and curative measures seems to be a more efficient way of coping with the situation than building more and more jails for those who have problems related to alcohol.

The Alcohol Abuser

For hundreds of years, attempts have been made to define problem drinking and problem drinkers. The task is extremely difficult because of the broad range of what is considered "acceptable" drinking behavior. One group may define an occasional "binge" as a problem. Another group may say that this is acceptable behavior.

Alcoholism is an illness and the alcoholic is a sick person who can and should be treated. This concept is accepted by the American Medical Association and the World Health Organization.

The American Medical Association defines alcoholics as those "excessive drinkers whose dependence on alcohol has attained such a degree that it shows a noticeable disturbance or interference with their bodily or mental health, their interpersonal relations, and their satisfactory social and economic functioning."

The World Health Organization describes alcoholism as a "chronic illness that manifests itself as a disorder of behavior. It is characterized by the repeated use of alcoholic beverages to an extent that exceeds customary dietary use or compliance with social customs of the community and that interferes with the drinker's health or his economic or social functioning."

Some problem drinkers are not well-adjusted. They are overwhelmed by vague feelings of uncertainty, anxiety, apprehension, inadequacy, and inferiority. As a result, they tend to consider themselves failures in everything they do. They fear testing situations and will do anything to avoid them.

Alcohol provides such a person with a false sense of security and confidence. When the effect of the alcohol wears off, the problem becomes magnified because feelings of fear, guilt, and rejection are added. The person tends to repeat the use of alcohol to regain the feeling of security and confidence.

The basic problem is an emotional one. Without assistance, the person's chances of recovery are poor.

Other problem drinkers seem to be well-adjusted at first. In this group, the individual's social life and business activity involve overdrinking. The person lets things slide and begins losing the sense of responsibility. This starts affecting relationships with people at home and on the job. Worries increase and the individual becomes defensive, and therefore drinks more. As people become impatient and irritated with the drinker, the drinker tends to blame problems on hard luck and lack of understanding on the part of others. The drinker thinks the only thing that helps is more alcohol.

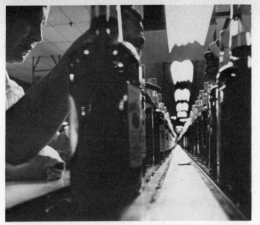
70,000,000 people in the U.S. drink.

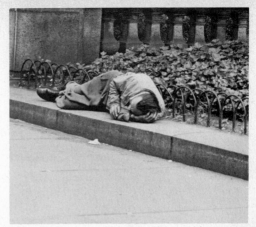
15% of the alcoholics are of the skid-row type.

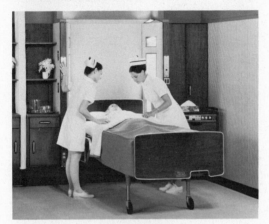
5,000,000 people are alcoholics.

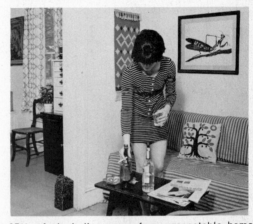
85% of alcoholics come from respectable homes.

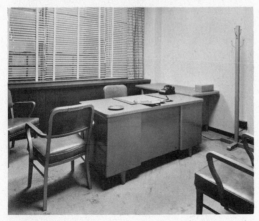
$432,000,000 is lost annually through absenteeism due to alcoholism.

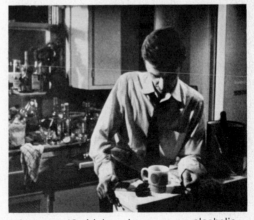
1 in every 13 drinkers becomes an alcoholic.

Figure 8-4 ● Facts about alcoholics.

Blood Alcohol Concentration and Part of Brain Affected

Behavior

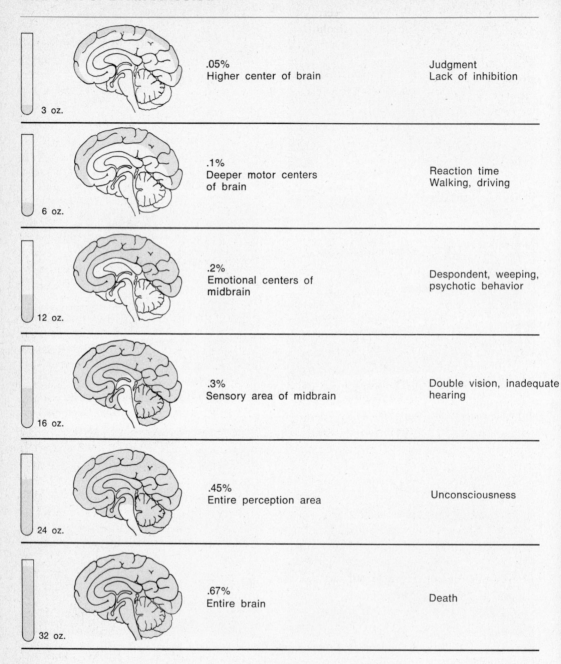

3 oz.	.05% Higher center of brain	Judgment Lack of inhibition
6 oz.	.1% Deeper motor centers of brain	Reaction time Walking, driving
12 oz.	.2% Emotional centers of midbrain	Despondent, weeping, psychotic behavior
16 oz.	.3% Sensory area of midbrain	Double vision, inadequate hearing
24 oz.	.45% Entire perception area	Unconsciousness
32 oz.	.67% Entire brain	Death

Figure 8-5 ● The effects of alcoholic beverage consumption on the brain and behavior.

How Alcohol Affects the Body and Behavior

All alcoholic beverages—wine, beer, and distilled spirits—contain ethyl alcohol in varying amounts. The alcohol acts principally on the central nervous system. The effects can be observed first when the alcohol reaches the brain after traveling through the bloodstream.

The amount of alcohol consumed and the concentration in the blood determine how much the brain will be affected. The first effect is on restraint and judgment. As the concentration in the blood increases, both mental and physical performance become impaired. Speech becomes blurred and the individual becomes clumsy and sleepy. The drinker may eventually sink into a coma. In a more subtle way, reflexes slow down, reaction time is longer, the ability to understand and learn is not so sharp, and loss of memory may occur.

About 10 percent of the alcohol consumed is eliminated unchanged from the body through the kidneys and lungs. The rest is destroyed by oxidation, a chemical process in which energy is released for the body. Generally, an individual can increase the rate of oxidation of food by increasing the amount of work. This cannot be done with alcohol. After alcohol has been consumed, nothing can be done to speed the rate at which it leaves the body or to destroy its effects. No amount of black coffee will do away with intoxication. The effect of coffee is to keep the intoxicated person awake. The symptoms become less pronounced as the concentration of alcohol in the blood becomes lower.

There are individual differences, still not clearly understood, that determine the effect of alcohol on a person. Some people remain apparently sober even though they drink large amounts of alcohol. Others are seriously affected by a very small quantity.

Symptoms of Problem Drinking

A number of symptoms indicate that people may be having problems with drinking. There may be signs quite early that these people are using alcohol to get over difficult situations and that the habit is growing.

One of the more obvious early symptoms is that the individuals drink more than is customary in their social group. They seek more and more opportunities to drink and, on each of these occasions, drink more. This might be an indication that they are developing a psychological dependence on alcohol.

As this tendency progresses, they may begin to have blackouts. This does not mean they lose consciousness, but that later on they cannot remember what happened after a certain point. If this happens repeatedly, it is a strong indication of developing alcoholism.

As the desire for alcohol becomes stronger, alcoholics gulp, rather than sip, the beverage. Drinking may be done secretly so that others will not know how much is being consumed.

Finally, the drinkers lose control of their drinking. They feel such a strong physical demand for the alcohol that they cannot stop. They have greater problems in trying to maintain good interpersonal relationships with others and this results in more alcohol being consumed. The drinking has now passed beyond the point where it can be used as a means of coping with problems. The individuals are alcoholics.

Prevention, Treatment, and Rehabilitation

Specific actions can be taken by the individual and society to reduce the misuse of alcohol.

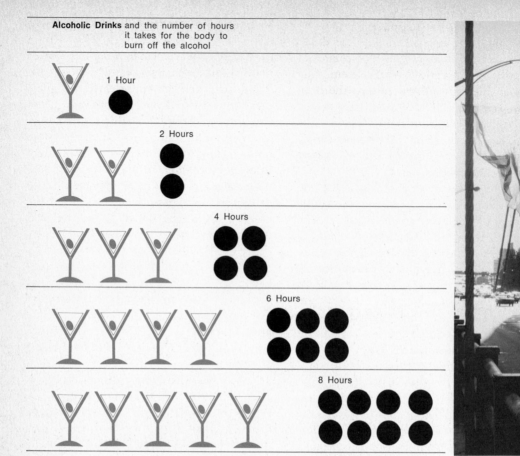

Alcoholic Drinks and the number of hours it takes for the body to burn off the alcohol

1 Hour

2 Hours

4 Hours

6 Hours

8 Hours

Figure 8-6 • This chart indicates how long it takes the body to reduce alcohol in the blood to a safe level. What implications does this have for driving?

More time and effort must be spent in preventing people from becoming problem drinkers. Young people can learn the proper use of alcohol in our society. They can learn that it is acceptable adult behavior not to use alcoholic beverages.

More time and effort also are needed to find and treat those with drinking problems as early as possible. Much is already being done through education. But much more needs to be done. Alcoholism is still known as the "hidden disease." However, progress is being made. The abuse of alcohol is now generally regarded as a medical

problem. This makes it easier for individuals to admit that they have a drinking problem. Once they have made this admission, it is easier for them to seek help from their doctor or from some organization specifically established for this purpose.

The primary goal of treatment is to help the problem drinker remain away from alcohol and at the same time handle his problems constructively. No one treatment program is effective for everyone. Treatment must be individualized.

The problem drinker often has medical problems that must be resolved. Doctors may use special drugs to help some patients stop drinking. Persons taking these drugs become violently ill if they drink alcohol while the medicine is in their system. The drugs are used primarily to keep the individual from alcohol while other forms of treatment are being carried out.

Some of the tranquilizing drugs are useful in treating the problem drinker. These drugs quiet the anxieties and tensions that bring about the improper drinking behavior.

It is important for you to make wise decisions now concerning the use of alcohol, because it is almost impossible for a person who has become dependent on alcohol to break away from it completely unless some form of emotional support is received. Psychological assistance can help the drinker to understand the problems. It can also provide guidance in working out solutions to problems without using alcohol. This kind of assistance can be provided on an individual or group basis.

A therapy has been developed whereby the alcoholic, the wife (or husband) and other members of the family work together to solve the problems that brought on alcoholism. Such a therapy helps establish a better home environment for the individual, thus speeding rehabilitation.

Alcoholics Anonymous

A great deal of success in helping alcoholics has been achieved by Alcoholics Anonymous. This is a group of rehabilitated alcoholics who have banded together to help themselves and others stay away from alcohol. The AA meetings have some of the advantages of group therapy. They make it possible for individuals to discuss their problems and get rid of their personal anxieties. The discussions take place in a friendly atmosphere and among persons who have had similar problems and have successfully overcome them. An attempt is made to give emotional support to all participating members. AA is not a complete therapy. Members often take additional treatment.

More recently, wives, husbands, and teen-age children of alcoholics have formed groups to discuss their common problems. This has enabled them to better understand and cope with alcoholism.

The spouses' group is called Al-Anon. The teen groups use the name Alateen.

Figure 8-7 ● Effective health education is an important preventive to problem drinking. If you were in the classroom pictured here, what would you list as advantages of not drinking?

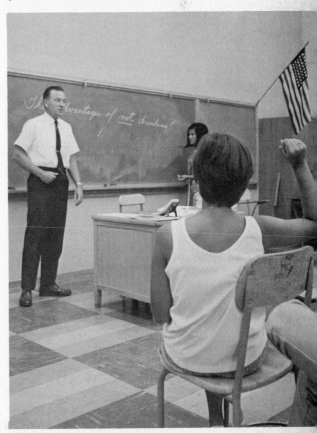

New Programs

Fewer communities are depending entirely on the jails and mental hospitals to handle alcoholism. More and more techniques of diagnosis, treatment, and rehabilitation are becoming available. Comprehensive programs to combat alcoholism are being developed in many parts of the United States. A number of the programs include the following services.

Early Casefinding

By finding persons with drinking problems and treating them early, it may be possible to intercept the process of alcoholism. Persons recognized early as potential alcoholics are more easily rehabilitated than long-term alcoholics, and are less likely to become community burdens. Some programs are taking a close look at children of parents who are alcoholics. It is believed that many of these children will follow the same pattern if something is not done to prevent it.

Diagnostic-Referral Centers

These centers receive referrals from community agencies, industry, police agencies and interested individuals. Here, persons with drinking problems are given an examination to determine the state of their involvement, physiologically and psychologically, with alcohol. Once a diagnosis has been made, the patient is either helped directly by the staff of the center or referred to another agency for treatment and rehabilitation. In many centers, an interdisciplinary approach is used. This means that a team of professional workers provides assistance. Usually, physicians and nurses will be concerned with restoring the physical health of the patient. Others, such as social workers and psychologists, will focus on the emotional needs of the patient and provide various forms of therapy.

Emergency Care

Severely intoxicated persons very often have illnesses or injuries that are masked by the effects of alcohol. They may also be in emotional or physical shock at the same time. These individuals need emergency care. In many communities there is no place to take them other than a jail or the psychiatric ward of the county hospital. To remedy this situation, all hospitals are encouraged to provide emergency care for those who are severely intoxicated.

Court Screening

Many admissions to state mental hospitals are for alcoholism. Each admission costs the taxpayers of that state hundreds of dollars. A large number of these individuals could be cared for by community services without being hospitalized. In many communities the courts are being encouraged to make referrals to community organizations, rather than to commit all alcoholics to the state mental hospitals.

Halfway Houses

Many problem drinkers have no permanent home or else need to be separated from their usual environment during part of their recovery period. The halfway house is an attempt to provide a residential facility with a friendly atmosphere to develop healthy social relationships. When necessary, the trained staff can provide help with personal problems. As a means of helping the residents back into the community, they are encouraged and helped to find employment.

Health Education and Information

Increased education and information are also a part of the developing programs. It is important to learn more about problem drinking, the kind of behavior that may identify persons who have a high risk of becoming problem drinkers, and additional ways in which help may be given. These activities provide a basis upon which all members of the community can participate in helping solve this complex and extremely serious problem.

What You Can Do

To drink, to drink moderately, or not to drink at all is a decision that is faced by everyone. Your attitude toward drinking has probably developed from attitudes and experiences in your family and among your friends.

Enough people have difficulties with alcohol to cause concern for their health and welfare and for the society in which they live. **In itself, alcohol is neither good nor bad; there are only good and bad uses of alcohol.** You will have to make a decision about the use of alcohol. This may mean that you will not use alcohol at all. You should be aware that a large number of people enjoy life and all its pleasures without drinking. It may mean learning the acceptable use of alcoholic beverages and how to avoid intoxication and dependency on alcohol. Everyone should learn how problems related to alcohol can be prevented or reduced.

Summary

Misuse of alcohol can have serious medical, economic, emotional, and social effects. It is one of society's most troublesome problems.
People's drinking practices are closely related to those of their parents. However, there are many influences other than parents.
Alcoholic beverages affect the body in a variety of ways. Most important is the effect on behavior, including restraint and judgment, and on mental and physical performance.
There are a number of symptoms which indicate a person may have a drinking problem. Early casefinding, diagnosis, treatment, and rehabilitation can help those who have drinking problems.
In itself, alcohol is neither good nor bad; there are only good and bad uses of alcohol. You must make the decision regarding the use of alcohol. Be aware of the problems related to drinking. Do not be afraid to decide that alcohol has no place in your life.

in making health decisions . . .

Understand These Terms:

Alcoholic beverages
Alcoholics Anonymous
alcoholism
court screening
dependency

diagnostic-referral centers
ethyl alcohol
halfway houses
intoxication
rehabilitate

Solve This Problem:

Juanita Johnson, a junior in high school, has a friend whose parents are
alcoholics. She wants to give advice to her friend as to what can be
done to help the parents. What recommendations should she make?
Juanita also is thinking about getting a job that would allow her to help
those who are alcoholics. Where could she look for jobs of this type?
Will she need any kind of special training?

Try These Activities:

1. Many arrests by law-enforcement personnel involve persons who have
   been misusing alcohol. Contact your local police agency. Inquire as to
   the number of arrests per year that involve the direct or indirect use
   of alcohol. Be prepared to make a classroom chart and discuss your
   findings with the class.

2. From among the following categories, identify those which you feel
   represent the greatest harm resulting from the unwise use of alcohol:
   a. Damage to the body
   b. Damage to property
   c. Damage to society
   d. Damage to the family
   e. Damage to others
   f. Damage to the brain
   How would you defend your choices?

3. Make a survey of your community to determine the facilities and other
   resources available for helping those who have problems with alcohol.
   Determine whether any of these programs focus on helping young
   people. Be ready to make a verbal report to the class on your findings.

Interpret These Concepts:

1. Misuse of alcohol can have serious medical, economic, emotional, and
   social effects.

2. One can live a normal, full and happy life without misusing alcohol.

3. Alcoholism is an illness.

Explore These Readings:

"Business Drinking: A Health Hazard," *U.S. News & World Report,* Vol. 72 (Mar. 13, 1972), pp. 70–71.

"Forgotten Addiction," *America,* Vol. 126 (Jan. 15, 1972), pp. 32–33.

Holden, Constance, "Alcoholism: On-the-Job Referrals Mean Early Detection and Treatment," *Science,* 179:363–365 (Jan. 26, 1973).

"Latest Teen Drug: Alcohol," *Newsweek,* Mar. 5, 1973.

Wolff, P. H., "Ethnic Differences in Alcohol Sensitivity," *Science,* Vol. 179 (Jan. 26, 1973), pp. 363–365.

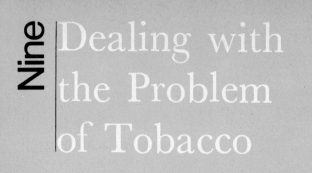

Nine

Dealing with the Problem of Tobacco

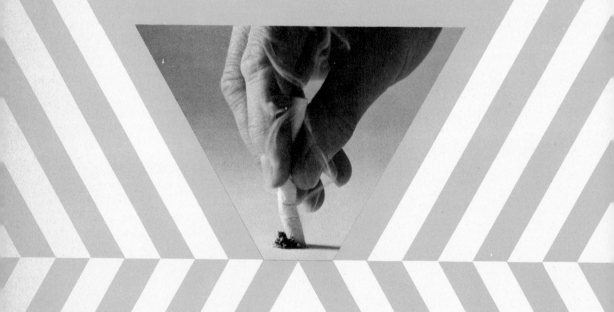

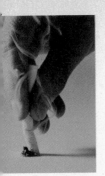

Cigarette smoking continues to be a major health problem in the United States and in many other countries of the world. While the evidence is quite conclusive that cigarette smoking is harmful to health, some persons reject this evidence. They reject the many studies which clearly indicate that:

- Deaths from all causes are higher for smokers than for nonsmokers.
- The increase in lung cancer and emphysema parallels the increase in cigarette smoking.
- Deaths among smokers increase as the number of cigarettes smoked increases.
- Giving up smoking reduces the danger of many diseases.
- Tobacco smoke serves as a source of pollution and irritation for the person who does not smoke.

Those who reject this evidence think that all the results that have been presented are purely statistical and therefore circumstantial. They argue that a cause-and-effect relationship between smoking and disease has not been definitely established. In addition, it is their view that some of the increase noted in lung cancer and other diseases may be due to better diagnosis and casefinding. Further arguments suggest other possible causes, such as air pollution from industry and automobile exhaust emissions.

In considering whether or not you should smoke, examine the evidence. Make an intelligent decision based on this evidence, rather than following the example of others.

Cigarette Smoking and Health

Present evidence indicates that there is a relationship between smoking and ill health. The most critical factors seem to be the kind of smoking that is done (cigarettes and small cigars), whether the smoker inhales, the amount smoked, and the number of years an individual has continued the habit. All these factors considered together emphasize the increased risk of acquiring many health problems. Reasons for this were originally given in a report in 1964 by the Surgeon General of the United States. Since that time, additional reports have been released by the Surgeon General. These, together with hundreds of new studies that have been completed in many countries of the world, emphasize that cigarette smoking is hazardous to the health of the smoker and may harm the nonsmoker.

Various types of research have been conducted to find the relationships between cigarette smoking and health. The research included the following procedures.

Animal Experiments

In many studies, animals have been exposed to tobacco smoke and to the tars and chemical compounds contained in the smoke. A number of changes in the cell structure of the animals' lungs have been noted. Many of these chemical compounds have been shown to be cancer-causing. Other substances, although not cancer-causing themselves, seem to lower the resistance of the cells to cancer. Additional tests show that cigarette smoke paralyzes the cilia (hairlike projections of mucous-membrane cells) in the animal's respiratory system so that it cannot do its job of cleaning. Nicotine has been shown to increase the pulse rate and the blood pressure.

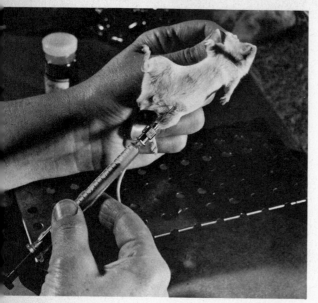

Figure 9-1 • Important evidence on the hazards of smoking has been obtained through animal experimentation. How do medical scientists relate such studies to people?

Clinical and Autopsy Studies

Examination of thousands of patients and autopsies of smokers and nonsmokers revealed damage of many kinds to the body. Evidence of the actual destruction of cells, as well as changes in the cell structure, was observed in smokers. In addition, the blood vessels of smokers thickened much more, indicating that an added strain may have been placed on the smokers' hearts.

Population Studies

Smoking histories of persons with a specific disease have been compared with those of persons without the disease. The studies showed that more cigarette smokers were found among the lung cancer patients than in the population without cancer. In addition, the more cigarettes smoked, the greater the risk of coronary heart disease.

Other studies revealed that symptoms such as chronic cough, sputum production, breathlessness, chest illness, and decreased lung function consistently appear more frequently in cigarette smokers than in nonsmokers.

Cigarette smoking is considered to be the major cause of lung cancer in males and a significant cause of lung cancer in females. While the difference in disease and death rates between smoking males and females has not been fully explained, there is growing evidence that the female is increasing her risk of a variety of diseases when she smokes.

In general, the greater the number of cigarettes smoked daily over a period of years, the greater the risk of ill health and death. For men who smoke fewer than 10 cigarettes per day, the death rate from all causes is about 40 percent higher than for nonsmokers. For those who smoke 10 to 19 cigarettes per day, it is about 70 percent higher; for those who smoke 20 to 39 per day, 90 percent higher; and for those who smoke 40 or more per day, it is 120 percent higher. Men who smoke a pipe or cigars do not seem to have the same increased risk of ill health or death. This is probably due to the fact that these smokers do not inhale. Giving up the habit of cigarette smoking seems to have a significant effect upon reducing the risk of various health problems.

An outcome of this concern has been the following warning that is required to be printed on all cigarette packages and all advertising for cigarettes:

"Warning: The Surgeon General Has Determined That Cigarette Smoking Is Dangerous to Your Health."

A more recent Public Health Service report directly states that, if it were not for cigarette smoking there would be fewer deaths from lung cancer, other respiratory diseases, and cardiovascular diseases.

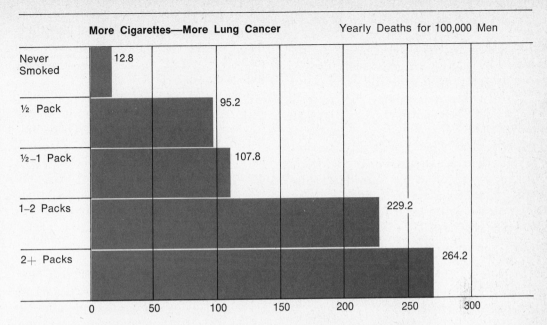

Never Smoked   12.8

½ Pack   95.2

½–1 Pack   107.8

1–2 Packs   229.2

2+ Packs   264.2

0   50   100   150   200   250   300

Figure 9-2 ● Your chance of getting lung cancer increases the more you smoke.

Physical Complaints of Nonsmokers and People Who Smoke a Pack or More of Cigarettes a Day

Complaint	Cigarette Smokers (Percent)	Nonsmokers (Percent)	Ratio Smokers to Nonsmokers
Chest Pains	7.0	3.7	1.9
Shortness of Breath	16.3	4.7	3.5
Cough	33.2	5.6	5.9
Hoarseness	4.8	2.6	1.8
Difficulty in Swallowing	1.4	1.0	1.4
Tendency to Fatigue Easily	26.1	14.9	1.8
Abdominal Pains	6.7	3.8	1.8
Stomach Pains	6.0	3.8	1.6
Loss of Appetite	3.3	0.9	3.7
Diarrhea	3.3	1.7	1.9
Loss of Weight	7.3	4.5	1.6
Insomnia	10.2	6.8	1.5

The Effects of
Cigarette Smoking

❈ **The effects of cigarette smoking on the body vary with individuals.** Some smokers find pleasure in the taste and smell of the tobacco. Others report that they seem to feel calmer when they smoke. Certain effects are so slight that it is extremely difficult to measure them. These effects may last only a short time and may not seem to involve the general health of the individual. However, the ability of the individual to undertake certain types of activity may be affected by smoking.

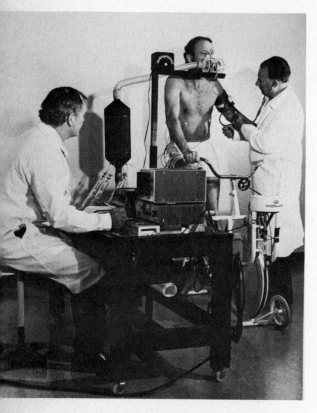

Figure 9-3 ● Recent research indicates that there are immediate effects on health from smoking cigarettes. The test illustrated was used to measure the effects of smoking on human performance. It was found that smoking tends to reduce work efficiency.

Immediate Effect

Research studies on healthy young males under the age of 22 indicate that the heart rate of cigarette smokers is significantly higher than that of nonsmokers. The smokers' blood pressure also seems to be affected. Increased amounts of fatty acids in the smokers' blood were also noted. These findings may account for the increase in coronary heart disease among smokers. Other immediate effects include nausea, shortness of breath, dizziness, irritation of the throat, chronic cough, and interference with the appetite.

Various parts of the body are also affected in numerous ways.

Circulatory System. There is a great deal of variation in how individuals respond to cigarette smoking. Most people, as indicated earlier, experience some constriction of the small arteries, a rise in blood pressure, and an increase in the heart and pulse rates. These changes take place in the beginning smoker as well as in one who has been smoking for many years.

A number of studies demonstrate that death rates from coronary heart disease increase with the amount of cigarette smoking. Autopsy reports show that the blood vessels of smokers are thickened much more than those of nonsmokers, indicating that there may be an added strain upon the heart.

Respiratory System. Cigarette smoke contains a number of products that irritate the respiratory tract. Coughing, hoarseness, and bronchitis are all related to smoking. A more important relationship involves the tiny hairlike filaments called cilia. The cilia cover the cells which line the trachea and bronchial tubes. Cilia act as cleaning brushes by moving in whiplike fashion to remove dirt, bacteria, and other foreign matter from the air passages. Cigarette smoke slows down and then completely

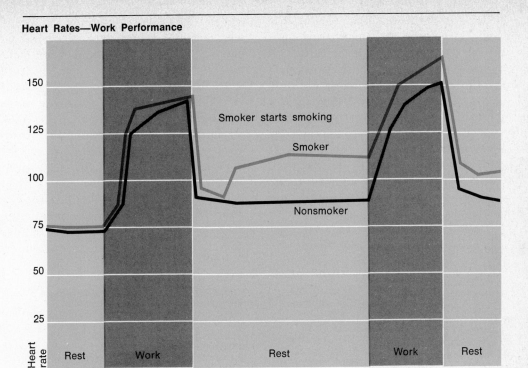

Figure 9-4 ● One of the immediate effects of smoking cigarettes is the dramatic increase in heart rate as shown in this graph. Note how much more the smoker's heart must work to accomplish the same task as the nonsmoker.

stops this action. After a time, many of the cilia are destroyed, allowing the harmful smoke particles, dust, and bacteria to invade the lungs. This weakens resistance to lung diseases. In lung cancer, the smoke particles may directly cause an abnormal growth of cells. In emphysema, cigarette smoking may cause the air sacs in the lungs to enlarge and lose their elasticity.

Digestive System. Cigarette smoking seems to irritate the digestive tract in some persons. Many smokers are known to have indigestion. In addition, smokers have more illness and higher death rates from peptic ulcers. The number of cases of peptic ulcer has been found to be almost 100 percent higher for male smokers and more than 50 percent higher for female smokers than for

those who have never smoked. Studies have also shown that smoking retards the healing of ulcers of the stomach.

Other Conditions

Many other problems are associated with cigarette smoking. Sometimes tremor and loss of control of the small muscles of the body occur. This interferes with activities that require fine hand-eye coordination. There are also some indications that vision itself might be affected.

Women who smoke cigarettes during pregnancy tend to have babies that weigh less than the babies of women who do not smoke. A newborn weighing less than 5½ pounds is considered premature and must have special care. Although more research is needed to determine the effects of smoking on babies of mothers who smoke, early findings suggest that these babies have a higher risk of stillbirth or early death.

It is also known that nicotine can cross the placental barrier and increase the heart rate of the fetus, thus making its heart work harder. More research is needed on the long-range effects of cigarette smoking on these babies.

Doctors have observed that many of their patients, although well, frequently complain of being constantly tired, nervous, and restless. Many of these individuals are smokers. Very often they feel better and perform their duties more efficiently when they give up smoking.

Tobacco smoke can contribute to the ill health of many individuals. Some smokers develop an allergic reaction to cigarette smoke. Even nonsmokers who are exposed to cigarette smoke show signs of ill health. Studies have shown that the carbon-monoxide level in a smoke-filled room is quite high. As a result, even nonsmokers have their vision and hearing affected and some have developed allergic reactions.

Normal Epithelium

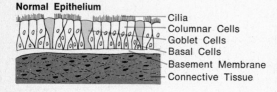

- Cilia
- Columnar Cells
- Goblet Cells
- Basal Cells
- Basement Membrane
- Connective Tissue

Figure 9-5 ● How continued smoking has a damaging effect on the mucous lining of lung tissue. (1) Normal cells with cilia and basal cells intact. (2) The swelling of basal cells. (3) Loss of cilia needed to sweep foreign substances from the lung. It is at this time that the lung tissue is most susceptible to infection. (4) Tissue in disorderly growth. (5) Cancerous growth.

Hyperplasia Increased basal cells

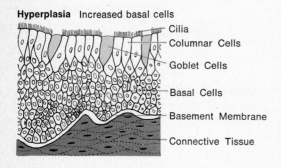

- Cilia
- Columnar Cells
- Goblet Cells
- Basal Cells
- Basement Membrane
- Connective Tissue

Carcinoma in Situ Atypical nuclei and disorderly growth

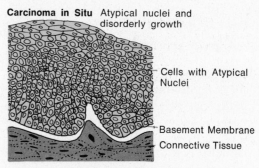

- Cells with Atypical Nuclei
- Basement Membrane
- Connective Tissue

Squamous Cells Loss of Epithelium Cells become flattened

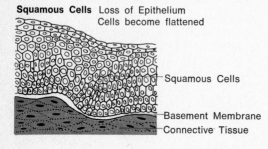

- Squamous Cells
- Basement Membrane
- Connective Tissue

Invasion Cells break through the basement membrane and spread to the rest of the body

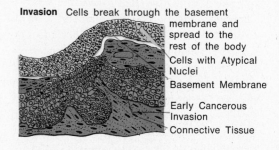

- Cells with Atypical Nuclei
- Basement Membrane
- Early Cancerous Invasion
- Connective Tissue

Teen-Agers and Cigarette Smoking

More and more young people are becoming aware of the dangers of cigarette smoking. They are raising a number of questions. Many of these questions and their answers have been summarized in material prepared by the U. S. Department of Health, Education and Welfare.

Why is there so much concern about teen-age smoking?

The younger people are when they start smoking, the greater the risk that they may become ill at an earlier age. Statistics show that smokers who take up the cigarette habit before they are 20 are the ones who go on to smoke more cigarettes for more years and who inhale more deeply. This is also the description of smokers who are more likely to be disabled or killed by cigarettes. So, young smokers are the ones most likely to become the steady, fairly heavy smokers during their twenties, thirties, and forties. And these steady, heavy smokers are the ones who face the greatest health risks.

Why is there such concern about diseases that are caused by cigarettes? We all have to die sometime.

First: Cigarettes shorten a smoker's life expectancy. Smokers face serious risks that they will die younger than nonsmokers, that they will die prematurely—before they would have died if they had not smoked.

Second: Cigarettes are linked with disabling illnesses. Lung diseases and heart diseases make smokers invalids, unable to work or lead normal lives. More and more, these illnesses are striking people who are quite young, parents of small children. Young people who begin to smoke in their middle teens may show irritating symptoms in their twenties and may develop disabling diseases in their thirties.

What reasons do teen-agers give for smoking cigarettes?

There are many reasons, researchers have found. Here are some typical answers.

"Because the rest of my crowd smokes."

"It.makes me look big."

"To be a big shot."

"To feel sophisticated."

"I was curious about it."

"Because I was tense and nervous."

"Because I enjoy smoking."

"Because I wasn't supposed to."

The answers at the top of the list were given more often than the ones at the bottom. Cigarettes seem to be a symbol that proves something to the individual, that helps him belong.

Does anyone know how many teen-agers smoke cigarettes?

A rough estimate would be that about 30 percent of American teen-agers smoke. It is difficult to give a precise figure because smoking habits vary so much from town to town, even from school to school.

Researchers do know that very few young people smoke in their early teens, but that more and more take up the habit as they go on to the upper grades of high school.

Why call it the cigarette habit? Does smoking always become a habit?

It usually does; and this is how the habit-forming process develops:

Young people take up cigarettes to satisfy the desire to belong, to feel big. They will usually continue to tie in those good feelings with the act of smoking.

Later, when they are anxious or nervous about anything, they are likely to recall those good feelings that they tie in with cigarettes; and they find themselves reaching for that pack. They probably won't be aware of this tie-up, any more than most of us are aware of developing the daily habits that become part of our personalities. But this is how a habit takes hold of us.

Suppose teenagers have experimented by trying one or two cigarettes. Will this make them ill?

It won't make them ill in the sense of causing a disease. It may give them a feeling of nausea—of being sick to their stomach—because their system is not used to the nicotine in the tobacco smoke. But this will be purely a temporary reaction. It will have no lasting effect if they do not continue to smoke.

What about all the adults who lecture us about not smoking—while they're lighting their own cigarettes?

These people probably began smoking many years ago, before we had today's evidence on the tie-up between cigarettes and disease. Many adult smokers are working hard to become ex-smokers—either on their doctor's orders or after reading the facts themselves. But it is far from easy for people to give up a habit on which they have depended for 20 or 30 years.

What about filters? Can't they make cigarettes safe?

No, filters do not make cigarettes safe. Researchers have not yet found and tested all the ingredients in cigarette smoke, so there is no way of knowing exactly how many harmful substances must be filtered out.

Many filter-tip cigarettes have a lower tar and nicotine content. Smokers who choose brands with the lowest tar and nicotine content can reduce their exposure to the harmful effects of smoking, if they do not compensate by smoking more.

The Decision Is Yours

You have to make your own decision. No one can keep you from smoking. By the same token, no one can make you smoke. It is important for you to weigh all the evidence so that you can make an intelligent decision. If you are interested in reducing the risk of various kinds of health problems, consider the following possible approaches to the situation:

- Limit the amount you smoke, either by smoking fewer cigarettes or by smoking less of a cigarette.
- Don't inhale—or smoke a pipe or cigar instead of a cigarette (this kind of smoke is more difficult to inhale. However, you have to consider other hazards associated with this kind of smoking).
- Remember, the surest way to reduce risk is to avoid it by not smoking at all.

How Can a Smoker Stop Smoking?

Perhaps you are a smoker and you have decided that the cigarette you just put out is the last one you will ever smoke. Or perhaps you feel that you can stop any time, so why bother to do it now? Perhaps you have already tried to stop but haven't succeeded. Or perhaps you are undecided.

Smoking is something you enjoy, but you still wonder. Is it worth giving up the enjoyment in order to improve your chances of living a more healthy life? No one likes to stop doing something he enjoys. But millions of smokers are stopping because the evidence from medical researchers has become so overwhelming. **You can stop smoking if you really want to.** Consider the following suggestions made by young people who have successfully stopped smoking. These suggestions were compiled by the Department of Health, Education, and Welfare.

When you decide to stop smoking, you have two moves ahead of you:

STOP:

You may choose to quit cold, immediately and completely. Today. If this method seems right for you, toss out your pack right now and you're on your way.

Or you may prefer another method: tapering off. Three days is the limit here—72 hours. You may take less time, but not more.

Taper off this way: Each day, smoke less than half of what you smoked the day before. If you smoked a full pack yesterday, cut back to nine cigarettes today, four tomorrow, and one on your third and final day of smoking.

STICK BY YOUR DECISION:

You often need morale boosters during the first few weeks after quitting. Every ex-smoker knows that, and may have depended on the suggestions outlined here.

You can help yourself by:

■ Sorting out your reasons for quitting.
■ Enjoying yourself.
■ Keeping busy.

■ Finding new things to do.
■ Letting people help you.
■ Putting up stiff resistance if you're ever tempted to smoke.
■ Changing your way of thinking about cigarettes.

Relax and Pamper Yourself

Make your life without cigarettes as comfortable and pleasant as possible. There is no need to grit your teeth and feel as if you were fighting a disagreeable battle. Instead, try to do the following:

■ Look for enjoyment. Set up a relaxing schedule for the next few weeks. Include a few good movies, a ball game. Plan a party. Do things you particularly enjoy.
■ Burn your bridges behind you. Throw away your cigarette case, lighter, matchbooks, favorite ashtray. Get rid of everything that reminds you of smoking. Don't test yourself with temptations.
■ Avoid the smoke screen. This isn't always easy, but it is especially important in the very beginning. Stay out of the smokers' section at the movies and other places where the smoke will be thick. If possible, spend more time with non-smoking friends than with smokers.
■ Find something to do with your hands. Try playing the harmonica or sketching cartoons or knitting socks or painting the kitchen or whittling. Anything to avoid feeling empty-handed just because you're not fingering a cigarette.
■ Reach for chewing gum, peppermints, sourballs. Pop something into your mouth whenever you think you want a cigarette. Give yourself this break for awhile, even if you are dieting. Later you can work off those extra pounds.

■ Change your daily routine. For instance: eat new foods for breakfast or dinner; walk to school a different way; study in a different place; find an after-school job; find a new hobby (try volleyball if you like to read, or carpentry if you are a swimmer).

The point here is that after you have smoked for some time, cigarettes become a habit. You reach and light up automatically. Smoking becomes tied in with all the other automatic, habitual moves you make during the day. You need a different habit pattern now. Making different moves will jolt you out of the habit routine and help you avoid the desire to smoke.

Take Advantage of the Money Saved

Each week, put away the money you would have spent on cigarettes. It is a matter of simple arithmetic: a pack a day for a year can total over $175—even more, if you have friends who make a habit of scrounging cigarettes from you.

Plan how you will spend that money after you have hoarded your dimes and quarters for 10 or 12 months. Whether you set your mind on a camera, a new coat, or an electric guitar—or plan to save toward a car or a college education—you will be astonished to see how this goal strengthens your decision to stay away from cigarettes.

Figure 9-6 ● There are many good reasons to stop smoking.

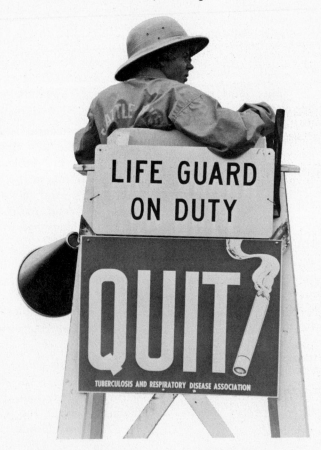

Don't Slip, Even Once

We can all find excuses—very clever ones—for starting to smoke again; that is easy. What takes strength is sticking by your decision to stop.

Don't let yourself be taken in by your own excuses. Find a good solid answer to every thought that tempts you to smoke.

Reinforce Your Decision

People who have successfully stopped smoking are those with strong satisfying reasons for staying away from cigarettes. Keep reminding yourself that within a very short while you'll have proof positive of the advantages of not smoking. Put your reasons down on paper:

- You will have far better wind for swimming, cycling, tennis, and other ball games.
- Your food will taste better. Cooking, flowers, and perfume will smell better.

- Your breath, clothes, and hair will lose that stale tobacco smell.
- You will have no more ugly yellow stains on your teeth and fingers.
- You will need no more annoying throat-clearing.
- You will have no more arguments with the nonsmokers in your life—your parents and your girlfriend or boyfriend.
- You will have more money for other things.
- You will have satisfaction, because you have the strength to stop and stop permanently.
- You will have pleasure, because you are setting a fine example for younger brothers and sisters and for other youngsters who admire you.
- You will have pride, because you are no longer dependent on cigarettes.
- You will have relief, because you stopped smoking when you were young enough to avoid permanent damage to your lungs and heart.

Summary

The overwhelming evidence supports those who think there is a relationship between smoking and ill health.

The effects of cigarette smoking upon the body vary tremendously. While some smokers find pleasure in the taste and smell of tobacco, most others report immediate effects such as nausea, shortness of breath, dizziness, irritation of the throat, and chronic cough. In addition, medical research reports a variety of effects upon the circulatory system, respiratory system, digestive system, and other parts of the body.

More and more young persons are becoming aware of the dangers of cigarette smoking. Many are deciding not to smoke at all. Others are changing their smoking behavior or deciding to quit entirely.

The decision is yours. You must weigh all the evidence and make an intelligent decision.

in making health decisions . . .

Understand These Terms:

bronchitis	irritating symptoms
cause and effect	nicotine
cilia	Surgeon General
constriction	trachea
emphysema	ulcers

Solve This Problem:

Cigarette smoking is said by some to be a method of coping with anxiety, social pressure, and control. Interview five cigarette smokers. Find out their reasons for smoking. Determine whether their reasons fall into the categories listed on page 137. Summarize your findings in a brief written report.

Try These Activities:

1. Ask five people who are nonsmokers to describe the relationship between cigarette smoking and ill health. Do the same for five smokers. Compare the responses. Be prepared to report to the class the similarities and differences between the responses of the two groups.

2. There is great concern about young people smoking. Make a list of the risks young people run if they start smoking at an early age. Compare your list with those of others in the class.

3. In this chapter a number of suggestions have been made as to what a smoker can do to stop smoking. Talk to several smokers and ask whether they have tried any of these methods. Be prepared to report your findings to the class.

Interpret These Concepts:

1. Present evidence indicates that there is a relationship between smoking and ill health.

2. The younger a person is when he or she starts smoking, the greater the risk that she or he may become ill at an earlier age.

3. You can stop smoking if you really want to.

Explore These Readings:

"The Continuing Cigarette Problem," *The Nation,* Vol. 216 (Apr. 2, 1973), p. 422.

Corwin, Emil, "Roses, Music, Misocapnists, and Smoking," *Health Services Reports,* Vol. 87 (June–July, 1972), pp. 491–495.

Irwin, Theodore, "Those Smoking Statistics: Fact or Distortion?" *Today's Health,* Vol. 48 (April, 1970), pp. 34–37.

Ross, W. S., "High Cost of Smoking," *Reader's Digest,* Vol. 100 (March, 1972), pp. 105–108.

Terry, Luther, "Pushing the Anti-Smoking Crusade in New Directions," *Today's Health,* Vol. 51 (June, 1973), pp. 12–13.

Ten | Preventing Drug Abuse

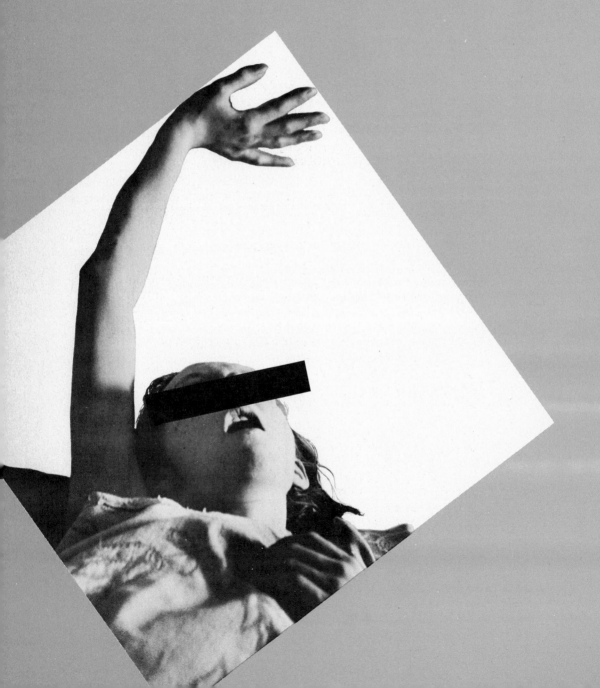

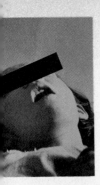

The general public, it seems, is now aware that we are living in a drug-oriented society. Radio and television commercials, along with advertisements in various other media, inform us that there are drugs available to help us sleep, to help us wake up, to slow us down, to pep us up, to help us lose weight, and to help us gain weight. The implication of the drug-oriented society concept is that there is a drug-related solution for every problem known to humanity, and perhaps even for some problems that we are unaware of.

Ever since history has been recorded, people have experienced pain, fear, unhappiness, and disappointment. These unpleasant feelings play a part in everyone's life, and it is not surprising that some attempt should be made to escape from them.

Most individuals choose acceptable ways of escaping from these problems. For example, sleep is nature's way of providing rest from physical exertion and mental activity so as to leave you refreshed and better able to cope with your problems. A number of persons, however, attempt to find a substitute for the more acceptable ways of easing their difficulties. Some find it in the various drugs which partly imitate nature's way of relieving care and fatigue.

Why You Should Be Concerned

The total number of persons who misuse drugs in the United States is not known. Because people hide their dependency on drugs, it is doubtful that the extent of the problem can be estimated with any degree of accuracy. The best information available usually deals with estimates made of those dependent upon the opiate-type drugs such as morphine and heroin. Sometimes these estimates include the use of hallucinogens (drugs that produce imaginary visions or hallucinations such as marijuana, mescaline, and Lysergic Acid Diethylamide (LSD). The figures usually given indicate that there are some 60,000 addicts in the United States. Other figures suggest that many more individuals are involved and the number is closer to 100,000. When other types of drugs such as barbiturates and amphetamines are considered, the difficulty of estimating the problem becomes even greater. Very little statistical research along these lines has been done. However, it has been suggested by a number of researchers that the amount of drugs produced is far greater than that needed for proper medical treatment.

Whatever the number of drug users, the difficulties brought about by drug abuse are much greater than might be implied simply by counting individuals dependent upon drugs. The effect, physically and emotionally, upon the individual and the impact upon society give rise to great concern. President Nixon, in March, 1970, said: "Drug misuse is a growing national problem. Hundreds of thousands of Americans—young and old alike—endanger their health through the use of drugs of all kinds. More than a hundred thousand of these Americans lead totally unproductive lives because of their addiction to narcotics."

More is known about individuals who are dependent upon opiate-type drugs and marijuana than about other drug users. This information shows that such individuals are predominantly concentrated in the largest cities of the United States. It is also noted that the problem is not limited to the socially and economically disadvantaged sections of these cities. The characteristic pattern of this type of dependency appears to have undergone a change since World War II. Before 1940, individuals dependent on drugs were older and a higher proportion were women. Today, the problem is considered to be more of a behavioral disorder of youth. There is now a large concentration of cases in your age group, with an estimated 10 times as many boys as girls involved. One explanation for this shift may lie in a change from the use of drugs as physical pain-killers to their use for "kicks."

Figure 10-1 ● This graph shows the estimated number of active narcotics addicts reported in several selected cities as of 1973. Explain why these figures do not represent a true picture of the drug problem.

Estimate of Active Narcotics Addicts Reported in Several Selected Cities 1973

Total Estimated Active Addicts 500,000

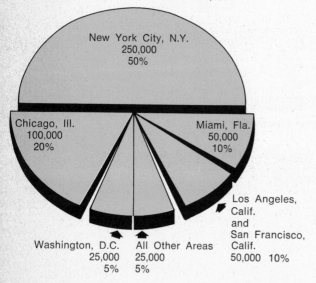

New York City, N.Y.
250,000
50%

Chicago, Ill.
100,000
20%

Miami, Fla.
50,000
10%

Washington, D.C.
25,000
5%

All Other Areas
25,000
5%

Los Angeles,
Calif.
and
San Francisco,
Calif.
50,000 10%

Drug Abuse Is a Social Problem

Drug abuse and all the destruction that goes with it—physical, mental, moral, occupational, and social—is plainly a problem that cannot be solved by its victims alone. **Drug abuse is a social problem which should concern everyone.**

Large numbers of young people have no decent home life, drop out of school early, do not develop occupational skills or do not have satisfactory work experience, and are exposed at an early age to drug abuse as a way of avoiding reality. These social situations seem to contribute to the misuse of drugs by young people.

Much more research must be completed before it is possible to understand what can be done to prevent drug abuse. However, improvement of social situations may be an important way of reducing the number of drug abusers.

Drug Abuse Is a Law-Enforcement Problem

Some persons use drugs that are banned by law. Others take properly prescribed drugs and use them illegally. In this respect, drug abuse is a legal problem that requires law enforcement.

Crimes of violence are often committed by persons suffering under delusions from stimulant drugs. Use of other drugs and dependence on them lead individuals to commit crimes to obtain money to support their habit. Part of society's duty is passing necessary laws and upholding law-enforcement activities to curb these situations.

Drug Abuse Is a Psychological Problem

Many individuals who abuse drugs have personality problems. They are unhappy and are not able to face their life situations. Some of these persons begin taking drugs before they are old enough to develop adequate strength to face reality.

Figure 10-2 ● The solution to the problem of drug abuse requires the cooperative efforts of individual groups and agencies. How can you help?

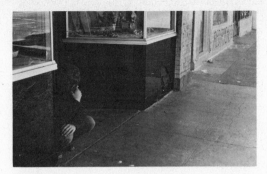

Social Problem

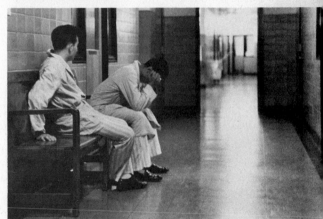

Law-Enforcement Problem

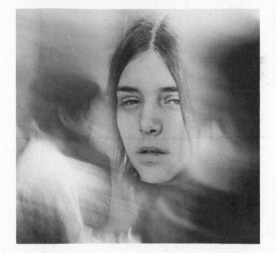

Psychological Problem

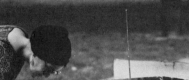

Public-Health Problem

Medical Problem

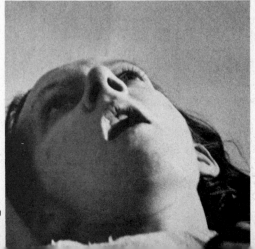

Individual Problem

Various types of inadequate persons misuse drugs. Many of them are antisocial, at war with society, defiant—although drugs may mask the defiance and make them seem passive. These persons take drugs for a thrill, and they do not care about anything or anybody else.

These inadequate persons seem to be addiction prone, but research still has not told us why only some of them become drug abusers. Neither has research indicated whether drug abuse is different psychologically from misuse of other types of products.

Drug Abuse Is a Medical Problem

Medical science has the necessary ability to prevent the severe withdrawal illness associated with certain drugs. Physical treatment alone, however, is not enough. Social and psychological treatment with a long period of supervised rehabilitation is necessary.

Not all authorities are willing to consider drug abuse as an illness. The relationship to crime and antisocial behavior makes the problem seem to many to be one of law enforcement only. However, even those who prefer to treat drug abuse as a social condition rather than as a disease must agree that the individual involved is a seriously disabled person who needs treatment.

Drug Abuse Is a Public-Health Problem

It is only natural that drug abuse be attacked as a public-health problem through studies of the kinds of people who become dependent upon drugs and the environment and circumstances in which they do so. In addition, research could be conducted to compare various methods of treatment, rehabilitation, and control.

Drug abuse can be considered a chronic disease because it lasts for months or years and leaves some disability or handicap.

Drug abuse can be considered communicable as well as chronic, because the typical user introduces the habit to others, causing it to spread as a process of social contagion.

Historical Background

Narcotic drugs have been used to relieve pain and induce a feeling of well-being as far back as historical records exist. Opium is listed on Assyrian medical tablets written during the 7th century B.C. Egyptian records mention opium as early as the 16th century B.C. By the beginning of the Christian Era, opium and its uses were well-known.

For many years the Greeks and Romans used it in the practice of medicine. Opium was humanity's principal medication. So little was known about the causes of illness that doctors concentrated on the symptoms, and opium could dull the pain and discomfort of almost any disorder. During the 9th and 10th centuries, in the Far East, extracts were prepared from the poppy. Arab camel trains carried the products to other parts of the world, particularly India and Persia. There the drugs were widely recommended for the relief of such disorders as dysentery and diseases of the eyes.

Opium later became a very profitable article of trade after the sea route to the East was developed in the 15th century.

The drugs produced from opium became widely used. This occurred in spite of many governments' laws prohibiting the transport of such drugs.

In the United States, opium began being a problem during the 18th and 19th centuries. Large quantities of medicine containing opium or opium derivatives were manufactured and widely distributed. These medicines were available at very low cost and were utilized as pain-killers.

During the middle of the 19th century, doctors learned to inject drugs through the skin with a needle. This hypodermic method, invented by the French physician Charles Pravaz in 1853, became a much more efficient way of administering morphine (opium's principal ingredient) to relieve pain more rapidly.

The occurrence of the Civil War just a few years after the introduction of this method increased the need for drugs offering rapid relief from pain. Injections were used more frequently. The resulting increase in the use of morphine created many problems. Some wounded soldiers who were given injections of morphine to ease their pain became dependent on it. This dependency was so prevalent that the condition was described as "army disease."

Many civilian patients, too, were given morphine injections for any one of dozens of disorders. Numbers of these patients found that they had to keep on taking the drug. Gradually, a number of physicians and other observant people began to realize that medicines containing opium were not safe. Used excessively or over a long period of time, these medicines proved to be dangerous to people's physical and emotional health. In addition, they led to social problems. Unfortunately, the addicting dangers of these drugs were not agreed on by all physicians and the drugs continued to be taken freely by many people.

The introduction of opium smoking by the Chinese who were brought to the United States to help build the railroads of the West also contributed to the problem. The habit was taken up by Americans and gradually passed from the western to the eastern United States.

Today, there is concern about the possible addictive effect of many drugs in addition to opium and its by-products, morphine and heroin. **A variety of drugs produce dependency and thus create problems for the individual and society.** Among these other drugs are the barbiturates (depressant sedatives), cocaine (a stimulant), amphetamines (stimulants), marijuana and other hallucinogens, and minor miscellaneous products.

Drugs of Dependence and Their Effects

We can not overestimate the value and importance of drugs in the alleviation of pain, the prevention and treatment of disease and illness, and the general improvement of personal and public health. All medicines are drugs. Not all drugs, however, are medicines. For example, heroin and marijuana are illegal drugs, are not used for medical purposes in this country, and their use may result in dependence. Morphine, amphetamines, and barbiturates are legal drugs when used for medical purposes. When misused, even medically valuable drugs may produce dependence.

When properly used, drugs are extremely valuable to modern medicine. We would all have a difficult time getting along without them. But drugs are harmful when misused. When trying to understand these drugs, one can frequently be confused or misled by the use of terminology concerning them. When physicians and law enforcement officers talk about addiction, they usually mean addiction to morphine, heroin, and other opiates or opiate-type drugs. However, other drugs such as marijuana and cocaine, while not physically addicting, are associated in the public mind with the "drug menace." Drugs such as barbiturates, amphetamines, tranquilizers and other intoxicating or hallucinating-type products may present an even greater problem. Still other drugs, such as those present in glue, bring about different problems.

A newer descriptive term, "drug dependence," which is medically and scientifically valid, has been proposed by the World Health Organization. The term more properly covers the various types of drug abuse. It is defined as "a state arising from repeated administration of a drug on a periodic or continuous basis." This seems to be a better way of looking at the situation. **Different drugs produce different types of behavior and states of dependency.**

Opium, morphine, and heroin have caused concern because of the tendency to regard them as addictive. It is to be hoped that a new approach, examining the problem of drug abuse on the basis of psychological dependency rather than physiological addiction alone, will cause more drugs to be regarded as potentially dangerous. You should be concerned about any drug that is misused. Some of those most frequently misused are discussed in the following paragraphs.

Narcotic Analgesics

Opium and its extracts and preparations such as morphine, codeine, paregoric, and heroin are considered narcotic analgesics. Their major resemblance to one another is that all give relief from pain. They have a

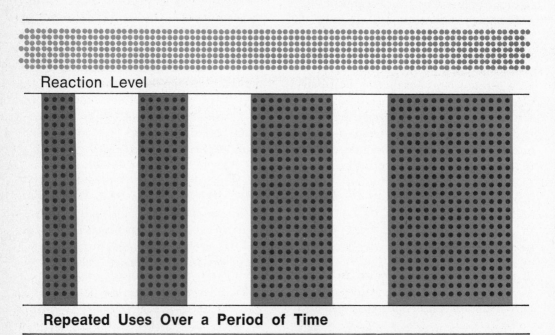

Reaction Level

Repeated Uses Over a Period of Time

Figure 10-3 ● As the body develops tolerance, the user requires increasing amounts of drugs to satisfy the addiction. Can you explain why the tolerance factor should be of major concern to the drug user?

narcotic (producing sleep or drowsiness), deadening, or numbing effect on consciousness. In larger doses, they produce stupor and coma. When misused, these drugs can kill.

Sometimes these narcotic drugs seem to act as stimulants because they produce active or excited behavior. Actually, such symptoms are misleading. The reason such drugs seem to be stimulating is that they depress or lower the mental controls that usually keep such behavior in balance.

When properly used under the guidance of a physician, the narcotic analgesics provide us with great relief from pain. The danger lies in improper use. If doses of these drugs are taken regularly, users develop a tolerance to the effects of the drugs. When this happens, they have to take a larger dose to meet the demand created in their body or to bring about the feelings they desire.

In addition, once dependent upon these drugs, if users stop taking them they become ill (withdrawal illness). Symptoms of withdrawal illness include excessive groaning and sweating; dripping eyes and nose; cramps in legs, back, and stomach muscles; and painful muscle-twitching. These symptoms are accompanied by vomiting, diarrhea, loss of appetite, fever, and rapid loss of weight. As you can see, it is a very distressing illness.

Barbiturates and Other Sedatives

Barbiturate drugs, also known as "sleeping pills" or "goofballs," are sedatives manufactured from chemicals. There are many on the market and their names usually end in -al. Taken in small amounts and under the direction of a physician, these depressants of the central nervous system can be extremely helpful in the treatment of hypertension and other health problems. However, when taken in uncontrolled quantities and at frequent intervals, they may cause as great a dependency as heroin and morphine.

Like alcohol, the barbiturates are intoxicating. Individuals involved with these drugs may become drowsy and confused, unable to think clearly, and unable to coordinate muscular action when they stand or walk. They become depressed, irritable, morose, and quarrelsome. They show poor judgment and find it difficult to perform simple tasks or take simple psychological tests.

The use of alcohol with barbiturates is very dangerous and may result in death. In this kind of mixture, the effect of each drug is intensified by the presence of the other. This intensification of effects is called synergism.

Sudden, complete withdrawal of barbiturates from a person dependent on them may result in convulsions and in a temporary psychosis resembling delirium tremens (a violent reaction of acute trembling and visual hallucinations caused by excessive use of alcohol). Certain tranquilizers also bring about similar dependency and associated problems.

Nobody knows precisely how many persons are dependent upon this type of drug today. However, the number appears to be many thousands and is continuing to grow.

Amphetamines

The amphetamines are the so-called "pep pills." When properly used, these drugs have many benefits. They act as a powerful stimulant on the central nervous system. Physicians find them useful in treating patients who are depressed. In addition, when applied to the mucous membrane of the nose (usually through an inhaler), they reduce the swelling caused by colds and allergic reactions. They are also used by physicians to decrease the appetite. Although these drugs are necessary for medical purposes, they should be used only under a physician's supervision. When they are used without proper supervision, you run the risk of developing a dependency on them. This dependency, in turn, may expose you to such dangers as elevated blood pressure, rapid pulse, sweating, tremors, spasms, and sometimes a psychosis.

Cocaine

Cocaine is a dangerous drug. People may develop such a strong desire for cocaine that they are unable to stop using it. It does not cause typical physical dependence or withdrawal illness. The drug causes some individuals to experience feelings of power, pleasure, or exhilaration. However, as these feelings wear off, users try to recapture them by taking more and more of the drug. Eventually, they develop dangerous hallucinations and may assault people in the belief that people are persecuting them or about to attack them. While once a major problem in the United States, cocaine is now used much less frequently.

Marijuana

Another intoxicating drug is marijuana. While it does not create physical dependency, an individual may become emotionally dependent on the drug and have an insatiable desire for its effects. Just as people who get drunk on alcohol have a number of varying reactions, people who get drunk on marijuana display a variety of behavior. Some are remorseful and quiet; others are happy and gay. Some are reckless and others are cautious.

People under the influence of marijuana tend to lose their sense of reality. As a result, they may have hallucinations and delusions. Some individuals believe they can perform certain tasks better when under the influence of marijuana. Studies suggest that they only *think* they do better, instead of actually doing better.

The effects of marijuana depend on the strength of the drug, the amount used, and the person who uses it. The active drug ingredient in marijuana is called Tetrahydrocannabinol, often shortened to THC. Studies indicate that marijuana grown in Mexico and the Far East contains higher concentrations of THC than that grown in the United States. Hashish and other forms of concentrated marijuana have greater THC content and, therefore, are more dangerous and unpredictable than the usual "street-grade" marijuana which causes serious problems for thousands of people every year.

In many cases, heroin addicts say that they started on marijuana. This does not mean that everybody who uses marijuana goes on to use heroin. The heroin addicts generally agree that once you start to use an illegal drug (marijuana or pills), you come into contact with people who have other illegal drugs available. You can see how this can then lead to the use of heroin.

Other Hallucinogens

Misuse of these drugs can bring about changes in mood and perception, and also cause visual and auditory hallucinations. Some tolerance is developed through repeated use of peyote, but physical dependence is not acquired. Individuals who give up the drug have no withdrawal symptoms.

LSD seems to affect that part of the brain where the input of information from the senses is decoded and processed. What takes place at this point varies greatly, depending upon the person and the circumstances involved. It appears that an extremely small dose of LSD will produce mental confusion and a variety of perceptual disturbances. For some users, lights swirl and dance and objects seem to move about. For others, shapes of flowers change; walls and ceilings sway. Unfortunately, these descriptions of the effects of LSD provide only a partial understanding of what happens to an LSD user.

The psychological implications are great. Some persons have a complete loss of identity and control and, as a result, their thoughts become chaotic. These reactions may continue for several hours and then lessen, with a return to normality. However, the same feelings may return spontaneously for a period of a year or longer. This may occur even though the individual does not take any more LSD.

Although the drug is not addicting in the physical sense, a strong psychological dependence is created. The user tends to increase his dosage to obtain the feelings he desires.

The indiscriminate, unsupervised use of LSD is clearly dangerous. Many hospitals report case after case in which persons are in a state of mental disorganization. Sometimes they are unable to distinguish their bodies from their surroundings. Other investigations have revealed that the use of LSD by an epileptic will trigger a seizure. This is of particular danger to those who have "hidden epilepsy" (where the problem is present but not yet diagnosed).

There also is evidence that LSD may cause chromosomal damage that can be transmitted from generation to generation for an indefinite period of time.

Other Problems

We are constantly learning about new drugs and new abuses. Although ether "sniffing" led to the important development of a general anesthesia, other kinds of experimentation have not been so successful or fortunate. Blindness and paralysis have often followed the use of radiator antifreeze, hair tonic, and many other substitutes for alcohol. The inhalation of these various products seems to give some people the brief feeling that they are walking on air. But they also run the risk of severe body damage.

Sniffing model airplane glue has aroused much concern because of its damage to the kidneys, bone marrow, liver, heart, and nervous system. In addition to the risk of damaging various parts of the body, the user also runs the risk of behavior changes. These may range from a feeling of being "high" to depression, delirium, muscular incoordination, and unconsciousness.

Glue sniffing does not lead to physical dependency, since the body does not require these chemical vapors. However, a strong psychological desire seems to be established in the user.

There are other dangerous substances which are not legally classified as narcotics or drugs. They are being abused, and their abuse is causing many personal and social problems. This group of substances is generally referred to as volatile substances. The fumes of these substances carry active ingredients which are harmful to the organs of the body, including the brain. These substances include paint, paint thinner, gasoline, kerosene, and similar products. Sniffing these substances may result in psychological dependence. The abuse of volatile substances over a period of time can result in permanent damage to the brain, as well as other organs of the body. Sniffing volatile substances has resulted in a number of deaths over the last few years.

Nature and Effects of Narcotics and Other Dangerous Drugs *

Drug	Properties	How Used	Effects
Narcotic Analgesics (Opiates) Opium	Sticky brown substance from opium poppy.	Smoked	Deadens feeling, saps energy, causes drowsiness and/or stupor. Forms strong addiction.
Morphine	Derivative of opium in white crystal form. Sold in powder, pill, capsule, or package.	Injected or swallowed	Relieves pain. Induces sleep. Is quickly addicting. Withdrawal symptoms.
Heroin	Derivative of morphine. White powder resembling powdered sugar. Sold in capsules. Outlawed medically in U. S.	Injected	Gives sense of well-being which is lost quickly. Highly addictive. Almost impossible to cure. Withdrawal symptoms.
Codeine	Derivative of morphine with similar properties.	Orally	Reduces pain. Is addictive and causes withdrawal symptoms.
Amphetamines Benzedrine Dexedrine Methedrine ("Speed")	Amphetamine sulphates. Powder in white or colored tablets or capsules. Commonly known as "bennies." Ingredient in some weight reduction preparations.	Orally	Stimulate. Lower muscle control; cause nervousness; decrease appetite. Overdose may lead to mental illness or death. Dangerous when driving.

* Adapted and reprinted with permission of The Macmillan Company from *Narcotics and Hallucinogenics* by J. B. Williams. Copyright © by Glencoe Press, a division of The Macmillan Company.

Drug	Properties	How Used	Effects
Barbiturates Pentobarbital Secobarbital Amobarbital Phenobarbital Barbital	Synthetic salts of barbituric acid. White powder sold in colored capsules or pill form (called yellow jackets or "goofballs").	Orally	Induce sleep, symptoms of drunkenness. Users in groggy state may take fatal overdose. Considered addicting. Serious withdrawal symptoms.
Tranquilizers Miltown Equanil	Meprobamates. White powder sold in tablets or capsules.	Orally	Calm nerves. Often used in combination with other drugs and alcohol. Become extremely dangerous. Dangerous when driving. Can be addicting.
Cocaine	Leaves of coca plant of South America (no relation to cocoa). Flaky, snowlike substance resembling epsom salts. Sold in capsules.	Sniffed	Kills pain, constricts tissues, dilates pupil of the eye, gives sense of elation. Quickly habit-forming. Mental and physical deterioration follow.
Marijuana	Leaves and stems of *cannabis sativa* (hemp) plant. Rolled into cigarettes.	Smoked	Unpredictable responses. Complete loss of time and space. Loss of inhibitions often leads to crime.
Hallucinogens Mescaline (Peyote) Psilocybin L S D	Alkaloids. From mescal cactus buttons. From mushrooms. From rye and wheat fungus.	Orally	Produce a variety of perceptual disturbances and mental confusion, particularly visual hallucinations. Not addictive.

Aerosols are all those products that are packaged in cans under gaseous pressure and are released for use by pressing a trigger-button. Aerosols are not harmful when they are used properly. When they are misused or abused, they can be dangerous and sometimes deadly. Aerosols should be used in exactly the way they were intended to be used. Directions for use should be read carefully, and followed exactly. The intentional abuse of aerosols can lead to psychological dependence. It can result in damage to the brain and other organs of the body. Abuse can result and has resulted in death.

Remember: **Drugs and other chemical substances should be used only for purposes for which they were intended.**

The Drug Abuser

It is difficult to develop a simple explanation for those who misuse or become dependent upon drugs. Most information about such individuals has been based almost exclusively on observation of users who have been arrested. However, it is possible to make some broad statements concerning the type of individual who abuses drugs, although more research will be necessary before absolute confidence can be placed in these generalizations.

Many persons who become dependent and abuse drugs have been generally characterized as having inadequate personalities with a low frustration tolerance. They need continued reassurance in any threatening situation and seek to avoid stress. Escape to a world of fantasy by means of drug abuse is to them one way of avoiding the constant demands of life around them. These individuals have also been described as being childishly pleasure-seeking.

Unfortunately, the present state of knowledge does not permit full under-

standing of the beginnings of personality disorders that might lead to drug abuse. Much research along these lines is being carried on, and may prove helpful in the future.

A common, but unsubstantiated, belief held by many people is that dependency is spread through society by the pusher who lures people under his influence and then entraps them with drugs against their strongest wishes. Virtually all informed observers agree that drug abuse habits spread from user to user and the pusher actually plays a somewhat minor role in the spread of the problem. New users are usually recruited from among individuals who come into social contact with those who are already drug abusers. The new users are individuals whose own personalities and social setting lead them to seek this type of society rather than to try to fit in with those who are already well-adjusted in their community. As a result, the spread of dependence is primarily through social contact. Thus you should be selective in choosing your friends.

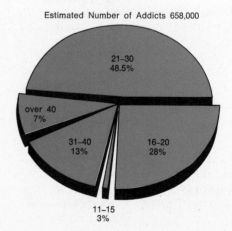

Age of Active Narcotics Addicts in the United States, 1971

Estimated Number of Addicts 658,000

Figure 10-4 • This graph shows the estimated percent of addicts by age group for 1971. How would these percentages differ for the age groups if all drug users, as well as addicts, were included?

Prevention, Treatment, and Rehabilitation

Prevention of addiction and treatment and rehabilitation of the dependent individual have been hampered by conflicting theories regarding the problem itself.

Sociologists see the problem of drug abuse in terms of specific environments. They point to minority groups who form a visible part of the problem and who are concentrated in a few big-city neighborhoods. These areas are usually economically depressed and culturally deprived, and have a high rate of delinquency.

Psychologists, on the other hand, interpret dependency as an expression of the frustration and hostility people feel and cannot express in any other way. These individuals represent the entire range of the socioeconomic spectrum.

Psychiatrists see the problem developing out of a specific kind of family situation. Obviously, this point of view transcends social, cultural, ethnic, and economic considerations.

And there are those who believe that drug abuse is strictly a problem of law enforcement. They think that, if the smuggling rings were smashed and the pushers thrown into jail, drug dependency would disappear, because illegal drugs would not be available.

Today, all of these theories are being merged and, as a result, newer concepts of prevention, treatment, and rehabilitation are being developed and put into practice.

It is far better to prevent health problems than to treat them. Therefore, programs are being developed to improve mental health and eventually reduce the number of individuals susceptible to drugs. Such advances as better housing and recreational facilities, which improve the mental outlook of the people, are being established in many areas. Since most dependent persons have been introduced to drugs by someone who is also dependent or is heading toward dependency, the treatment and rehabilitation of such individuals will help prevent the spread of the problem.

Dependency is also being fought by reducing the availability of illegal drugs. In a limited way, rehabilitation can be considered a form of prevention.

Some of the many programs aimed at the rehabilitation of the drug abuser are described in the paragraphs that follow.

Hospitalization

The Federal government, through the Public Health Service, provides hospitalization for narcotic addicts in Lexington, Kentucky and Fort Worth, Texas.

The treatment program at the hospitals endeavors to prepare the patient to return home and live without being dependent upon drugs. The first step, called withdrawal, consists of treating the physical dependence on the drugs. This is accomplished by substituting another drug for the one the patient has been using, and then gradually reducing the dosage of the substitute drug.

The withdrawal period varies, depending on the patient. At the end of this period, the patient is interviewed by members of the vocational, correctional, social service, and psychiatric staffs. A course of treatment is then outlined by a physician, who will supervise the program until the patient is discharged.

All activities of the hospital are designed to have therapeutic value for persons who have never quite grown up, distrust everyone in authority, and have substituted drug-taking for practically everything that occupies other people.

All physically able patients are assigned to jobs. For almost all types of work there is a training program that helps prepare the patient for getting and holding a job after discharge. The primary purpose of this work, however, is to help the patient learn to put some self-controls on and also to accept authority.

While the program described sounds as though it should be successful, there have been a number of disappointments and setbacks. Readdiction rates among those who leave the hospital against medical advice are high. One of the reasons for this is that more than one-third of the voluntary patients leave within two weeks—as soon as they have completed the withdrawal period or shortly afterwards. By the end of the first month, more than half the patients return to their old haunts.

The hospital staff believes that, if patients are to recover completely and start a new pattern of life, they should remain in a drug-free environment for four months after receiving their last drugs.

An After-Care Center Approach

Since hospitalization alone has not proved to be the complete solution, a number of additional approaches have been and continue to be tried to help the dependent individual learn to live without drugs.

New York City set up a Demonstration Center to help those released from the Federal hospital move back into the community. Selected patients returning to New York from Lexington were advised to go to the Center if they needed help. A social worker would listen to an individual's problems and then enlist the services of any community group that could help solve these particular problems. During the five years the Center was in operation, it had

more than 900 recent Lexington patients ranging in age from 16 to 72. While many of these individuals were not helped permanently—they went back to using drugs —a number did receive a great deal of benefit from the program.

In addition, several new ideas resulted from the work and these are being tried in other types of program. For example, it was learned that some individuals who were released from the hospital on probation or parole tended to do better than those who were released without parole. This was probably due to the constant attention they could receive as support for their efforts to remain free from drug dependence.

Parole Projects

Late in 1956 the New York State Division of Parole established a special narcotics project under which four parole officers who were trained social workers were each assigned 30 addicted persons newly paroled from reformatories and state prisons. Because the case load was lighter than that usually carried, each officer could see the parolees frequently and also visit their families. This provided many of the dependent persons with someone to whom they could turn for advice. Many of the families proved just as much in need of the counseling as the parolees.

Over a three-year period, the special project officers supervised approximately 350 parolees and of these 42 percent did not return to the use of drugs. This is an unusually high proportion of success. Unfortunately, these kinds of programs fluctuate in direct proportion to available funding, political attention, and public pressure. Various programs of this type have been initiated but have not expanded to any appreciable degree.

California established a somewhat similar program in 1962 in the California Rehabilitation Center for Addicts, operated under the State Department of Correction. This program is a combination of a confinement and parole approach.

When individuals are confined in the Center, they receive treatment consisting of physical conditioning, personal counseling, group psychotherapy, individual psychiatric care, academic instruction, vocational training, and religious guidance. The period of confinement may vary from six months to a number of years.

When released on parole, individuals are given close supervision to help them resist the urge to return to the use of drugs. This program is being continued and is being assessed to determine the actual implications for positive rehabilitation.

Treatment Centers

In 1967 a law was passed in the State of New York empowering judges to commit addicts for treatment of their addiction problem. The main focus of this law is upon the rehabilitation of the addict. Any individual convicted of a misdemeanor involving narcotics can be committed for treatment for up to three years. If the conviction is for a felony involving narcotics, the commitment can be for five years.

The most interesting part of this program is the concept of establishing treatment centers in various communities throughout the state. The facilities are operated as medical institutions, rather than as prisons. In these centers the program is concerned with the physical and psychological factors affecting addiction. In addition, provision is made for academic and vocational instruction.

Halfway House

In 1962 California established a Halfway House program for narcotic addicts. The purpose of such a facility is to provide an atmosphere of constructive living for narcotic-addict parolees during the critical months immediately following release. Past experience has shown that those individuals released from prisons or hospitals who return to their previous environment or a similar one are more likely to return to the misuse of drugs.

The Halfway House is an attempt to provide a new environment until the person is better equipped to resist permanently the return to drugs.

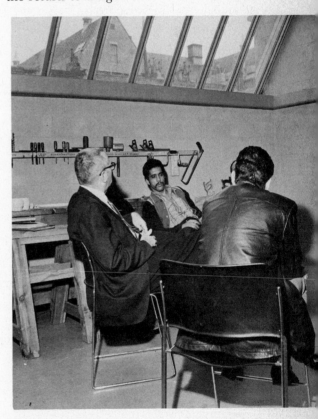

Figure 10-5 • Psychological factors of drug dependency are treated by various means of therapy, including group discussion, recreational activities, and vocational activities.

Methadone Treatment

In some cities, heroin addicts are provided with a synthetic narcotic drug called methadone. The use of this drug greatly reduces the physical reactions to the withdrawal from heroin. Over a sustained period of time, the methadone dosage is reduced and the addict more easily overcomes his physical dependence on heroin. The use of methadone does not help the addict overcome the psychological dependence. This phase of the dependence problem continues to require additional research and effort for an acceptable solution.

Methadone reduces the craving for heroin and prevents withdrawal illness, but methadone is addicting itself. It is sometimes argued, therefore, that the substitution of a lesser problem is not a real solution to the heroin-dependence problem. Others feel that the methadone maintenance treatment program could be a very important step toward a positive solution if the program were conducted on a hospital-confinement basis rather than as an outpatient treatment activity. The shortage of hospital beds and trained personnel for this specialized health problem seems to preclude the possibility of any large-scale methadone hospital-confinement program, at least at this time.

Other Efforts

Many efforts are being put forth to help the addicted or dependent individual. In addition, intensive research is going on all over the United States to develop new and better programs. Current efforts worthy of mention include the development of Narcotics Anonymous, an organization similar to Alcoholics Anonymous. It seems to be providing some help, but the program is still comparatively new and no definite information as to its degree of success is as yet available.

In the Los Angeles area, an organization called Synanon has enabled a number of addicted persons to help themselves. It is a residential organization in that once people are accepted, they agree to live in the residence for a considerable period of time.

During the first six months or longer, they live and work within the building. Then they get a job on the outside but continue to live at Synanon. During the entire

Figure 10-6 • The problem of drug abuse—whose responsibility?

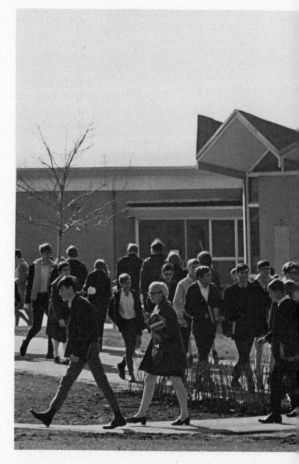

time they remain at Synanon, they participate in group discussions to gain insight into themselves as a first remedial step.

The basic approach of the organization is that only ex-addicts know enough about the problem of addiction to help others. Through a constant self-searching, it is hoped that the individual will become motivated to find a new way of facing life without dependence upon drugs.

The organization is growing and is establishing additional centers in other parts of the United States. The ultimate success of the organization has not yet been firmly established.

What You Can Do

Everyone needs to be informed about drug abuse and to lend support to efforts aimed at finding the solution to the problem. Some of the specific things you can do are:

- Do not let anyone persuade you to experiment with drugs.
- Help others understand that it is dangerous to fool with drugs.
- Disprove false claims about the harmlessness of drugs with facts.
- Be selective in choosing your friends.

Summary

Some people attempt to ease their difficulties by misusing drugs. The misuse is a social problem that should concern everyone.

The term "drug dependence" is being used to describe various types of drug abuse. As a result, an increasing number of drugs are being regarded as potentially dangerous.

There is no simple explanation for those who misuse or become dependent upon drugs. However, most authorities agree that drugs pose serious psychological as well as medical, public-health, and law-enforcement problems.

Attempts at prevention of addiction and treatment and rehabilitation of the dependent individual have had limited success. However, discovery, early diagnosis, treatment, and rehabilitation, together with law enforcement as a means of isolation and quarantine, are the approaches we can use now until research gives us the knowledge we need for preventing dependence.

in making health decisions . . .

Understand These Terms:

aerosol
addiction
depressant
drug abuse
habituation
hallucinogen
methadone

narcotic
physiological dependence
psychological dependence
rehabilitation
stimulant
tetrahydrocannabinol
volatile substance

Solve This Problem:

You have been asked to talk to a seventh-grade class about drug abuse. How would you answer the following questions:

1. "My parents take a drink now and then—so why shouldn't I smoke marijuana, if I want to?"
2. "If pills aren't good for you, how come they make so many and advertise them so much?"
3. "A friend of mine said she uses heroin, and she is not hooked—can some people use it and never become addicted?"

Try These Activities:

1. Prepare a report indicating
   a. How the individual and society benefit from the use of drugs when they are prescribed and used correctly.
   b. How the individual and society may be harmed by the abuse of drugs.
2. Itemize as many valid points as you can for both the pro and con sides of the question: Since cigarettes and alcohol are drugs, why are they legal?
3. It is often stated that drug abuse is not the problem—rather, it is a symptom of underlying problems. Identify what some of those underlying problems might be and suggest solutions that exclude the use of drugs.

Interpret These Concepts:

1. A variety of drugs produce dependency and thus create problems for the individual and society.
2. Different drugs produce different types of behavior and states of dependence.
3. It is far better to prevent health problems than to treat them.

Explore These Readings:

Bloomquist, Edward R., *Marijuana.* New York: The Macmillan Company (Glencoe Press), 1968.

Cohen, Sidney, *The Beyond Within: The LSD Story.* New York: Atheneum Publishers, 1967.

————, *The Drug Dilemma.* New York: McGraw-Hill Book Company, 1969.

Houser, Norman W. and Julius B. Richmond, *Drugs: Facts on Their Use and Abuse.* New York: Lothrop, Lee & Shepard Co., Inc., 1969.

Hyde, Margaret O., ed., *Mind Drugs.* New York: Pocket Books, Inc., 1972.

Louria, Donald B., *The Drug Scene.* New York: McGraw-Hill Book Company, 1968.

Nowlis, Helen H., *Drugs on the College Campus.* Garden City, N. Y.: Doubleday & Company, Inc., 1968.

O'Donnell, John A. and John C. Ball, eds., *Narcotic Addiction.* New York: Harper & Row, Publishers, 1966.

Stearn, Jess, *The Seekers.* Garden City, N. Y.: Doubleday & Company, Inc., 1969.

Eleven

Preventing
and Controlling
Communicable Diseases

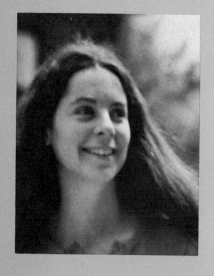

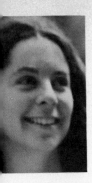

In the United States, as well as many other countries of the world, the reduction in the incidence of certain communicable diseases can be pointed to with pride. Excellent progress has been made in reducing such diseases as typhoid fever, smallpox, malaria, yellow fever, diphtheria, whooping cough, measles, and scarlet fever, to name a few. The death rates from diseases have declined to such an extent that in a number of states there have been no deaths reported from these diseases for several years.

These remarkable advances have been achieved through the application of scientific discoveries aimed at intercepting disease before a person becomes infected. In addition, new techniques of diagnosis and treatment of disease have been developed to help those who become infected (for example, the use of penicillin).

The advances have prevented great suffering and death. In addition, the cost of medical care and the loss of time from work because of specific communicable diseases have been dramatically reduced. Infant death rates have been reduced and life expectancy has increased.

However, it is not wise to be complacent. Some microorganisms have developed a resistance to antibiotics. This has created a serious problem in treating certain diseases such as staphylococcal infections. Gonorrhea continues to increase in spite of the availability of adequate treatment. New strains of viruses develop and spread across the world with great rapidity in a fashion similar to the pandemic (widespread epidemic) of Asian flu in 1957 and 1958. A new strain, Hong Kong flu, created widespread health damage in 1968. Still another strain, London flu, affected large numbers of persons in 1972 and 1973.

We can take pride in what has been accomplished. However, we must be constantly alert to continue advancing in the fight against communicable diseases. Everyone has responsibility for the prevention and control of disease. Techniques of prevention, such as immunization, are of no use unless many people take advantage of these preventive techniques. New methods of protecting water supplies and disposing of human wastes cannot be of any assistance in decreasing the spread of germs unless governmental agencies take the proper action and the citizens vote for adequate funds to provide these needed facilities.

You as well as other members of our society have a number of responsibilities in preventing and controlling communicable diseases. You should understand how diseases affect the body. You should know the principles of disease prevention and control. In addition, you should be able to put this understanding and knowledge into action.

The Concept of Disease

There is a constant interaction between the individual (host) and agents of disease. The interaction takes place in the environment in which the host and the agents reside. It is directly related to all aspects of the environment—physical, biological, social, and economic. The environment also contains a number of forces affecting this interaction. These include climate, temperature, housing, sanitation, living organisms, and other people. All these forces —and many others—may affect the host and the agents of disease, favoring one or the other or helping them live together without any problems. **The occurrence and distribution of diseases are affected by a person's heredity and environment.**

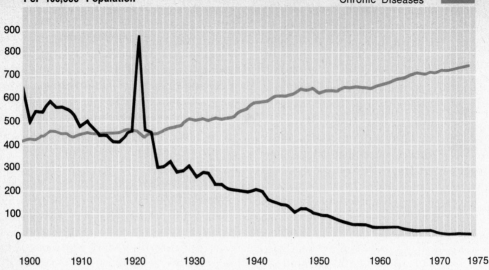

Figure 11-1 • The number of deaths resulting from communicable diseases has dropped sharply over the last 40 years. What are some of the factors that have contributed to the decline?

Definition of Disease

The American Public Health Association defines a communicable disease as:

> . . . an illness due to a specific infectious agent or its toxic products, which arises through transmission of that agent or its products from reservoir to a susceptible host, either directly or through the agency of an intermediate plant or animal host, a vector, or an inanimate environment.

When the body is invaded by an infectious agent or its toxic product, defense mechanisms start working. The condition called disease results when there is evidence of a struggle between the defense mechanisms and the infectious agent (for instance, a fever might develop).

Disease may be defined as the detectable reaction of the host to invasion by a specific agent or its toxic product in a particular environment.

The Host-Agent Relationship

The host (an individual) reacts to invasion through a variety of forces, including the body defenses; heredity and constitution; habits and customs; age, sex, and race characteristics; techniques of increasing resistance; and power to control the agents of infection.

The infectious agent affects the disease process by its ability to grow and reproduce; its resistance to attack by body defenses and heat, cold, moisture, sunlight, and chemicals; its ability to adapt itself to the host and cause a tissue reaction; and its virulence or strength.

A host and an agent of disease can often live together in harmony. This is called a symbiotic condition. Both the host and the agent live together without apparent ill effect on each other.

In other conditions, the agent of disease invades the host and causes severe illness and even death. The host may be destroyed at the same time as the agent is.

In still other conditions, the host may destroy the invader because immunization has increased the defense mechanisms or antibiotics have been used to kill the agent.

Development of Disease

Infectious disease develops in the following manner. First, there is an incubation period in which the agent of disease is growing, developing, and overcoming the body defenses. Second, there is the onset of the disease, when the signs and symptoms first appear. Third, there is a progressive stage during which the disease develops fully.

More information is needed on how agents of disease affect the body. However, certain knowledge is available. Some agents invade the tissues directly and actually destroy cells or rob them of food and blood. Some agents block the work of specific cells, tissues, and organs, interfering with their function. Others secrete a toxin or poison that is carried by the bloodstream to the nerve cells and interferes with the central nervous system.

Diseases usually bring about general changes in the body which are reflected in a variation of the total number of white blood cells as well as in differences in the blood chemistry. Various laboratory tests are of great assistance to the physician in making his diagnosis.

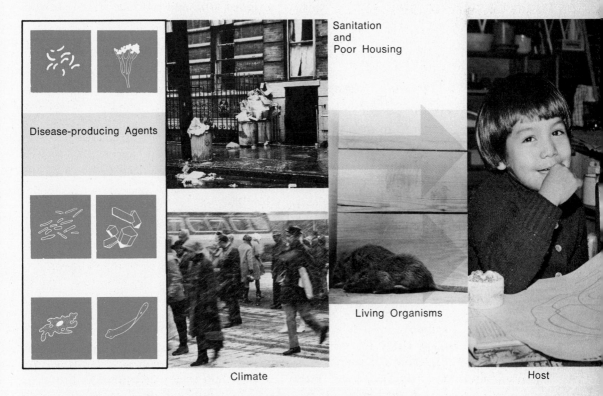

Disease-producing Agents

Sanitation and Poor Housing

Living Organisms

Climate

Host

Figure 11-2 • Interaction between host, environment, and microorganism. The environment plays an important part in the process of transmitting disease. How do the various environmental factors influence susceptibility to disease?

The Infectious Disease Process

For an infectious disease to occur, a series of events must take place. A change or interruption in the series usually means that the disease will not develop. Prevention and control of any single infectious disease depends upon thorough knowledge of this process.

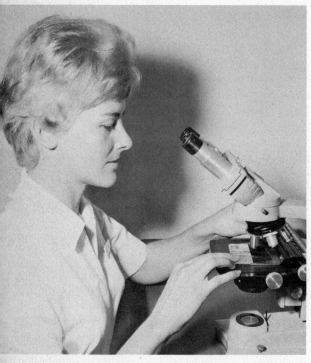

Figure 11-3 • The number of white blood cells stays at a fairly constant level in a healthy person. What are some of the conclusions that might be drawn, if the laboratory technician in the photo finds the white blood cell count to be substantially above normal?

Causative Agent

For an infectious disease to occur, there must be a causative agent. The agents may be bacteria, fungi, rickettsiae, viruses, protozoa, or helminths. Most of these may be classified as microorganisms.

Bacteria. Bacteria are unicellular (one-celled) organisms of varying size that may be viewed through a microscope. Not all bacteria are dangerous to man. In fact, some are quite beneficial. Those that can cause disease are called pathogenic. Tuberculosis is a disease caused by bacteria.

In a favorable environment, bacteria reproduce rapidly. Even under the best conditions, bacteria do not live too long, and under unfavorable conditions they die very quickly.

Unfortunately, some bacteria change to spore forms that are resistant to some unfavorable environmental conditions. In this state, the bacteria can live almost indefinitely. When the environment is favorable, the bacteria can return to their original form and continue their reproductive cycle.

Figure 11-4 • Organisms that cause diseases in people.

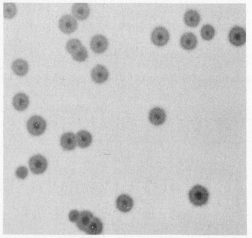

Bacteria

Fungi. Fungi are also plant forms that may be helpful or harmful to man. Molds are the greatest source of antibiotics in use today. The drug penicillin, produced by mold found on bread and cheese, is an example of how important certain fungi are to human beings.

Pathogenic fungi can cause problems. Fungous infections of the skin are quite common. Many people suffer from athlete's foot or ringworm of the scalp. Two serious diseases caused by fungi are coccidiodomycosis (valley fever) and histoplasmosis. Both are respiratory illnesses.

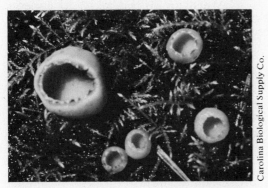

Fungi

Rickettsiae. Rickettsiae are disease-producing organisms that look like bacteria. They are barely visible under the microscope, being somewhat larger than viruses, yet smaller than bacteria.

Rickettsial diseases are transmitted by certain insects, such as lice and ticks. Typhus fever and Rocky Mountain spotted fever are examples of diseases caused by these microorganisms.

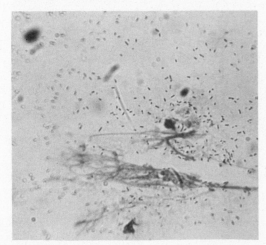

Rickettsiae

Viruses. Viruses are so small that they cannot be seen with the ordinary microscope. They must be seen and photographed through the electron microscope.

When a virus comes in contact with a cell, the protein coat of the virus attaches to the cell like a parasite. The cell is then invaded and the virus begins to rob it of nourishment. The reproduction of new viruses takes place within the cell. Some of these escape and invade other cells. Colds and influenza are diseases caused by viruses.

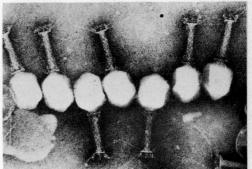

Viruses

Protozoa. Protozoa are unicellular animal organisms. Only a few are pathogenic. Like bacteria, they vary greatly in size and have the ability to reproduce rapidly.

Two common diseases caused by protozoa are malaria and amoebic dysentery.

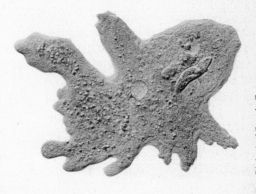

Protozoa

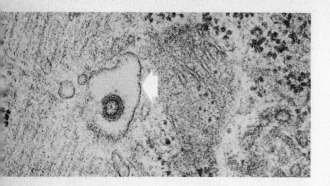

Figure 11-5 • Medical science can now isolate and identify certain forms of virus. How does this benefit you?

Helminths. Helminths are parasitic worms. They are multicellular (many-celled) animal forms and include tapeworms, hookworms, and trichinae.

Human beings become infected with tapeworms when they eat meat or fish that has not been sufficiently cooked to kill the cysts of the tapeworm that may be present in the muscles of the animal. In the human being, they affect the intestinal tract.

Hookworms are capable of piercing the skin and entering the body. This generally occurs when a person walks barefoot on soil contaminated by fecal material containing the hookworm. Once inside, hookworms reach the intestines and injure the individual by sucking blood, eating certain tissues, and producing a toxin.

Trichinae are small round worms that cause trichinosis. People acquire the disease by eating infested pork that has not been cooked sufficiently to kill the trichinae. Cysts eventually form in the muscles of the individual and cause extreme pain.

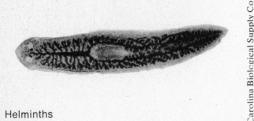

Helminths

Carolina Biological Supply Co.

Sources of Causative Agents

The source of causative agents is often called the reservoir of infection. This refers to the place where the causative agents live, grow, and multiply.

Human beings are an important reservoir. When an individual is sick, microorganisms are growing and multiplying within the body. Some persons may be healthy carriers in that they are not sick themselves, yet they carry organisms that may cause disease in others. Some individuals have subclinical diseases. This means that they are slightly sick, but do not have obvious signs and symptoms. At the same time, microorganisms are growing and multiplying within them and they can transmit the disease to others.

A number of diseases are acquired by human beings from animals. Rodents serve as a reservoir for plague. Dogs and squirrels (and many other animals) are common sources of rabies.

The environment, in a limited fashion, also serves as a reservoir of infection. Soil and dust may contain the spore form of some pathogenic organisms.

Mode of Escape

For the infectious disease process to continue, it must be possible for the causative agent to escape from the reservoir. This escape depends on where the organisms are located in the reservoir and on the available exits. If the organisms are located in the respiratory system, breathing, sneezing, coughing, and spitting will help expel them through the mouth and nose.

If the organisms are located in the intestinal tract, they may be expelled with the waste material. The urinary tract acts as a similar means of escape.

Body lesions (open sores) serve as a mode of escape for some diseases, which can thus spread to other people.

Mode of Transmission

The mode of transmission is one of the most important steps in the spread of infectious disease. Microorganisms may escape from a reservoir, but unless they are transmitted to a new host, disease cannot progress. It is at this point that many diseases are susceptible to attack.

There are two main modes of transmission, direct contact and indirect contact.

Direct Contact. Not all causative agents have the ability to live outside the reservoir for any length of time. As a result their transmission is limited to direct contact. Direct contact implies fairly intimate association but not necessarily actual physical contact. Microorganisms expelled from the mouth and nose may be transmitted by droplets through the air to a new host. Certain diseases such as syphilis and gonorrhea usually require direct physical contact of a specific nature.

Indirect Contact. There are a number of ways of transmitting agents of disease in an indirect manner. For this to occur, the agent of disease must be capable of living outside the reservoir for a period of time, and some vehicle of transmission must be available. Water, milk, other food, and insects commonly serve as vehicles of indirect transmission of disease-causing agents.

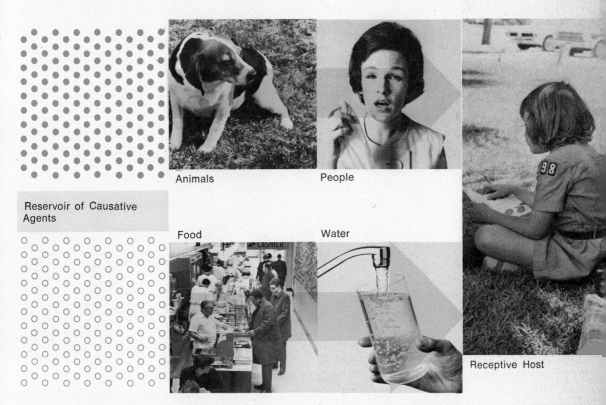

Reservoir of Causative Agents

Animals

People

Food

Water

Receptive Host

Figure 11-6 ● The cause of diseases could be eliminated if the reservoir of causative agents could be controlled. What might some of these controls be?

Mode of Entry

Once a causative agent has been transmitted, it must still gain entrance into a new host if it is to grow and produce infection. The natural openings of the body are the main portals of entry. A break in the skin caused by a scratch or the bite of an insect may also serve as a mode of entry.

Most causative agents must enter the body in a specific way to cause disease. They must reach a site which is favorable to their growth. Tetanus organisms are effective only if they can enter the body through a break in the skin. If these organisms are taken into the body through the mouth and enter the intestinal tract, the disease tetanus will not be able to occur.

The Susceptible Host

The final stage in the infectious disease process involves the new host. If the host is susceptible, disease will occur. If the host has immunity or has great enough resistance, the body will be able to ward off disease.

Resistance is a relative term. It refers to all the body defenses that prevent the progress of invading causative agents. These defenses include the skin, the stickiness of mucous membranes, the cilia of the nose, the acidity or alkalinity of parts of the digestive system, white blood cells, and antibodies. In addition, many other factors affect the resistance of the new host. These include the host's adequacy or inadequacy of nutrition, hormone balance, fatigue, chilling and exposure to low temperature, age, sex, and general physical condition.

The skin plays a major role in protecting the body. Many causative agents are found on the skin, but they are unable to penetrate unless there is a break in the

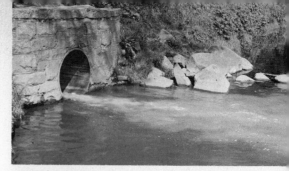
Polluted Water

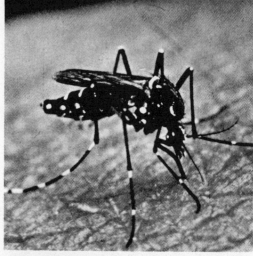
Mosquitoes

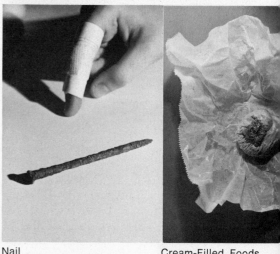
Nail   Cream-Filled Foods

Figure 11-7 ● Disease-causing organisms can be transmitted by indirect contact. What preventive measures can you take for each contact illustrated above?

surface. As a result, they must find other ways of reaching the inner tissues where they can grow and develop.

The moist, sticky mucous membranes trap microorganisms. The cilia or hairs in the nose keep causative agents from penetrating into the deeper tissues of the body. Many disease agents are destroyed in the stomach by the high acid content of the gastric juices. The intestinal tract rids itself of microorganisms by discharging them with waste material.

The white blood cells and antibodies constitute other important lines of defense. The white blood cells surround, kill, and digest invading organisms. These cells, however, cannot always destroy all invading agents. In such cases, the body must use another defense, antibodies.

Antibodies are chemical substances that are specific in origin and function. They are found in the plasma portion of the blood at the time the agent for any disease enters your body. Some antibodies act directly on bacteria by dissolving them. Others act upon toxins by neutralizing them, much like an antidote for poison. Once the antibodies reach a high enough level in the blood (for example, following recovery from a specific disease), you usually become immune to that particular disease.

Methods of Prevention and Control

For disease to occur, the causative agent must escape from its source, be transmitted to a new host, enter, and overcome any resistance that might be present. This process is quite specific for each and every communicable disease. Successful control comes from finding some weak spot in this sequence of events and applying an effective measure against it.

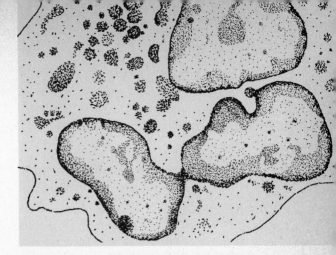

Figure 11-8 ● White blood cells constitute one of the body's natural defenses against disease organisms. What are the similarities and differences between the function of white blood cells and the function of antibodies?

Generally, prevention and control can be directed at four areas: eliminating the source of infection, upsetting the modes of transmission, increasing resistance, and early diagnosis and treatment.

Eliminating the Source of Infection

For some communicable diseases, it is possible to destroy the source of infection. Animals that serve as reservoirs of disease for human beings can be eliminated. This approach is used in preventing the spread of diseases such as the bubonic plague, rabies, and bovine tuberculosis.

Another approach used in eliminating the source of infection is removing the sick person from contact with other people, so that there is less chance that the infection will be passed on. This is accomplished by means of isolation or quarantine.

Isolation is the complete separation of infected persons from other persons for the period of time during which the disease may be transmitted.

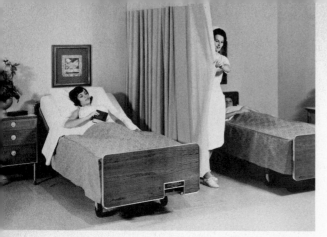

Figure 11-9 ● In some cases, isolation of an infected person is accomplished best in a hospital. In what other ways can valid isolation be accomplished?

Quarantine refers to the limitation of freedom of movement of persons who have been exposed to a communicable disease for a period of time equal to the incubation period of that disease.

Usually, procedures of isolation and quarantine are carried out by personnel from health departments after certain diseases have been reported to the health agency. There are specific rules followed by the health department for each disease requiring this approach.

Upsetting the Modes of Transmission

A number of measures have been devised that effectively interfere with the transmission of various types of disease agents.

The treatment and purification of water can control a number of diseases such as typhoid fever, cholera, and various types of dysentery. Proper disposal of human waste helps control the spread of various intestinal diseases by reducing the possibility of contamination of water, milk, and other food.

Inspection of animals to be used for human consumption and all other food products helps prevent the transmission of many diseases through food. The inspection of restaurants, bakeries, and other food-serving and food-processing establishments by health department personnel (sanitarians) also reduces the possibility of disease transmission.

Many techniques have also been developed to control carriers of disease agents, such as insects and rodents. By eliminating breeding places and by spraying, mosquito populations have been kept under control. As a result, malaria and yellow fever are no longer serious health problems in the United States. By ratproofing buildings; by properly disposing of garbage and trash; and by poisoning, trapping, and fumigation, rodent populations are kept small. This reduces the possibility of diseases such as the bubonic plague.

Other measures that interfere with the transmission of disease agents are the pasteurization of milk, proper washing of dishes in restaurants, washing the hands after using the toilet, keeping certain foods under refrigeration when they are not being served, and keeping other foods above a specified temperature to kill disease agents that might be present.

Figure 11-10 ● Health department personnel contribute a great deal to the control of communicable diseases. If you were this inspector, what would you examine more closely?

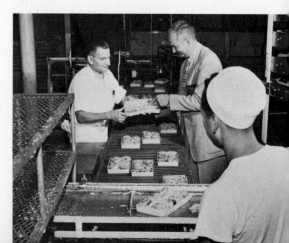

Increasing Resistance

One of the most effective ways of protecting a person from communicable disease is to increase that person's resistance. A high degree of resistance is called immunity. However the term immunity is a relative one and does not imply absolute protection. It reflects a high degree of resistance on the part of an individual to a particular disease. It depends on the various antibodies within the individual and the ability to produce new or additional antibodies when a disease agent enters his body.

Immunity may be either of two general types, active or passive.

Active Immunity. Natural active immunity is acquired by having a specific disease and recovering. Artificial active immunity is acquired by immunization with specific material that causes the body to produce antibodies similar to those produced in natural active immunity. The material used for immunization is actually a form of the disease agent.

In developing both natural and artificial active immunity, an antibody generator (antigen) stimulates the body to produce specific antibodies. When enough antibodies develop, the individual has produced its own immunity. As a result, if the same disease agent enters the body at a later date, sufficient antibodies are present or can be produced rapidly to overcome this invasion.

The duration of immunity varies with each disease. For some, immunity lasts a long time. For others, it is necessary to repeat immunization at regular intervals.

It is now possible to provide artificial active immunity against a number of diseases such as diphtheria, pertussis (whooping cough), tetanus, poliomyelitis (polio), smallpox, measles, German measles, and typhoid fever.

Passive Immunity. Passive immunity provides a high resistance immediately, but for only a short time—weeks or months. This is because the individual does not produce his own antibodies. Instead, the antibodies are produced in animals or taken from the pooled blood (gamma globulin) of other people and injected into the individual needing this protection. The procedure is called artificial passive immunity. It is effectively used in fighting diphtheria, scarlet fever, rabies, botulism, and tetanus. Protection against tetanus can be acquired both actively and passively. Figure 11-11 illustrates the conditions under which the different forms of immunity are provided.

Natural passive immunity also occurs. The mother transfers antibodies across the placenta to her unborn child during pregnancy. When the child is born, it has the same immunity as its mother. However, this immunity wears off in a few months and the child must start developing active immunity for itself.

New immunizing agents, active and passive, will continue to be produced. As a result, increasing the resistance to specific diseases will continue to be an effective technique of stopping the infectious disease process.

Figure 11-11 ● The use of polio-immunizing agents has been responsible for a dramatic decrease in the incidence of this dreaded disease. What are some of the diseases for which successful immunizing agents have not yet been found?

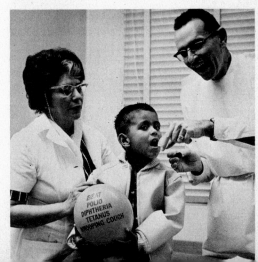

Early Diagnosis and Treatment

By finding disease early and treating it early, the spread of communicable disease can be minimized in population groups. The earlier a case is found and brought under control, the more it is possible to reduce the number of contacts between sick and susceptible persons. This approach to prevention and control is called casefinding and is an important part of the process of communicable disease control.

Some Important Communicable Diseases

Despite spectacular advances in the United States against many communicable diseases, certain ones still persist and others have become more of a problem. Some communicable diseases are responsible for the loss of a great deal of time from work, others cause a number of deaths each year, and still others reduce vitality and enjoyment of life. **Diseases may have both a personal and an economic effect on individuals and society.**

Venereal Diseases

The principal venereal diseases in the United States are syphilis and gonorrhea. They are two different diseases caused by two different organisms. They have different effects on the body and are treated differently. However, their mode of transmission is similar. These diseases are transmitted directly by an infected person during sexual intercourse or intimate bodily contact involving the sex organs, the mouth, or the rectum.

Figure 11-12 • This chart shows the number of reported cases of some communicable diseases in 1971.

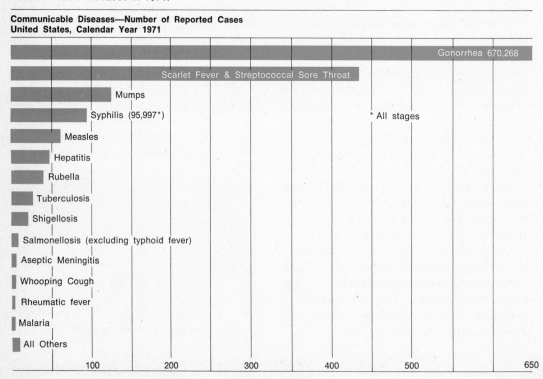

Communicable Diseases—Number of Reported Cases
United States, Calendar Year 1971

Gonorrhea 670,268
Scarlet Fever & Streptococcal Sore Throat
Mumps
Syphilis (95,997*)   * All stages
Measles
Hepatitis
Rubella
Tuberculosis
Shigellosis
Salmonellosis (excluding typhoid fever)
Aseptic Meningitis
Whooping Cough
Rheumatic fever
Malaria
All Others

100   200   300   400   500   650

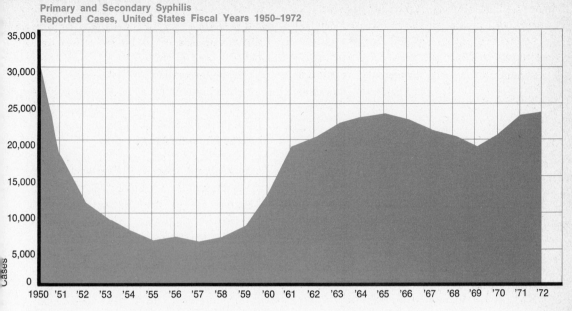

Primary and Secondary Syphilis
Reported Cases, United States Fiscal Years 1950–1972

Cases

Fiscal Year

Figure 11-13 ● This chart shows the change in the number of reported cases of
syphilis between 1950 and 1972.

Three other diseases are also classified as venereal diseases. They are chancroid, lymphogranuloma venereum, and granuloma inguinale. Each of these is different, is caused by different organisms, has different effects on the body, is treated differently, but has a similar mode of transmission.

Syphilis and gonorrhea are major health problems. They are among the leading communicable diseases in the United States. They cause a great deal of suffering, both emotional and physical. It is estimated that one out of every 13 persons with an untreated syphilis infection will develop heart disease; one in 25 will become crippled or incapacitated; one in 44 will develop paresis (syphilitic insanity); and one in 200 will become blind. A number of babies are born each year with congenital syphilis; many others are stillborn.

More than 60 percent of infectious syphilis and gonorrhea occurs in persons 24 years of age or younger. Many of these cases could have been prevented. Syphilis is easy to diagnose and relatively simple to treat and cure. Gonorrhea presents a few more problems, particularly in the female.

If these diseases are to be overcome, all young people must have knowledge about them. It is no longer safe or appropriate to maintain a "hush-hush" attitude. Syphilis and gonorrhea must be considered as intolerable diseases that present a threat to every member of society. If this can be accomplished, the chances of reducing the threat are greatly enhanced.

Syphilis. The human being is the only known host of syphilis. Everyone is susceptible to the disease because any immunity that might be present is very slight. After a cure, one may again be infected.

Chart of Venereal Diseases

Figure 11-14.

Disease	Causative Agent	Incubation period	Diagnostic procedures	Treatment
Syphilis	Treponema pallidum	7-90 days (usually 3 weeks)	Darkfield examination Serologic tests for syphilis Spinal fluid test X-ray of longbones of infants Clinical and contact histories	Penicillin Broad spectrum antibiotics
Gonorrhea	Neisseria gonorrhoeae	2-14 days (usually 3 days)	Culture Smear Clinical and contact histories (serologic test for syphilis)	Penicillin Broad spectrum antibiotics
Chancroid	Hemophilus ducreyi	2-6 days	Microscopic for Ducrey bacillus Clinical and contact histories (serologic test and darkfield examination for syphilis)	Broad spectrum antibiotics, including streptomycin
Lymphogranuloma Venereum	LGV virus	5-30 days	Frei skin test Serologic test for LGV Clinical and contact histories (serologic test and darkfield examination for syphilis)	Broad spectrum antibiotics
Granuloma Inguinale	Donovania granulomatis	Probably 8-90 days	Tissue scraping or biopsy Clinical and contact histories (serologic test and darkfield examination for syphilis)	Broad spectrum antibiotics

THE SKELETAL SYSTEM

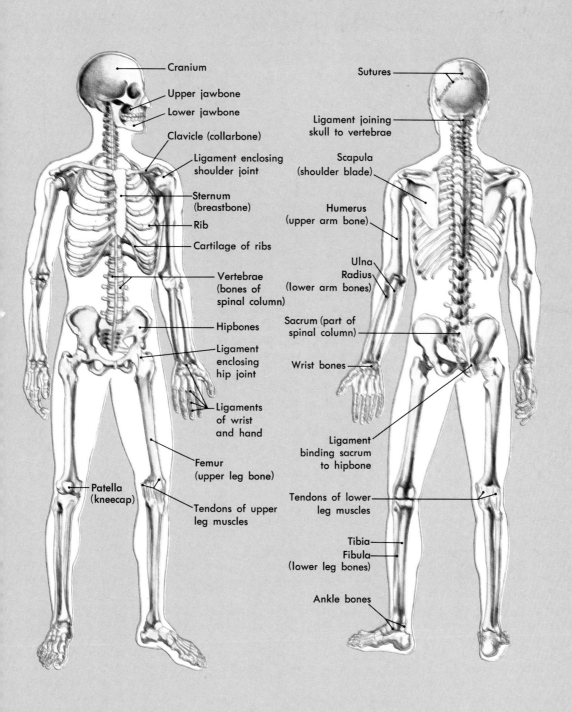

Cranium

Upper jawbone

Lower jawbone

Clavicle (collarbone)

Ligament enclosing
shoulder joint

Sternum
(breastbone)

Rib

Cartilage of ribs

Vertebrae
(bones of
spinal column)

Hipbones

Ligament
enclosing
hip joint

Ligaments
of wrist
and hand

Femur
(upper leg bone)

Patella
(kneecap)

Tendons of upper
leg muscles

Sutures

Ligament joining
skull to vertebrae

Scapula
(shoulder blade)

Humerus
(upper arm bone)

Ulna
Radius
(lower arm bones)

Sacrum (part of
spinal column)

Wrist bones

Ligament
binding sacrum
to hipbone

Tendons of lower
leg muscles

Tibia
Fibula
(lower leg bones)

Ankle bones

THE MUSCULAR SYSTEM

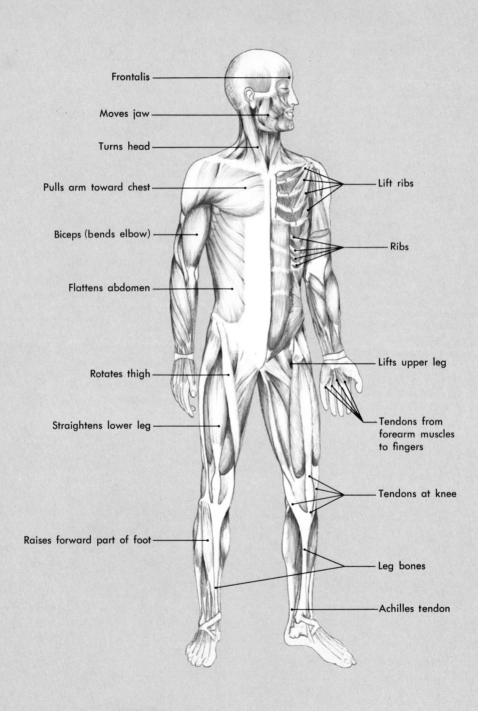

Frontalis

Moves jaw

Turns head

Pulls arm toward chest

Biceps (bends elbow)

Flattens abdomen

Rotates thigh

Straightens lower leg

Raises forward part of foot

Lift ribs

Ribs

Lifts upper leg

Tendons from forearm muscles to fingers

Tendons at knee

Leg bones

Achilles tendon

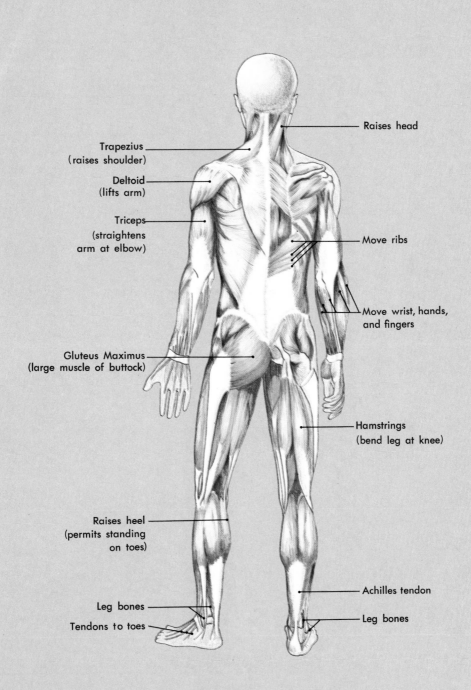

Raises head

Trapezius
(raises shoulder)

Deltoid
(lifts arm)

Triceps
(straightens
arm at elbow)

Move ribs

Move wrist, hands,
and fingers

Gluteus Maximus
(large muscle of buttock)

Hamstrings
(bend leg at knee)

Raises heel
(permits standing
on toes)

Achilles tendon

Leg bones

Leg bones

Tendons to toes

THE BONE-MUSCLE RELATIONSHIP

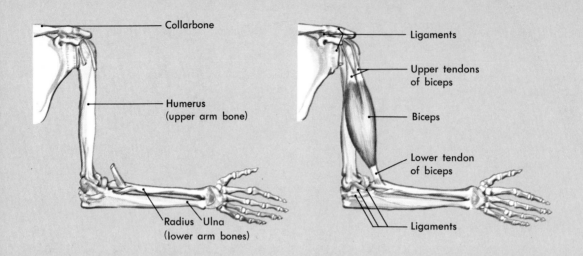

Collarbone

Humerus
(upper arm bone)

Radius   Ulna
(lower arm bones)

Ligaments

Upper tendons
of biceps

Biceps

Lower tendon
of biceps

Ligaments

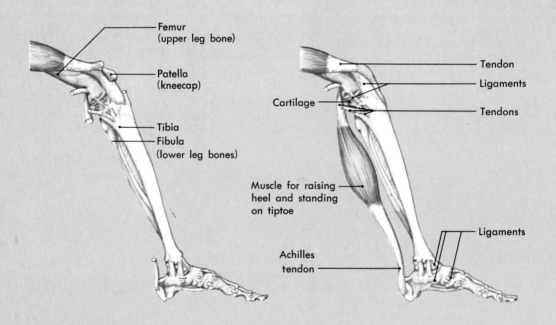

Femur
(upper leg bone)

Patella
(kneecap)

Tibia
Fibula
(lower leg bones)

Muscle for raising
heel and standing
on tiptoe

Achilles
tendon

Tendon
Ligaments

Cartilage

Tendons

Ligaments

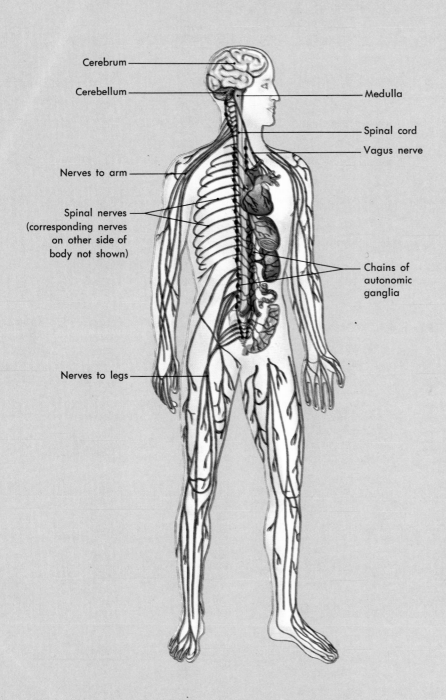

Cerebrum

Cerebellum

Medulla

Spinal cord

Vagus nerve

Nerves to arm

Spinal nerves
(corresponding nerves
on other side of
body not shown)

Chains of
autonomic
ganglia

Nerves to legs

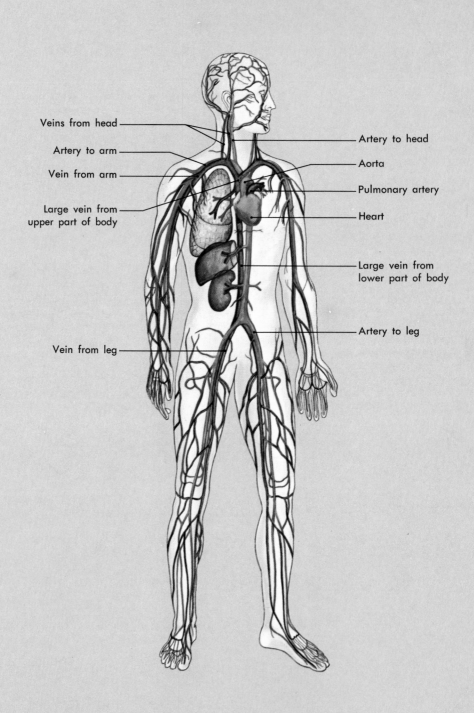

Veins from head

Artery to head

Artery to arm

Aorta

Vein from arm

Pulmonary artery

Large vein from
upper part of body

Heart

Large vein from
lower part of body

Artery to leg

Vein from leg

THE RESPIRATORY AND DIGESTIVE SYSTEMS

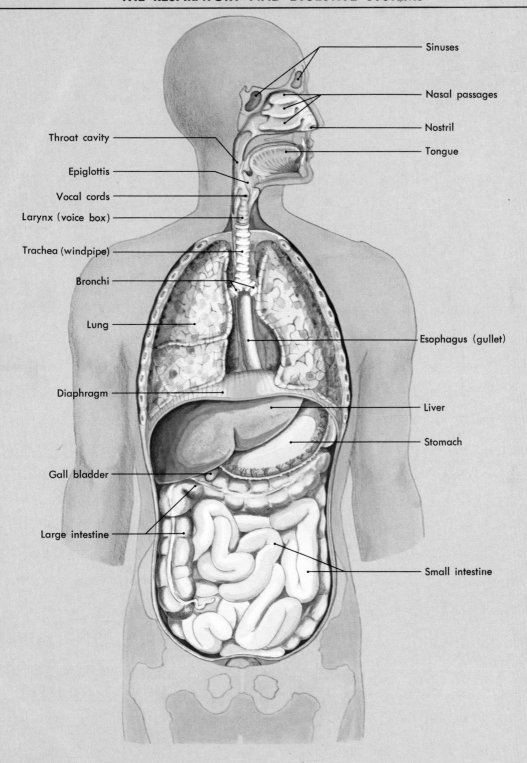

Sinuses

Nasal passages

Nostril

Tongue

Throat cavity

Epiglottis

Vocal cords

Larynx (voice box)

Trachea (windpipe)

Bronchi

Lung

Esophagus (gullet)

Diaphragm

Liver

Stomach

Gall bladder

Large intestine

Small intestine

PARTS OF THE RESPIRATORY SYSTEM

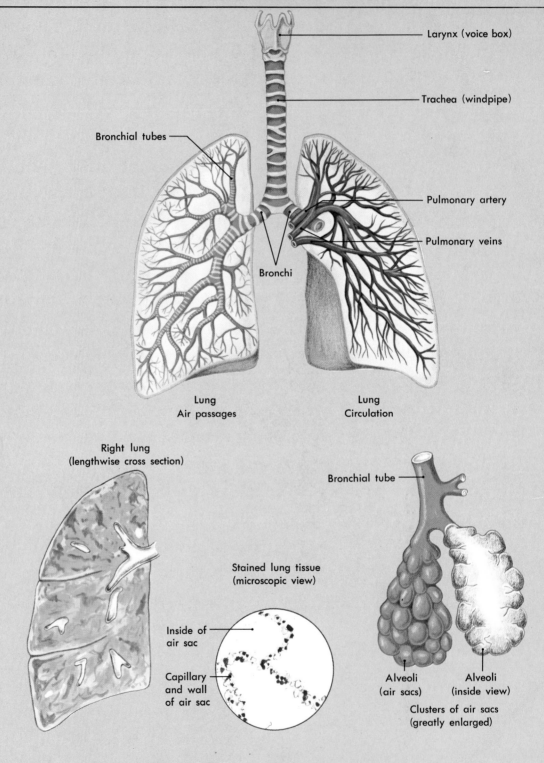

Larynx (voice box)

Trachea (windpipe)

Bronchial tubes

Pulmonary artery

Pulmonary veins

Bronchi

Lung
Air passages

Lung
Circulation

Right lung
(lengthwise cross section)

Bronchial tube

Stained lung tissue
(microscopic view)

Inside of
air sac

Capillary
and wall
of air sac

Alveoli
(air sacs)

Alveoli
(inside view)

Clusters of air sacs
(greatly enlarged)

Syphilis is caused by a spirochete, a form of bacteria. The organism is delicate and is easily destroyed by drying or by soap and water. It survives only a short time outside the human body. As a result, the only mode of transmission is by direct, intimate bodily contact with someone who has the disease. This contact usually occurs in sexual intercourse (either heterosexual or homosexual) and rarely through other means such as kissing. The spirochete enters the body through a minute break in the skin or through unbroken mucous membranes. It enters the bloodstream about 24 hours after infection. There is no evidence of the transmission of the disease through toilet seats, drinking glasses, towels, or other inanimate objects.

The main exception to the mode of transmission described above is the passing of the disease from the infected mother to her unborn child during pregnancy. This is called congenital syphilis. It occurs when the unborn baby is infected by the transmission of the spirochete through the placental blood system. These infections often cause the death of the baby before delivery (stillbirth) or the birth of an obviously diseased child. Infection occurring late in pregnancy may result in the birth of a diseased but apparently normal infant. Later, such children may become blind or deaf, or show other signs of syphilitic infection. Most states have a law (prenatal blood test) that requires a physician to give an expectant mother a blood test. If she is infected with syphilis, she can be treated to reduce the risk of infecting the unborn child.

Syphilis passes through several stages: primary, secondary, latent, and late. The most infectious periods are the primary and secondary stages. This is the time when the disease can be transmitted to others. The primary stage of the disease is characterized by a lesion called a chancre, that is

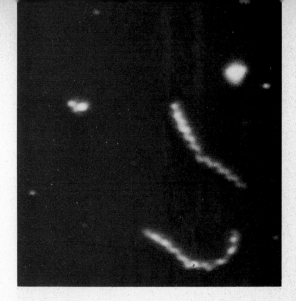

Figure 11-15 • The spirochete organism that causes syphilis can be detected only by trained medical personnel with specific laboratory tests. Self-diagnosis and treatment is foolish and dangerous.

usually painless. It may appear from 10 to 90 days after contact with an infectious person. Most frequently it appears 21 days after contact. At first the chancre may have the appearance of a pimple. Later it may develop into an open sore. This usually takes place at the point where the organism has entered the body. At this time, syphilis may be diagnosed by taking material from the chancre and looking at it through a microscope that has special lighting. This allows the spirochete to be seen, if it is present. The diagnostic procedure is called a darkfield examination.

Because the male has external sex organs, he will usually notice this symptom. In the female, this painless lesion may be internal and hidden from view, hence it goes undetected.

It is important to note that all chancres of syphilis do not have the appearance just described. Therefore, any "sore" on or in the sex organs should be looked upon with suspicion until it can be examined by a physician.

In either sex, the lesions may disappear in two to five weeks, even without treatment. Some persons are then misled into thinking that they have somehow become healed. Unfortunately, this is not true. The disease is not cured; it has merely progressed to the next stage. At some time during this stage, it becomes possible to diagnose syphilis by means of a special blood test.

Secondary-stage symptoms usually appear in about four to six weeks after the appearance of the first lesion. A skin rash may appear on any part of the body. Since the rash may look like rashes caused by other diseases, a physician's advice should be sought as soon as possible. Lesions of the mucous-membrane surfaces are often found. Other symptoms at this time may include a sore throat, fever, headache, swollen lymph glands, pains in the bones and joints, and falling hair. These symptoms will also disappear without any treatment. But the disease still infects the body. It passes to the latent stage, when its presence can be detected only by specific blood tests.

The latent stage of syphilis may last only a few months or may continue to the end of a person's life. During this time, the infected person seems to be disease-free. However, the spirochetes are proceeding into the deep tissues of the body. Although there are no visible signs or symptoms, various laboratory tests can be used to aid in making a diagnosis. This stage is usually noninfectious.

Following months or years of latency, the disease may become active and progressive again. A chronic inflammation of almost any tissue of the body may develop. Progressive degeneration of the brain and spinal cord may take place. The heart, blood vessels, and joints of the body may be attacked. Blindness, paresis, and death are not uncommon. These end results of an untreated syphilitic condition may not take place until 20 to 30 years after the appearance of the original chancre which was the first sign of infection. The late stage of syphilis is usually noninfectious.

Modern treatment of syphilis is very effective. Most individuals who are diagnosed early can be cured in approximately 10 days through massive injections of penicillin. Alternative antibiotics are available to persons sensitive to penicillin. Treatment stops the progress of the disease, and the infected persons no longer transmit it.

However, treatment cannot restore tissues or cells that have previously been destroyed. Therefore, the earlier the disease is discovered and properly treated, the less chance there is of permanent damage.

Gonorrhea. The human being is the only known host of gonorrhea. There is no known immunity and an individual may become reinfected after a cure.

Gonorrhea is caused by the gonococcus, a bacterium which is extremely delicate. It will die very quickly after leaving the human body. The bacteria are very easily destroyed by soap and water.

The mode of transmission is by sexual contact (heterosexual or homosexual) with an infected person. In the case of an infected mother, the disease may be transmitted to a newborn infant during its passage through the birth canal. In such instances, the infant's eyes might become infected and if nothing were done blindness could result. However, the practice of putting silver nitrate or an antibiotic into the eyes of newborn babies has eliminated nearly all infant blindness due to gonorrhea.

The gonorrhea organism enters the body through the mucous membranes of sex organs or rectum. It affects men and women in quite different ways because of the differences in their anatomical structure.

Syphilis Outbreak at a U.S. High School

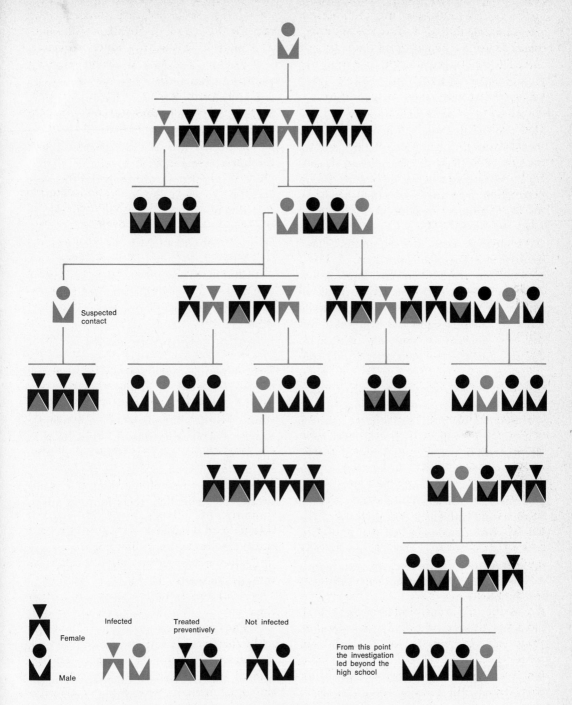

Suspected contact

Female

Infected   Treated preventively   Not infected

Male

From this point the investigation led beyond the high school

Figure 11-16 ● This chart is adapted from an epidemic that actually occurred.

In the male, usually two to six days after sexual contact with an infected person, the disease begins with a painful inflammation of the urethral canal (passageway for the urine). The inflammation causes a thick puslike discharge from the penis. Along with the discharge a sharp burning pain develops when urine is passed. These symptoms usually subside after two to three weeks. The infection may then extend to other parts of the male reproductive system. If the disease is not checked, sterility may result because sperm production is blocked. In recent years, an increasing number of gonorrhea cases have been discovered in men who do not have these obvious signs and symptoms. These men are still infectious for others.

Women usually do not know when they are infected with gonorrhea. Approximately 80 percent of the infected women have no obvious signs and symptoms, yet they are able to transmit the disease to others. Within a few days after sexual contact with an infected person, the individual may or may not experience the first symptom of the disease, a mild burning in the genital area. A puslike discharge may or may not be present. After one or more menstrual periods the infection moves to the uterus and into the Fallopian tubes. Pus forms and leaks out into the pelvic cavity and onto the ovaries. These tissues become swollen and inflamed. At this time, the woman may feel pain. If the Fallopian tubes become blocked, sterility results. The egg cell (ovum) that is released each month by one of the ovaries cannot travel through the Fallopian tube.

If diagnosed early, most cases of gonorrhea can be cured by appropriate treatment with penicillin during a single visit to the doctor. Some persons may require extended treatment. Penicillin still is effective treatment for gonorrhea as long as the proper dosage is given. This is why it

is so important for a person who is infected to be under a doctor's care. If a person is allergic to penicillin, other antibiotics can be used.

The most effective way to prevent syphilis or gonorrhea is to avoid sexual contact outside of marriage. Indiscriminate sexual behavior increases the opportunity for the individual to develop a serious venereal infection.

A person who is exposed should seek prompt treatment from a reliable source. Only a physician can properly diagnose and treat venereal disease. Prompt casefinding, diagnosis, and treatment will reduce the effects and spread of these diseases. Self-treatment should not be attempted. It is dangerous and useless. A physician's advice should be sought on effective preventive measures for syphilis and gonorrhea.

Infectious Mononucleosis

Infectious mononucleosis (glandular fever) is often referred to as the "students' disease" because it occurs so frequently among young people of high school and college age, or the "kissing disease" because it is spread by direct contact. However, it is by no means confined to this age group.

The diagnosis of the disease is sometimes difficult because the symptoms are so similar to those of other diseases. There is usually a fever, sore throat, swelling of the lymph glands, headache, fatigue, and loss of energy. A specific blood test is necessary to help diagnosis.

Deaths or serious complications from infectious mononucleosis are rare. There is no specific cure. Recovery usually takes place within two or three weeks with proper rest and diet. Some individuals require a longer recovery time. Some of the symptoms, such as exhaustion, headaches, and lethargy, may persist for months.

The Common Cold

The most common disease is the cold. It is responsible for more school absences and loss of time from work than all other diseases combined.

Colds are caused by a number of viruses. They are spread from person to person by direct contact. Coughing, sneezing, and talking send into the air droplets that transfer the virus to susceptible persons.

The common cold is not a serious disease, but it may lower the body's resistance so that other infections may gain a foothold. The cold is most contagious in the early stages, usually the first day.

Many factors influence the catching of a cold. The resistance of the host is affected by overfatigue, malnutrition, other illnesses, and the physical environment.

The best treatment for the common cold is rest. This allows the body defenses time to mobilize. The cold sufferer should maintain adequate nutrition by eating light meals containing nourishing food.

There are no remedies against the viruses of the common cold. Most of the widely advertised treatments are worthless. Vitamin C (or ascorbic acid) does not prevent colds. Penicillin and antihistamines do not cure colds. Little help, other than relief of symptoms, can be expected from drinking juices or from using gargles, applying hot compresses, or inhaling vapors.

A cold is usually a self-limited infection lasting from two to seven days. If it persists longer than usual, call a physician.

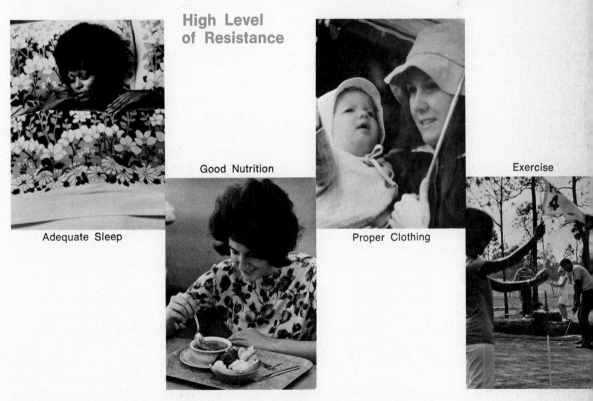

High Level of Resistance

Good Nutrition

Exercise

Adequate Sleep

Proper Clothing

Figure 11-17 ● The incidence of colds could be lowered substantially by using common sense and reasonable health practices. How effective are cold vaccines for immunization against this disease?

Hepatitis

Infectious hepatitis has increased markedly in the United States. It is commonly found among children and young adults.

The disease is usually transmitted through water, milk, shellfish, and other foods that have been contaminated by human waste containing the virus of infectious hepatitis. In some cases, disease will occur through the transmission of human waste directly from one person to another.

Infectious hepatitis is characterized as a viral infection with fever, nausea, abdominal distress, and enlargement of the liver. In some cases, the patient may have a jaundiced (yellowed) appearance.

There is no specific treatment. Most patients recover simply with bed rest and proper diet.

Another type of hepatitis infection is called serum hepatitis. It is transmitted through human blood taken from an infected person and used for transfusion. It may also be transmitted by needles, syringes, and other instruments that have been contaminated with the virus.

The symptoms of the disease, the effect upon the body, and the treatment are the same as those of infectious hepatitis.

Infectious Diseases of the Eye

Some diseases of the eye affect vision, while others are merely irritating.

Conjunctivitis. This condition is an inflammation of the conjunctiva, the membrane that lines the eyelid and covers the front of the eyeball. It may be brought about by any one of a number of causes, such as bacterial or viral infection, irritation, nutritional deficiency, or an allergic reaction. The irritation usually goes away by itself, but in some cases medication prescribed by a physician may be needed.

A form of conjunctivitis that is caused by a bacterium is commonly called pinkeye. It is highly contagious and often becomes epidemic in school populations. The disease usually causes the eyes to become inflamed and bloodshot. They feel itchy and irritated. Often, after a night's sleep, a crust forms on the eyelids and the eyes cannot be readily opened until the crust has been washed off.

Because conjunctivitis of this type is so contagious, it should be called to the attention of a physician.

Stye. A stye is an infection of the root of an eyelash and the glands lining the margin of the eyelid. Styes which recur repeatedly usually are a reflection of poor general health. It is also possible that the styes may be associated with uncorrected errors of refraction and eyestrain. If styes occur frequently, consult with your physician.

Infectious Diseases of the Ear

Middle-Ear Infections. The efficiency of sound conduction may be affected by inflammation of the middle ear. The Eustachian tube, which equalizes pressure on each side of the eardrum, also permits the entry of microorganisms into the middle ear from the nose and throat. Infection of the middle ear may follow a head cold, tonsillitis, influenza, scarlet fever, measles, and other diseases involving the upper respiratory tract.

The invasion of the middle ear may cause an inflammation (otitis media) resulting in a severe earache, fever, dizziness, and difficulty in hearing. The pressure set up by the pus from the inflammation causes the eardrum to bulge outward. If not taken care of, the eardrum may become ruptured, leaving a large or jagged hole. Such conditions tend to heal slowly and may result in hearing loss. Scar tissue from middle-ear infections may contribute to hearing loss.

Many middle-ear infections can be properly treated with antibiotic drugs. Sometimes the physician finds it necessary to relieve the pressure by making an incision near the edge of the eardrum to permit drainage. This type of incision heals quickly and there is no loss of hearing. Prompt treatment of middle-ear infections prevents complications.

Athlete's Foot

The skin is subject to a number of diseases. One of the most common is ringworm of the foot—athlete's foot.

The causative agents of athlete's foot are fungi. These agents cause scaling and cracking of the skin, especially between the toes. Blisters containing a thin watery fluid are also common. Once the disease takes hold, it can become a tough, persistent foe.

There is some suggestion that fungous infections are caused by decreased resistance of the human being to pathogenic fungi lying dormant on the skin. Over the years, it was thought that the infections were brought about by contact with contaminated sources such as floors and locker rooms or public bathing facilities.

Past measures to prevent fungous disease that emphasized the use of foot baths in shower and locker rooms are outmoded. The best approaches are those that raise or maintain the resistance of the individual's skin. The following procedures may be helpful in preventing fungous diseases:

- Use well-ventilated shoes during the hot periods to reduce foot moisture.
- Wear moisture-absorbing hosiery, such as wool and cotton socks.
- If your feet tend to perspire profusely change your shoes and socks frequently.
- Dust your feet with talcum powder to help keep them dry.
- Dry your feet thoroughly after bathing, especially between the toes.

Summary

Scientific progress has brought about the control or potential control of a number of communicable diseases. Much is still to be accomplished. You have the responsibility of applying scientific knowledge to your everyday life. If you understand the infectious disease process and the ways in which this process can be interrupted, the prevention and control of many communicable diseases become possible.

Each year communicable diseases take an enormous toll of health, vitality, and money. They also take a great many lives and some inflict irreparable damage to health. Some, like the common cold and athlete's foot, are persistent, seeming to be with us always. Some, like polio, are "conquered" and become relatively unimportant.

As these diseases become less important, others increase in importance. Infectious hepatitis and infectious mononucleosis were little heard of until a few years ago. Syphilis and gonorrhea appeared to be almost conquered, only to have a resurgence, probably because medical authorities and the public relaxed their vigilance too soon.

Some diseases may be prevented by killing the causative agent. Others are prevented by controlling ways in which they are transmitted. Still other diseases may be prevented by increasing the resistance of the host.

You should take advantage of the many immunizations that can increase your resistance to specific diseases.

Some of the more prevalent communicable diseases that concern young adults are syphilis, gonorrhea, infectious mononucleosis, the common cold, and infectious hepatitis. Prevention and control of these and other communicable diseases requires your intelligent decisions and actions. These must be based upon accurate, up-to-date information.

in making health decisions . . .

Understand These Terms:

antibodies	resistance
casefinding	quarantine
conjunctivitis	self-limited infection
immunity	stye
latent	subclinical
otitis media	symbiotic condition
pandemic	toxic
pathogenic	virulence
reservoir of infection	

Solve This Problem:

Susan Anderson will be graduated from high school in June. During the past year, she has been working as a volunteer in a youth clinic. The youth clinic has had a great deal of success in helping young people solve problems related to syphilis, gonorrhea, and the misuse of drugs. Susan is interested in continuing this type of work after she leaves high school. She is considering going to a community college or a four-year college to help her in this work. What skills and knowledge should she have? What kind of courses or major should she select in college?

Try These Activities:

1. What common childhood communicable diseases have members of your family had? Use the following chart to gather information.

	Yes	No	Don't Know
Chicken pox			
Diphtheria			
German measles (rubella—3-day)			
Measles (rubeola—10-day)			
Mumps			
Polio			
Rheumatic fever			
Scarlet fever			
Whooping cough			

Compare your chart with those of other members of the class. Make a composite class list and arrange the diseases in order of incidence, with the most common disease at the top and the least common disease at the bottom.

2. Some communicable diseases are reportable. This means that when doctors diagnose one of these diseases, they must report it to the health department. Find out what communicable diseases are reportable in your state. Why is it necessary to report communicable diseases to the health department?

3. Make a list of similarities between gonorrhea and syphilis. Make a list of differences between the two diseases. Compare your lists with those of others in the class. Help make a composite class list and be prepared to post it on the bulletin board.

4. Using the following chart, fill in information about the following diseases:
   a. The common cold
   b. Gonorrhea
   c. Measles

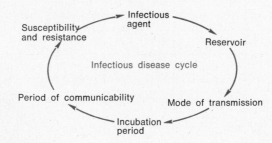

Interpret These Concepts:

1. You, as well as other members of our society, have a number of responsibilities in preventing and controlling communicable diseases.

2. For an infectious disease to occur, there must be a causative agent.

3. One of the most effective ways of protecting a person from communicable diseases is to increase that person's resistance.

4. The occurrence and distribution of diseases are affected by a person's heredity and environment.

5. Diseases may have both a personal and an economic effect on individuals and society.

Explore These Readings:

Control of Communicable Diseases in Man. New York: American Public Health Association, 1970.

"Defending Against Disease," *Time,* March 19, 1973.

"Some Surprising Setbacks in the War Against Disease," *U.S. News & World Report,* Vol. 73 (Dec. 25, 1972), pp. 65–68.

Today's VD Control Problem (booklet). New York: American Social Health Association, annual.

"The VD Epidemic," *Newsweek,* Jan. 24, 1972.

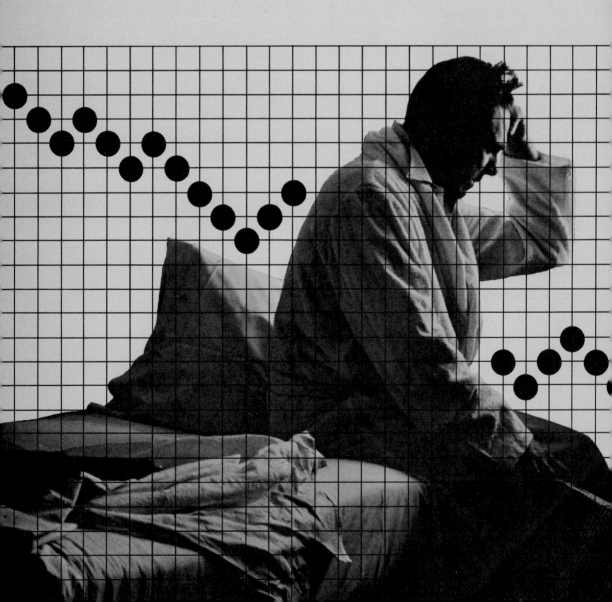

Twelve | Understanding the Nature of Chronic Illness

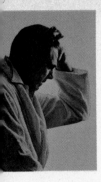

Today, infectious diseases are pretty well under the control of modern medical technology. Typhoid fever, smallpox, diphtheria, and tuberculosis are no longer the leading causes of death, as they were during the early years of the 20th century. Today, nine of the ten leading causes of death are chronic illnesses.

As the years of life expectancy increased, chronic illnesses began to replace infectious diseases as the primary causes of death. The entire category of chronic illnesses is often referred to as *chronic and degenerative illnesses*. This generally raises the question of "Why add the word 'degenerative'?" One of the best answers to this question is found in the definition of chronic illness proposed by the Commission on Chronic Illness of the National Health Council:

". . . all impairments or deviations from normal which have one or more of the following characteristics: are permanent, leave residual disability, are caused by nonreversible pathological alterations, require special training of the patient for rehabilitation, may be expected to require a long period of supervision, observation or care."

Most of the changes between 1900 and today reflect two basic facts. Many infectious diseases are now under control and other types of diseases tend to become more common as the number of older people in the population increases. The increase in life expectancy suggests that the number of persons over 65 will continue to grow. As a result, one can expect an increase in long-term or chronic illness. This is an increasingly important public-health problem.

Causes of Death

One of the best indications of the change in importance of health problems is the listing of leading causes of death for specific years. Figure 12-1 shows the 10 leading causes of death in the early 1900's as compared to today.

While chronic or long-term ailments generally afflict those over 65 years of age and are considered part of the aging process, many of these diseases also affect young adults and often begin early in life.

Cancer and other malignant neoplasms (tumors) are the second leading cause of death for your age group; diseases of the heart rank fifth.

You should also remember that **a number of long-term illnesses may begin during young adulthood.**

Causes of Illness

It is best to examine causes of illness as an index of health problems, because there are many health problems that do not result in death. Accurate information regarding the extent of illness is difficult to obtain. However, national and local health surveys, along with information from insurance companies, do provide some useful information. Reports of the National Health Survey indicate that half the persons with a chronic illness or impairment are below 45 years of age.

One of the characteristics of long-term illness is limitation of activities. The long-term illnesses, besides causing physical and emotional problems, also have economic consequences. Many chronic conditions that involve extended disability bring about loss of earning capacity and heavy medical expenses. To minimize these problems, you should plan to obtain health and hospital

Death Rates for the 10 Leading Causes of Death 1900 and Today

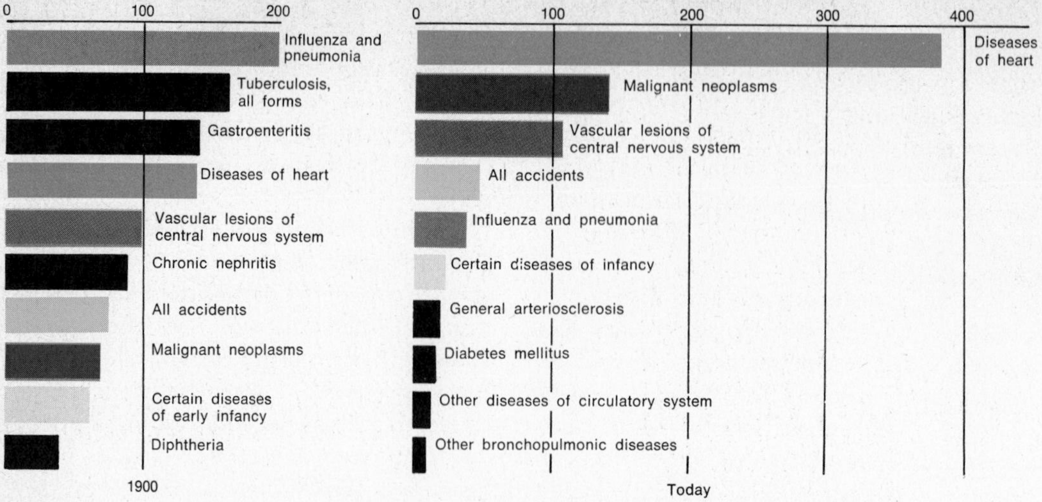
0
100
200
Influenza and pneumonia
Tuberculosis, all forms
Gastroenteritis
Diseases of heart
Vascular lesions of central nervous system
Chronic nephritis
All accidents
Malignant neoplasms
Certain diseases of early infancy
Diphtheria
1900
0
100
200
300
400
Diseases of heart
Malignant neoplasms
Vascular lesions of central nervous system
All accidents
Influenza and pneumonia
Certain diseases of infancy
General arteriosclerosis
Diabetes mellitus
Other diseases of circulatory system
Other bronchopulmonic diseases
Today

Figure 12-1 • How do you account for the change in causes of death over the years?

insurance while you are still healthy. This will help you meet the costs of medical care when professional services are necessary. (See Chapter 15.)

Prevention of Long-Term Illness

The diseases and disorders that are responsible for long-term illness are quite varied. Each chronic illness must be analyzed separately to find a basis for its control and prevention. It is possible, however, to consider several approaches that might be applied in the prevention and treatment of all chronic illnesses.

Promoting Health

Many activities and habits have an effect on health and well-being. **The types of chronic illness you are likely to have in the future are influenced by many of your current health practices.** Proper nutrition, a proper balance between work and play and between rest and exercise, and continuing health supervision all contribute to your general welfare. Some illnesses are less likely to occur if you follow these practices.

Preventing Disease and Disorders

As more is known about specific diseases it often becomes possible to put into practice certain measures that intercept a disease before people become affected. For example, most authorities accept the relationship between cigarette smoking and lung cancer and coronary heart disease. One method of reducing the risk of these diseases, or preventing them, is to change the smoking behavior or stop smoking.

Similar approaches are possible for other long-term illnesses. There is some evidence that a reasonable amount of physical activity will help prevent coronary heart disease if the activity is carried on throughout a person's lifetime. Appropriate nutri-

Selected Chronic Conditions Causing Limitation of Activities, 1969–1970

Tuberculosis, all forms	156 *
Malignant neoplasms	358
Benign and unspecified neoplasms	204
Diabetes	865
Mental and nervous conditions	1,033
Heart conditions	3,609
Cerebrovascular disease	604
Hypertension without heart involvement	1,059
Varicose veins	169
Hemorrhoids	44
Other conditions of circulatory system	694
Chronic bronchitis	219
Emphysema	566
Asthma, with or without hay fever	1,010
Hay fever, without asthma	149
Chronic sinusitis	105
Other conditions of respiratory system	451
Peptic ulcer	320
Hernia	434
Other conditions of digestive system	589
Diseases of kidney and ureter	243
Other conditions of genitourinary system	357
Arthritis and rheumatism	3,265
Other musculoskeletal disorders	914
Visual impairments	1,115
Hearing impairments	431
Paralysis, complete or partial	817
Impairments (except paralysis) of back or spine	1,613
Impairments (except paralysis and absence) of upper extremities and shoulders	431
Impairments (except paralysis and absence) of lower extremities and hips	1,551

* Figures in thousands.

Figure 12-2 ● This chart shows the number of cases of chronic conditions causing limitations of activity in 1969–1970.

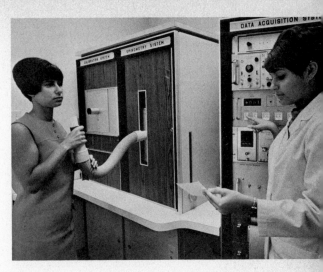

Figure 12-3 ● The spirometer is one technique which can be used in the early detection of respiratory conditions.

tional habits will prevent vitamin-deficiency diseases. Dental caries can be prevented by fluoridation of water.

As more knowledge is gained, it will be possible to prevent the occurrence of other chronic diseases. As soon as this knowledge is accumulated, it must be put to use. The appropriate application of knowledge will help eliminate some of the chronic illnesses, precisely as certain infectious diseases have been eliminated.

Detecting Disease

Early recognition of disease is of extreme importance. Prompt treatment can be given and thus lessen the disability or the possibility of complications.

A careful health examination, including selected laboratory tests, can be most helpful in finding the early signs of disease. It is your responsibility to place yourself under the supervision of a physician. The best diagnostic test in the world is of no value if it is not used.

Some chronic diseases lend themselves to screening tests that aid in early detection. Some of the screening tests are so simple that they can be used on a mass basis. Indeed, the trend today is to provide multiple screening tests (multiphasic screening) to various population groups to increase the possibility of early detection of disease. The tests themselves do not establish a diagnosis. They suggest the need for more definitive examinations because some suspicion of disease has been aroused.

Some diseases or conditions that can be screened are:

Cancer of the Cervix. The Papanicolaou vaginal smear test for cervical cancer is a most efficient screening technique. Through this test, cancer cells can be detected a number of years before a physician might see some clinical signs or symptoms. As a result, the treatment that is then started has a much better chance of being successful.

Diabetes Mellitus. Diabetes mellitus lends itself to screening through the use of several tests. Specific urine tests and blood tests have detected diabetes that had been previously unsuspected.

Anemia. Often that tired feeling is due to anemia. A fairly simple blood test can help diagnose the condition, and corrective action (usually medication and diet) can then be taken.

Tuberculosis. Mass X-ray studies of population groups have been used for years to detect unsuspected cases of tuberculosis. Today, it is common practice to use a tuberculin skin test for preliminary screening, followed by an X-ray of those who have a positive skin reaction. Both tests are well-accepted screening measures.

Figure 12-4 ● A commonly used screening procedure for tuberculosis is the skin test. A positive reaction (Top, right) does not necessarily mean a person has tuberculosis. When a positive reaction occurs, however, the individual will be referred for a chest X-ray for definite diagnosis. No further referral is necessary for negative reactions (Bottom, right).

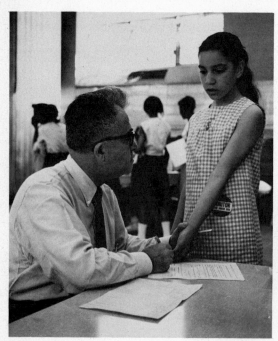

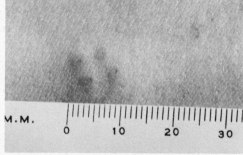

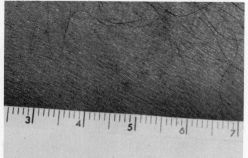

Sickle Cell Anemia. The National Sickle Cell Foundation in cooperation with the medical profession conducts screening clinics to identify carriers of sickle cell anemia. The testing procedure requires a small sample of blood. It is a simple, fast, and painless process. Those identified as having characteristics of the disease can be treated and counseled regarding their potential to transmit sickle cell anemia to their children. (Review Chapter 3.)

Vision Problems. One of the simplest screening tests involves the use of an eye chart hung on the wall. The individual to be screened stands at a specified distance from the chart, covers one eye, and attempts to read letters of varying sizes. The inability to read letters of a certain size may be an indication of either nearsightedness or farsightedness.

Hearing Problems. Good hearing consists of the ability to hear sounds of a loudness of about 15 decibels. An instrument called an audiometer is used for accurate measurement of a person's ability to hear.

These and many other screening procedures are available to you. Regular utilization of these techniques can help detect disease in the earliest possible stage. Treatment can then be given to halt or slow down the disease process. Your responsibility is to have regular examinations in which many of these tests can be performed.

Rehabilitating the Afflicted

Rehabilitation is also a form of prevention. Individuals with quite severe handicaps or long-term illness can often be returned to useful places in society. Through rehabilitation, complete disability is being prevented.

There are many examples of successful rehabilitation. Think of the individual who has lost an arm or a leg and has learned to use an artificial limb. Through physical therapy, some people with long-standing arthritis can be taught to do things for themselves. A number of individuals with mental illness have been successfully rehabilitated and restored to useful places in society.

Many long-term illnesses can be approached only through the process of rehabilitation because modern knowledge is not sufficiently advanced to permit the use of preventive measures. As knowledge increases, the approach to prevention changes. Poliomyelitis is a good example of this change. Not too many years ago, rehabilitation was the only approach to the solution of the paralytic polio problem. Today, polio is no longer a problem because it is possible to prevent the disease through widespread immunization.

Cardiovascular Diseases

The circulatory system of the body is designed to distribute blood to all the cells. Nourishment and oxygen are provided and wastes are removed. The heart, a muscular pump, keeps the blood circulating and a system of valves helps regulate the flow of blood. Arteries carry nutrients and oxygen to the body cells. In the lungs, the blood releases carbon dioxide and receives a new supply of oxygen. Most other waste products are filtered out of the blood by the kidneys.

When any part of the circulatory system is impaired, the body cells may be deprived of their blood supply. If these cells are without blood for a sufficient period of time, damage will probably occur. This damage may take place in the heart itself, in the brain, the lungs, the kidneys, the skin, or any other part of the body.

Congenital Heart Disease

Some forms of heart disease present at birth may result from an inherited condition. However, it is more likely that something went wrong during the first trimester of pregnancy, while the baby was developing in its mother's uterus. If a mother-to-be has German measles or takes certain drugs during this three-month period, the risk of congenital heart disease in the embryo is increased. Additional research is needed to determine what other factors contribute to the development of congenital heart disease.

Figure 12-5 ● When blood vessels become constricted, there is a corresponding increase in blood pressure. Can you explain why? Hypertension results when the constriction is prolonged.

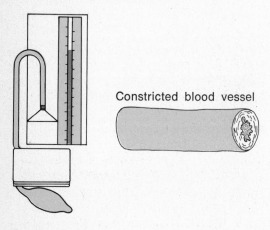

Constricted blood vessel

Sphygmomanometer

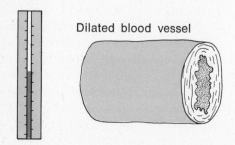

Dilated blood vessel

One familiar type of congenital heart disease causes the blue baby. The blueness means that the baby's blood is deprived of oxygen. Because of a hole in the wall separating the chambers of the heart, some blood is diverted into the circulatory system without passing through the lungs. This condition can now be corrected through surgery.

Other congenital defects can affect the valves of the heart. In recent years there has been excellent progress in diagnosis, surgery, and medical care for these and other types of congenital heart defects. Most patients can be restored to normal or near-normal health.

As more is learned about the actual cause of congenital heart defects, other preventive action will be taken. For example, immunization against German measles is now available. It is now possible to protect girls against German measles by injecting them with Hyper-Immune Gamma Globulin before they marry and have children. Congenital problems caused by this disease can then be avoided.

Hypertensive Heart Disease

Blood pressure is a measure of the pressure put on the walls of the arteries as the heart pumps blood to various parts of the body. In some people blood pressure remains higher than it should be. The defect is not in the heart but in the blood vessels. They become constricted and the heart must exert more pressure to push the blood through them. The heart must actually work harder. Over a period of time, the heart may weaken and the overworked circulatory system will not work as well as it should.

In about 10 percent of the cases, hypertension may be traced to some other disease.

Curing the underlying ailment usually means an end to the hypertension. The cause of most cases of hypertension is unknown. In spite of this, much can be done to keep the problem under control. There are many drugs that are helpful in reducing blood pressure. In addition, weight reduction, a change in diet, and avoidance of stress and anxiety will assist in solving the problem.

Rheumatic Heart Disease

Rheumatic heart disease is caused by rheumatic fever. The exact cause of rheumatic fever is not known. Doctors suspect it is the aftereffect of the invasion of the body by a germ of the streptococcus family. The streptococcus germs are also responsible for such serious conditions as the "strep" sore throat, scarlet fever, and "strep" ear infections.

When rheumatic fever occurs, it may affect any part of the body. The effects on most parts of the body are temporary. However, when the valves of the heart are affected, there may be a prolonged heart disorder. Rheumatic heart disease is the result of a scarring of the heart valves by rheumatic fever. The valves are designed to keep the blood flowing in one direction. When they are scarred, the valves cannot close properly and blood leaks back.

Heart valves damaged by rheumatic fever can be repaired by surgery in many cases. In some situations, the entire valve may be replaced by a nylon or dacron valve.

The main approach in the fight against rheumatic heart disease is the prevention of rheumatic fever. This can be done successfully by treating the various "strep" infections with antibiotics. Even if an individual acquires rheumatic fever, it can be kept under control with small protective doses of sulfa drugs or other antibiotics. This intercepts rheumatic fever and in turn prevents rheumatic heart disease.

Coronary Heart Disease

When a portion of the heart muscle is cut off from its blood supply, a heart attack will occur. The attack may seem sudden, but it is usually the result of a slow thickening that takes place along the inner lining of the coronary artery wall. The process begins early in life with the gradual deposit of fatty material. As more of the deposits are formed, the channel through which the blood flows becomes narrower.

If the blood supply is only mildly decreased, the symptoms of the heart disease will be relatively slight. There may be a pain (angina) radiating to the neck, jaw, and upper left arm. The pain is a symptom. It is a brief warning that the blood supply to a portion of the heart muscle is inadequate for the moment. The pain will not last long and the heart muscle will not be permanently damaged.

Sometimes angina pectoris (anginal pains) is a warning of an impending heart attack. Angina pains may, however, be the result of constriction of coronary blood vessels and may not lead to a heart attack. However, chest pains should be reported promptly to a physician. Very often the pain is due to other causes, such as heartburn or indigestion, but the diagnosis can be made only by a physician.

If the coronary artery is completely blocked by a thrombus (blood clot) or by fatty deposits completely filling the channel, the blood supply for a particular portion of the heart is cut off. This results in a heart attack. Some of the medical terms for heart attack are coronary thrombosis, coronary

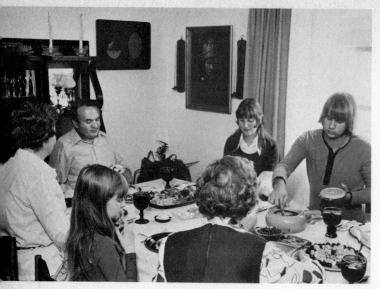

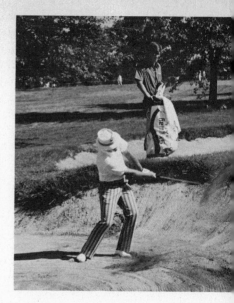

Figure 12-6 ● (Top) How to reduce the risk of heart disease: (1) Proper diet. (2) Regular exercise. (3) Seeing a doctor regularly and controlling high blood pressure. (4) Not smoking cigarettes. (5) Trimming down overweight.

(Bottom) Know these facts about heart disease: (1) Some forms of heart disease can be prevented; a few can be cured. (2) All heart cases can be cared for best if diagnosed early. (3) Most heart patients can keep on working— very often at the same job. (4) Almost every heart condition can be helped by proper treatment. Your "symptoms" may or may not mean heart disease. Don't guess; don't worry. See your doctor and be sure.

occlusion, and myocardial infarction. Serious as this is, most people who have an attack get well and resume their normal lives after a period of treatment and rehabilitation.

After a heart attack, healing begins almost immediately. Small arteries near the blocked area widen and deliver blood to the affected portion of the heart. Treatment is

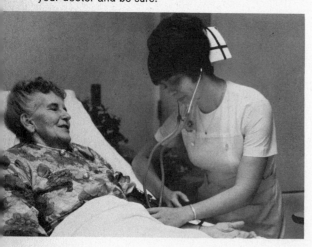

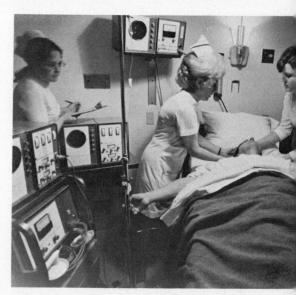

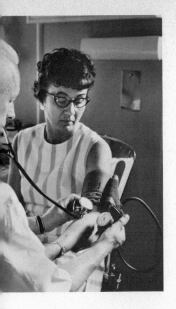 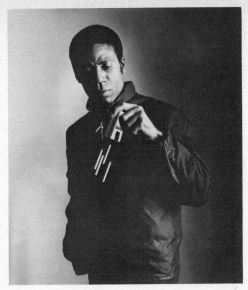 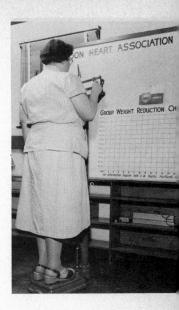

focused on giving the heart an opportunity to heal. Some patients receive anticoagulants (anticlotting drugs) to prevent the formation of new blood clots. Most patients require rest and a gradual return to normal physical activity.

Our knowledge of how to prevent coronary heart disease is somewhat limited. However, several procedures will be beneficial. Everyone should engage in regular physical activity. The heart is a muscle that needs to be exercised. Moderation in eating is important. Everyone should also avoid excessive consumption of animal fats. Smokers should cut down on smoking—or, better still, stop smoking. The risk of heart disease is greater for those who smoke cigarettes and inhale.

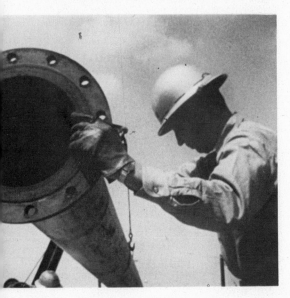 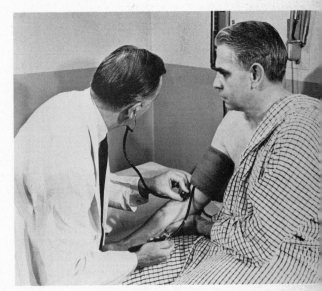

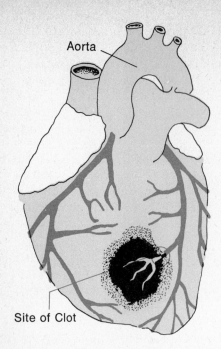

After a stroke, the damaged nerve cells may recover. Frequently their functions are taken over by other brain cells. Much can be done to help a person recover from a stroke. Through physical therapy a patient can learn to use the muscles that have been affected.

Some of the measures mentioned to reduce the risk of coronary heart disease may also be helpful in reducing the possibility of strokes.

Aorta

Site of Clot

Figure 12-7 ● A heart attack. Notice how the coronary blood supply is blocked, causing damage to a portion of the heart tissue. Explain how physical exercise can be valuable for the heart as a preventative or as treatment for heart attacks. (See Chapter 7.)

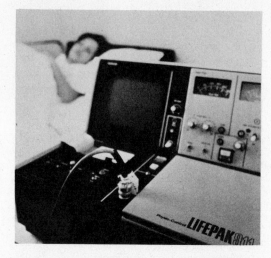

Figure 12-8 ● Medical science is constantly developing new techniques in the fight against heart disease.

Strokes

Strokes are not necessarily a problem of old age. They may occur at any time the blood supply to a part of the brain is reduced or completely cut off. When this takes place, the nerve cells in that part of the brain cannot function. As a result, that part of the body controlled by these nerve cells cannot function normally, either. A stroke may result in paralysis of one side of the body, loss of memory, or difficulty in speaking.

Some strokes are caused by a blood clot in an artery narrowed by fatty deposits. Other strokes are caused by a hemorrhage (bleeding) from an artery in the brain, by constriction of the blood vessel, or by a growth pressing on the blood vessel.

Cancer

The term "cancer" refers to an uncontrolled growth of abnormal cells. More than 200 different types of cell disorders have currently been classified. It is convenient to use the term "cancer" when discussing these abnormal cell growths.

Some cancers grow very slowly and destroy neighboring tissue by local invasion. Others are very aggressive and metastasize (travel to other parts of the body) rapidly. The bloodstream and the lymph system may help in this process.

Normal cell growth is characterized by order and control. Cells become differentiated into skin, bone, and other tissues in a regulated manner. Cell division is orderly, with one cell becoming two, two becoming four, and the process continuing in this regular and controlled manner.

Cancer cells do not have this order and control. When they divide, one cell may become three or four. These in turn continue to divide in an uncontrolled way. The cancer cells serve no useful function.

The terms "malignant" and "benign" are often associated with cancer. Benign tumors are usually considered harmless, depending on the location and whether they interfere with normal body functioning. In this type of tumors, the growth has stopped. Malignant tumors or growths are dangerous in that abnormal cell division is continuing. The greatest danger lies in the possibility of spread to other parts of the body. When this occurs, treatment is much more difficult.

Diagnosis of a malignancy is usually based on identifying the abnormal cells by microscopic examination. A small sample of the suspected tissue is surgically removed (biopsy) and cut into extremely thin slices. The slices are then mounted on a slide and stained with special dyes. This process can be carried out very rapidly, even while a patient is in surgery. The doctor can thus be provided with information that will help in making a decision regarding the extent of surgery necessary.

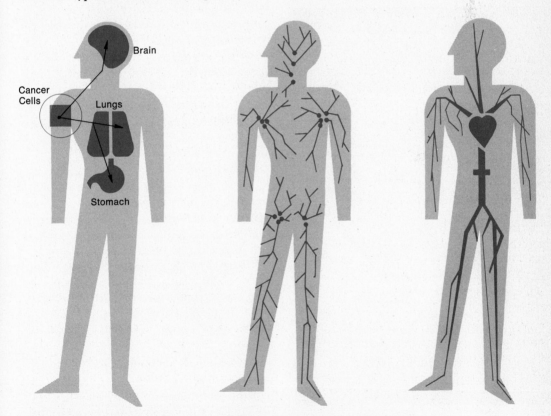

Figure 12-9 • Cancer can spread from the original site to other parts of the body through the blood and the lymph vessels. This process is called metastasis. Why is early detection of cancer so important?

Causes of Cancer

The exact trigger mechanism that causes a cell to begin growing in a wild, abnormal fashion is not known. But progress is being made. Research has produced information about the causes of some forms of cancer and how they may be prevented. Our modern environment presents a number of cancer hazards. In addition, some of our personal habits and customs increase the risk of acquiring a particular form of cancer.

Recent findings suggest the possibility that some forms of cancer are caused by viruses. While this has not yet been proved definitely, much research continues in this area of investigation.

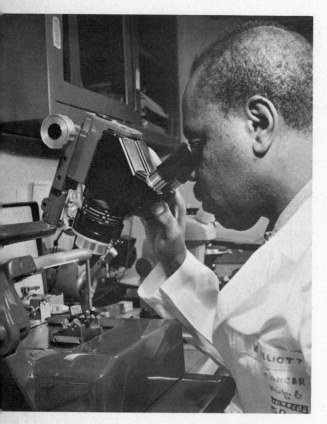

Figure 12-10 • Cancer research activities are resulting in important findings concerning the disease.

Environmental Factors

A number of environmental factors have been implicated in the development of various forms of cancer.

Air Pollution. Air pollution has increased greatly in the past few years. Smoke and fumes from furnaces, open fires, incinerators, automobiles, trucks, buses, and industrial plants are modern irritants that can adversely affect people.

Although the evidence of the long-range effects of air pollution on health is largely circumstantial, there is a strong indication that it is involved in the development of lung cancer as well as of heart disease, asthma, and bronchitis.

Government and industry have in recent years been concerned with instituting control measures to reduce the quantity of irritants in the air.

Radiation. Another potential problem has arisen from the widespread use of atomic energy. The development of industrial nuclear reactors and the atmospheric testing of nuclear weapons have increased public awareness of the hazards of radiation and radioactive fallout.

Much more is known today about the effects of large doses of radiation on human beings. An increased leukemia rate has been noted among groups exposed to relatively large quantities of whole-body radiation in nuclear accidents.

Not so much is known about the danger of small doses of radiation. However, most scientists now believe that for purposes of health protection it is necessary to shield people from even very small amounts of radiation.

Shielding of equipment and patients is becoming more common. Even dentists are beginning to shield their patients when taking X-rays of the teeth. It has become common practice for dentists to drape their patients with a lead-lined apron, so that the

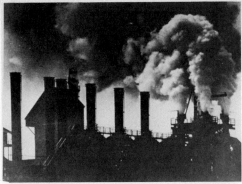

Air Pollution

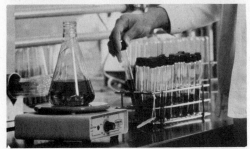

Viruses

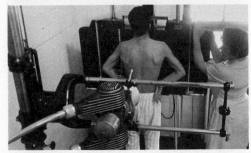

Radiation

Chemicals

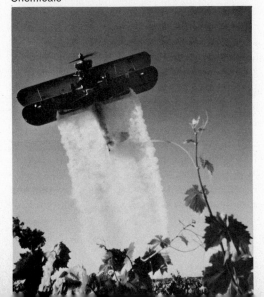

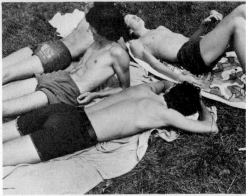

Exposure to Sunlight

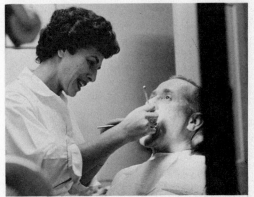

Dental Problems

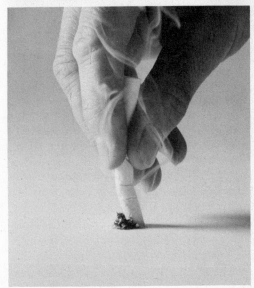

Cigarette Smoking

Figure 12-11 ● Environmental and personal factors that cause cancer.

only part of the body that will receive radiation is the teeth.

Chemicals. Much concern has been expressed over the widespread use of pesticides by farmers, gardeners, and fruit growers. Certain substances in the pesticides are suspected of cancer-causing activity.

Various government agencies protect the consumer through inspection programs. No residues of a chemical are permitted on foods if any amount of the substance is shown to cause cancer in laboratory animals.

Many chemicals are also added to foods to preserve them. By law, all of these chemical additives must be tested and proved safe before they can be used as food preservatives.

Viruses. As yet, no human cancer has been demonstrated to be due to a virus. Nevertheless, the findings that a number of cancers in animals do involve viruses continues to cause concern.

In recent years viruslike particles have been found in the blood of leukemia patients. This has caused an increase in research, with the goal of developing a vaccine that might possibly prevent leukemia.

Personal Factors

People are exposed to some cancer hazards through habits or practices that are essentially a matter of choice.

Smoking. Many studies have provided evidence that cigarette smokers have a higher death rate from lung cancer and many other diseases than nonsmokers do. While much research is now under way to discover methods of eliminating or reducing the potential cancer-causing elements in smoking, the best advice for you is: Don't smoke. If you smoke, stop. If you can't stop smoking, cut down on it.

Exposure to Sunlight. Many people deliberately expose themselves excessively to the ultraviolet rays of sunshine. Studies have shown that frequent and long exposure to sunshine can create skin problems. This can lead to skin cancers, especially among people with light complexions who live in very sunny regions.

Your best protection is to expose yourself gradually to sunlight. This will activate the protective mechanisms in your skin. Avoid excessive exposure, even after tanning. People who sunburn rapidly can get information from their doctor on the type of preparation that will help increase their skin's natural resistance to burning.

Oral Problems. Chronic irritation caused by broken teeth or poorly fitting dentures can lead to precancerous conditions in the mouth. Regular dental examinations will help detect any potential trouble spots, so that they may be corrected.

Diagnosis and Treatment

Many types of cancer can be controlled somewhat if they are detected early. By having regular medical examinations and by reporting unusual symptoms promptly to your physician, you can do your part to avoid or control cancer.

Unfortunately, pain is seldom an early sign of cancer. You should be aware of the danger signals that are stressed by the American Cancer Society (see Figure 13-11). The appearance of any one of these symptoms does not necessarily mean cancer. However, you cannot make the diagnosis yourself. Let your physician make the diagnosis.

Diagnosis. There is no single, simple test for detecting all types of cancer at the present time. The physician will use various procedures in the examination:

- Observing and feeling for growths
- Microscopic examination of cells from the lining of the respiratory and genital tracts
- X-rays of internal areas of the body
- Biopsy of suspected tissue

Treatment. The purpose of treatment is to destroy cancer cells completely with as little damage as possible to normal cells. This is accomplished by surgery, radiation, and chemotherapy (the use of chemicals in treating disease). All cancers do not respond to the same type of treatment. Physicians select the approach they feel will accomplish the most.

Surgical procedures are used to cut away the cancerous growth. Radiation destroys the malignant cells where they occur. Chemotherapy inhibits or controls abnormal cell growth where surgery or radiation is not possible. Combinations of treatments are often used.

People should not feel hopeless about cancer. Much can be done to prevent various types of the disease. Improvements in detection and treatment are saving many lives. Your awareness of the preventive measures available will help continue this trend.

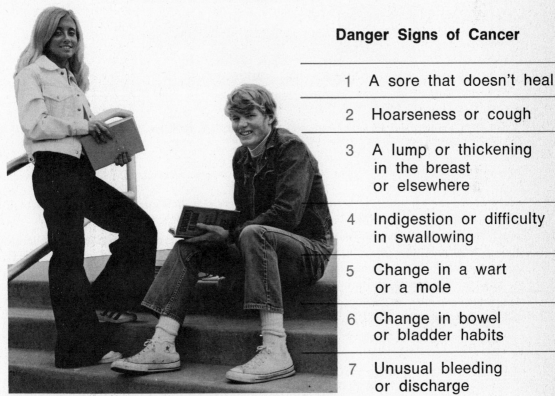

Danger Signs of Cancer

1	A sore that doesn't heal
2	Hoarseness or cough
3	A lump or thickening in the breast or elsewhere
4	Indigestion or difficulty in swallowing
5	Change in a wart or a mole
6	Change in bowel or bladder habits
7	Unusual bleeding or discharge

Figure 12-12 ● The seven danger signs of cancer. If a symptom lasts longer than two weeks, go to a doctor. Remember, pain is not an early cancer sign.

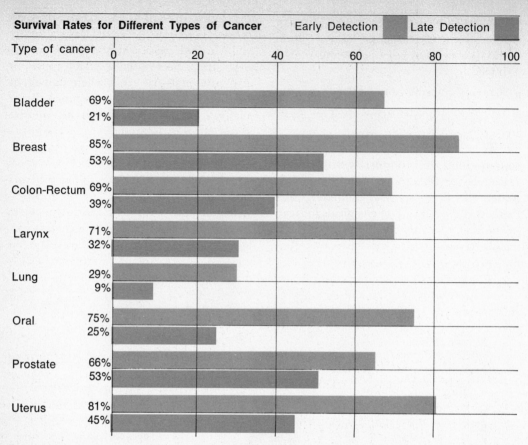

Survival Rates for Different Types of Cancer	Early Detection	Late Detection

Type of cancer

Type of cancer		
Bladder	69%	
	21%	
Breast	85%	
	53%	
Colon-Rectum	69%	
	39%	
Larynx	71%	
	32%	
Lung	29%	
	9%	
Oral	75%	
	25%	
Prostate	66%	
	53%	
Uterus	81%	
	45%	

Figure 12-13 • Notice how important early detection of cancer is. What would be the danger signs for each of the types of cancer in the graph?

Allergies

More and more attention is being paid to allergies today as chronic illnesses. In some cases allergies cause an impairment of efficiency. In others, they may bring about a severe disability. The economic loss in terms of time off from work and school and the cost of medical care for allergy further emphasize the problem.

Causes of Allergies

The reason some persons are allergic and others are not is not clearly understood. There may be some hereditary tendency or predisposition involved.

The substances responsible for allergic reactions are called allergens. Allergens may be taken into the body in a number of ways: by breathing dusts, feathers, and pollens; by eating various foods; by coming in contact with certain substances; and by using certain drugs.

When the allergens enter the body, antibodies are produced. These antibodies do not protect against disease. Instead, they react with more allergen to cause the body to release a chemical called histamine. Histamine produces the typical allergy symptoms. Drugs commonly used to combat allergic reactions are therefore called antihistamines.

Prevention and Control

Detecting an allergy is not always easy. The symptoms are similar to those of many other health problems, particularly colds. The eyes may itch and water. A rash may appear or the skin may scale and crack. Sometimes giant hives may erupt. Sometimes breathing may become labored and painful.

The diagnostic tools used by a physician include a detailed health history, a thorough study of the patient's environment, and allergy testing to determine sensitivity to one or more allergens.

Figure 12-14 • This physician is testing for sensitivity to allergens.

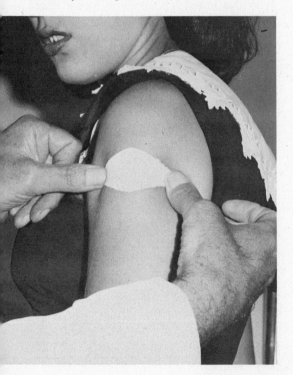

Once a diagnosis is made, the treatment involves avoiding the allergen responsible for the allergy symptoms. This may mean finding a new home for the household pet; eliminating certain foods from the diet; taking a vacation away from home during the pollen season; removing rugs or draperies from the home; or purchasing a device for filtering the air that comes into the home.

In some situations, avoiding the allergen is extremely difficult. Physicians can often provide relief by prescribing certain antihistamines, which alleviate the symptoms of some allergies.

Some allergies respond to a form of immunization. Specific allergens are injected under the skin in increasing amounts. After a time, a tolerance is developed which permits ordinary exposure without any allergic reaction.

Medical science is constantly discovering new forms of allergy and gaining new insights into its causes and treatment. While in the past allergy sufferers vainly sought relief from the discomforts and disabilities caused by their allergies, today they can get competent and sympathetic medical care.

There are many more elements in the environment to cause allergic reactions than were present in the past, and the pace of modern life heightens the possibility of "attacks." Modern science continues to seek answers to this problem.

Rheumatic Diseases

Rheumatic diseases have afflicted man for thousands of years. These include more than 100 disorders related to the joints of the body and the supporting structures. The most common of the rheumatic diseases are rheumatoid arthritis and gout.

Rheumatoid Arthritis

This disease can strike at any age, but it is most likely to occur between the ages of 25 and 50. The cause is unknown.

In most cases, the disease develops gradually. In the early stages, the person may have vague pains and stiffness in the joints upon awakening in the morning. In the later stages, the patient may develop a fever, fatigue, poor appetite, weight loss, enlarged lymph glands, and inflamed eyes. Destruction of tissues, resulting in swelling and deformity, is the common sign of the advanced stage of rheumatoid arthritis.

Early diagnosis of rheumatoid arthritis will enable the physician to start treatment to slow down the disease process and reduce the disability. Diagnostic procedures include blood tests, analysis of joint fluid, and X-ray.

There is no specific cure for the disease. Treatment includes proper diet, rest, and controlled exercise. Aspirin is commonly prescribed to reduce pain and inflammation. Physical therapy and special drugs help some individuals.

Because there is no cure for arthritis, its victims are particularly susceptible to the misleading claims of the quack. As a result, many waste money, delay seeking qualified medical advice, and frequently aggravate their condition.

When early signs of possible arthritis are present, proper medical advice should be sought as soon as possible.

Gout

This is a rheumatic disease generally thought to be due to a defect in the body chemistry. Individuals with gout have an above-normal quantity of salts of uric acid in the blood and tissues.

Attacks of gout are extremely painful. Inflammation usually occurs in the tissues at the base of the big toe. Drugs are now available to treat attacks of gout by causing the body to excrete the excessive uric acid.

Sickle Cell Anemia

Sickle cell anemia is the result of a mutation in the protein structure of the hemoglobin molecule in red blood cells. The abnormal cells become elongated and resemble crescents or sickles. The elongated cells clog blood vessels, causing destruction of nearby tissue. Symptoms of this disease include bone, joint, or abdominal pain which may or may not be accompanied by fever. When a person has both genes for this trait, this disease is serious, and it is often fatal.

Sickle cell anemia is prevalent among inhabitants of malaria regions of Africa. It is also found among those whose ancestral origin was Africa, no matter where they live at present. It is interesting to note that individuals with only one gene for this trait seem to have an increased resistance to malaria, a disease often fatal to inhabitants of tropical regions. (Review Chapter 3.)

As mentioned on page 35, screening procedures used to detect sickle cell anemia are simple, fast, and painless. Biochemists have developed laboratory procedures for identification of carriers as well as interception and medical management procedures for the treatment of infants born with sickle cell anemia.

Diabetes Mellitus

Diabetes results when the body does not produce enough of the hormone insulin or when the insulin is not utilized properly. As a result, the body does not use sugar efficiently. The consequences of this are as follows:

- The blood-sugar level is abnormally high.
- The kidneys excrete sugar in the urine.
- The excretion of sugar in the urine results in an excessive loss of salt and water.
- The body increases its utilization of protein and fat sources for heat and energy.
- The body is poisoned by products of incomplete combustion of proteins and fats.

Causes of Diabetes

No single factor causes diabetes. Heredity seems to be important. If both parents have diabetes, all their children are likely to develop the disease. If the parents are free of diabetes but carry recessive genes for the disease, some of their children may develop diabetes.

Obesity appears to be a contributing factor. Studies indicate that it precedes diabetes in a vast majority of cases. The exact reason for this is not known.

Detection

Most cases of diabetes develop after the age of 40. However, they have their beginnings much earlier. The disease can be detected long before there are obvious symptoms. This can be done through urinalysis and specific blood tests. Regular physical examinations should include a diagnostic test for diabetes.

Treatment

Diabetes is one of the most readily controlled of the chronic illnesses. In some cases, proper diet and exercise are all that is needed. In other cases, oral drugs may be given to stimulate the production of insulin or help the body use the insulin more effectively. In certain cases, insulin must be administered by injection.

Diabetes is not cured. It is controlled when the individual is able to maintain relatively sugar-free urine and avoid other symptoms. With the advice and guidance of a physician, a diabetic can expect to live a near-normal life.

Mental Illness

Although there is a tendency to discard the traditional classifications of mental illness, you may still hear individuals described as neurotic or psychotic.

Psychoneurosis

Psychoneurosis is considered to be a behavior disorder due to emotional tension. The individual finds it difficult to meet the demands of daily living and behavior becomes eccentric. However, the person still has some adjustive capacity and can function within society.

Some of the common forms of psychoneurosis are hysteria; unreasoning fears, obsessions, and compulsions; overwhelming anxiety; and hypochondriasis (morbid anxiety over health).

Many of these problems can be prevented early in a person's life by understanding parents. Treatment and correction can be achieved through professional assistance.

The individual who has this type of problem needs help, otherwise greater maladjustment may result.

Psychoses

Psychoses are serious mental disorders. A psychotic person cannot face reality at all and is unable to meet all obligations to society.

The behavior of some mentally ill individuals combines the symptoms of both psychoneurosis and psychosis. However, one does not generally lead to the other.

The psychoses may be classified into organic and functional types. An organic psychosis is caused by some physical or structural change in the brain because of disease or injury.

Those individuals who have a functional psychosis seem to have a normal-appearing brain, but they are still not able to function adequately. Two common types of functional psychosis are schizophrenia and manic-depressive psychosis.

Schizophrenia is the most common and the most important severe mental disease. Individuals with this problem become so disorganized that they have trouble thinking and feeling. Very often they have a complete disregard for living in society. Manic-depressive individuals become so disturbed in the way they feel about life and their experiences that their judgment and behavior are affected. As a result, they may experience periods of extreme depression or elation.

Prevention and Treatment

Some studies have reported that 1 person in 10 had some form of mental illness that was serious enough to require treatment to

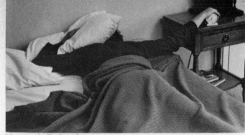

Normal Behavior
Turn off that alarm! Even if it is Monday, I'm going to snooze another hour.

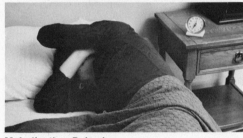

Maladjustive Behavior
Neurosis
I can't sleep—but I don't see any point in getting up. If I do get up, should I go to school or watch TV? Nothing is worth doing anyway!

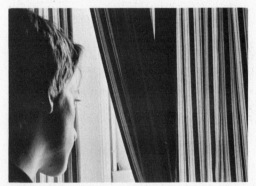

Maladjustive Behavior
Psychosis
Don't be ridiculous! The sun can't be up. I blew it out.

Figure 12-15 ● (a) Normal—Normal people occasionally play hooky from their duties, but not all day, every day. (b) Maladjustive behavior (Neurosis)—If people suffer from apathy, indecision, and unhappiness most of the time, they are displaying maladjustive behavior. (c) Maladjustive behavior (Psychosis)—These people live in their own private world. Their fantasies are real to them, but they are not actually in touch with reality.

achieve full recovery. Other studies report that there are more people in hospitals at any one time with mental illness than with all other diseases combined.

Great advances are being made in the treatment of the mentally ill. With modern care and treatment, 70 percent of the patients hospitalized for mental illness can be expected to return home partially or totally recovered.

As with physical problems and disorders, mental disorders should be brought to the attention of a competent specialist as early as possible for proper diagnosis and treatment.

There are four major types of treatment for mental illness. These treatments may be used singly or in combination. Not all forms of treatment require that the patient be hospitalized.

Individual and Group Therapy. Various forms of individual and group therapy are now available. The purpose of therapy is to help the individual develop solutions, confidence, and respect through discussions. The reasons for the illness are explored.

Some therapists try to probe for past experiences that may have contributed to the maladjustive behavior. Others place emphasis on the here and now, to help the individual develop a more appropriate manner of behavior. By talking things out and releasing pent-up feelings, the patient can make a more satisfactory adjustment to the problems of everyday living.

Drugs. Drugs have been extremely beneficial in making patients better able to participate in other forms of therapy. Some drugs slow patients down and keep them from becoming too excited. These are called depressants. Other drugs help bring patients out of extreme states of depression. These are known as stimulants.

Chemotherapy is widely practiced today in conjunction with other forms of therapy. Because of the success of drug ther-

apy, many patients can now be treated in their doctor's office or in an outpatient clinic. The need for hospitalization is being reduced. Where hospitalization is necessary, the length of time the patient has to remain in the institution is also being reduced. This is alleviating one of the major problems of the past, when patients were separated from society for a long period of time—they could not adjust when they were released. They no longer had the security of the hospital and, as a result, could not relate to other people. The use of drugs and other therapy has helped resolve this problem.

Hypnosis. Hypnosis has been used by some therapists in an attempt to communicate better with emotionally disturbed patients. By probing into the unconscious, the therapist may be able to get at the source of the patient's problem. Then, through other forms of therapy such as individual and group counseling, it may be possible to bring about a cure.

Hypnosis alone is not considered a cure for emotional problems. This type of treatment, in the hands of the unskilled or unqualified individual, poses a potential hazard. Hypnosis should not be considered a plaything or a form of entertainment. Only a competent psychiatrist or psychologist with special training in psychodynamics should use hypnosis as a form of treatment for physical or emotional problems.

Electrical Stimulation. Electrical stimulation of the brain (ESB) has been used for a number of years to help persons with emotional problems. It has been particularly useful with individuals who are suffering deep depression.

Exactly how stimulation works to alleviate depression is not fully understood. As with other forms of therapy, this form of treatment is not used alone. Individual and group counseling, along with drug therapy, is often involved in the treatment.

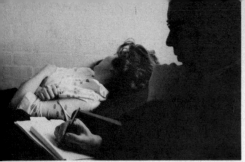
The Psychiatrist

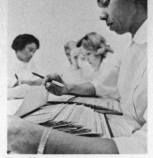
The Nurse

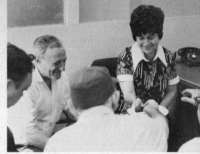
The Psychiatric Social Worker

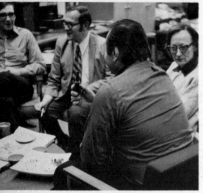
The Therapist

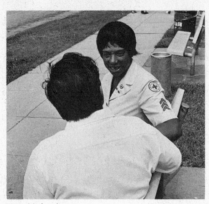
The Volunteer

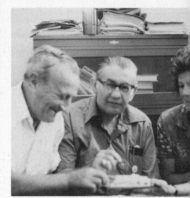
The Aide

Figure 12-16 ● Many people comprise the teams that help the mentally ill. Many more teams are needed. Would this be a good profession for you?

Visual Disorders

Refractive Errors

These disorders result when the visual image does not focus properly on the retina. Both far vision and near vision can be affected. The following are common problems in this category.

Myopia (Nearsightedness). A person who has myopia, can see close objects quite well, but has difficulty in seeing distant objects. In nearsightedness, the eyeball is too long from front to back. The light rays come to a focus in front of the retina rather than on it. Many individuals who are nearsighted may be able to do close work comfortably and show no symptoms except blurred vision when they look at a distant object. The problem is easily corrected by use of specifically prescribed lenses (concave) that properly focus the image on the retina. If a child has myopic vision, it usually becomes progressively worse until the eye has reached its full size (at approximately age 12 to 14 years). New lenses may have to be prescribed periodically until the eye has stopped growing.

Hyperopia (Farsightedness). Individuals who have hyperopia can see distant objects quite well, but have difficulty seeing close objects. Farsightedness occurs when an eyeball is too short from front to back. The light rays come to a focus behind the retina rather than on it. Children are usually farsighted at birth because their eyeballs have not yet reached their full size. As they mature, they may become less farsighted, normal-sighted, or even nearsighted. Hyperopia can be corrected easily by specifically prescribed lenses (convex) that correctly focus the image on the retina.

Presbyopia. This is a condition caused by the loss of the elasticity of the lens. It is part of the normal aging process. When the lens of the eye is normal, it enables an individual to see objects clearly by adjusting to whether they are near or far. When the object is near, the lens bulges or becomes thicker. When it is far, the lens flattens or becomes thinner. When a person has presbyopia, the lens cannot make these normal accommodations to near and far objects. Properly prescribed convex lenses will correct this condition.

Astigmatism. A person with astigmatism cannot see things clearly at any distance. Astigmatism is caused by some irregularity in the curvature of the cornea or of the lens of the eye. As a result, light rays cannot be brought to a sharp focus anywhere on the retina. This results in an unclear or blurry image. Lenses that are specifically prepared to compensate for the existing irregularity of the cornea can correct this condition satisfactorily.

Strabismus (Muscle Imbalance)

A common name for strabismus is crossed eyes or squint. This condition is caused by an imbalance of muscles that control the movements of the eyes. The muscles of one eye do not function simultaneously with the muscles of the other eye. As a result, both eyes cannot focus on the same object at the same time. A person with this problem may have double vision. Some individuals subconsciously compensate for this difficulty by suppressing the image from one eye. If the condition is left uncorrected, that eye will gradually lose its function.

The disorder is serious, but it can readily be corrected by eye exercises, properly prescribed glasses, and in some cases by surgery.

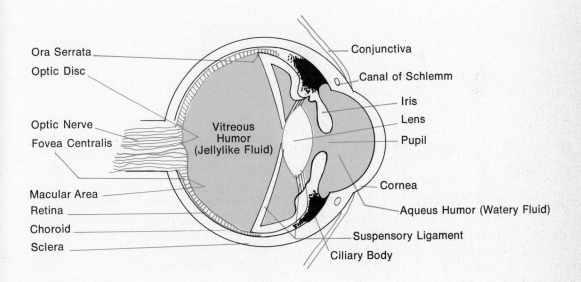

Figure 12-17 ● Diagram of the eye. Use this as a reference when reading about various eye disorders.

Diseases and Other Disorders of the Eye

Glaucoma. Glaucoma is a serious disease. It is the chief cause of blindness in the United States. The condition results from the buildup of fluids within the chambers of the eye. The increased fluids cause the development of excess pressure within the eye. If not corrected, the excess pressure causes a gradual loss of vision and ultimately results in the destruction of the optic nerve and the retina. Early diagnosis and treatment of this disease can help prevent serious and permanent damage. Symptoms that should be called to the attention of the physician include loss of side vision, seeing colored rings around lights, intense pain around the eyes, or inability to adjust to dark areas. Your physician can administer a simple, painless diagnostic test for glaucoma by means of an instrument (tonometer) that measures the pressure in the eye.

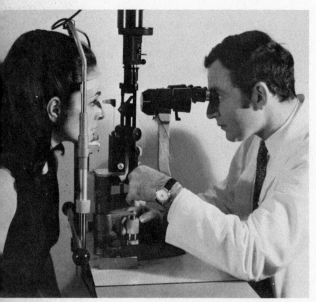

Figure 12-18 ● A tonometer is an instrument used to detect glaucoma.

Cataracts. Cataracts are serious disorders characterized by a cloudiness of the cornea or lens obstructing the passage of light. They may occur at any age. Some cataracts are congenital (present at birth). This may be due to a viral infection, possibly German measles, in the mother during the first three months of pregnancy. Cataracts may also be caused by radiation exposure, other kinds of injury, diseases of the eye, or the process of aging.

As the clouding condition progresses, the person's sight diminishes. The condition results in blindness unless it can be corrected by surgery. However, not all surgery for the removal of cataracts is successful. Much depends on the skill of the physician, the condition of the eye, and the general health of the patient.

Hearing Disorders

The importance of hearing in your daily life should be apparent to you. Hearing is one of the most important communicating senses you possess. Not only does it allow you to hear others, but it is also an important factor in your speech.

Hearing loss is a chronic ailment of many people in the United States. It is estimated that approximately 3,000,000 persons have a major hearing disability. Of these, approximately 200,000 cannot understand the loudest speech; they are deaf.

Hearing disabilities may occur at all ages. They are among the most complex, distressing, and handicapping health problems. Because of insufficient personnel, technical difficulties, and a lack of public awareness and interest, research in this area has been limited. In spite of this, progress is being made. Advances are being achieved in early diagnosis and treatment.

Conduction Defects

Otosclerosis. This is the most common cause of conductive deafness in young adults. Loss of hearing is brought about by bony growth that gradually closes the opening between the middle and inner ear. The sound vibrations cannot be effectively transmitted when this occurs. In a number of cases, the problem can be corrected by surgery.

Sensory-Neural Defects

Sensory-neural defects result in hearing loss because of degeneration of sensory cells, nerve fibers, or both. These can be classified into defects which are most prevalent in childhood and those which attack adults. In the former group, sensory-neural defects are usually inherited or result from problems that occur to the unborn child during pregnancy. If a woman has German measles during the first trimester (three months) of pregnancy, her child may be born with hearing difficulties. Other virus diseases and certain drugs given to the mother during pregnancy may also affect the hearing of that child.

A sensory-neural condition of concern to young adults results from the use of drugs that may cause damage to sensory cells and nerve fibers in the ear. A number of drugs that are commonly used to treat various infections (aspirin, quinine, and antibiotics) cause allergic reactions in some individuals. The allergic reaction may involve the ear, causing damage that results in hearing loss.

The relationship between noise and hearing loss is also cause for concern. Occupational groups confronted with abnormal noise during the work day have shown higher rates of hearing difficulties. More recently, it has been observed that many young people who constantly listen to loud music run the risk of hearing loss. Noise first affects a person's ability to hear extremely high tones. Since these tones are not heard in normal conversation, the hearing loss generally goes undetected for a time. Persons who work in a noisy environment should have periodic hearing tests.

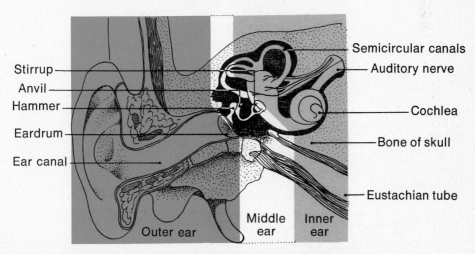

Figure 12-19 ● Diagram of the ear. Use this as a reference when reading about various hearing disorders.

Central-Neural Defects

Hearing loss from central-neural defects is caused by damage to the acoustic nerve or to the auditory center in the brain. Thus signals do not reach the brain, or if they do, they cannot be interpreted. These conditions are not common. When they do occur, they are readily apparent and demand the care of hearing specialists.

Summary

Chronic illnesses are becoming more common. You probably feel that they are a long way off for you. However, you should realize that many of the chronic diseases have their beginnings early in life.

Current knowledge permits the prevention of certain forms of cancer and heart disease. Through early diagnosis and treatment, still other forms of cancer and heart disease can be brought under control. Individuals with severe handicaps or long-term illness can often be returned to useful roles in society.

Most people with mental problems can be helped. It is important to remember that mental illness demands preventive measures and prompt care just as much as physical illness does.

Seek the advice and guidance of a physician on a regular basis to cope effectively with problems of chronic illness. Learn how you can develop personal habits that will help you avoid some of these illnesses.

in making health decisions

Understand These Terms:

allergen
angina pectoris
antihistamine
astigmatism
benign
biopsy
chemotherapy
chronic
coronary infarction
coronary occlusion
coronary thrombosis
degenerative
depressant
hyperopia

insulin
malignant
manic-depressive
metastasis
multiphasic screening
myopia
neurosis
otosclerosis
predisposition
psychodynamics
psychosis
stimulant
strabismus
thrombus

Solve This Problem:

You have been thinking about the possibility of preparing for a health career related to chronic and degenerative illnesses. Your school counselor has suggested that prior to making a decision, you might wish to learn more about job opportunities by exploring the following sources of employment:

a. Those advertised by local hospitals, clinics, and similar sources
b. Those available in doctors' offices, dentists' offices, and nursing homes
c. Those advertised in local newspaper want ads
d. Those available as civil-service positions with city, county, state, and federal agencies
e. Those advertised by commercial and industrial firms

1. What is the first thing you would attempt to determine in exploring these sources for career opportunities?
2. What are some of the other factors you would have to consider before making a decision?

Try These Activities:

1. List those personal characteristics that you feel would be of greatest importance for a person who is considering a health-related career in the field of chronic and degenerative illnesses.
2. Obtain job-application forms for health-related positions from your local county offices. Assess your personal characteristics, training, and experience in comparison to the criteria expressed or implied in the forms.
3. Medical advances in the treatment and prevention of chronic disorders are being made constantly. Select a recent development and
   a. Describe the medical discovery.
   b. Report on its degree of success at this time.
   c. Discuss its implications for you as a health-educated individual.

Interpret These Concepts:

1. Some chronic diseases lend themselves to screening tests that aid in early detection.
2. The types of chronic illness you are likely to have in the future are influenced by many of your current health practices.
3. As with physical problems and disorders, mental disorders should be brought to the attention of a competent specialist as early as possible for proper diagnosis and treatment.

Explore These Readings:

Burn, Harold, *Our Most Interesting Diseases.* New York: International Publications Services, 1969.

Graham, Marion F., *Prescription for Life.* New York: David McKay Co., Inc., 1966.

Maroon, Joseph C., *What You Can Do About Cancer.* Garden City, N. Y.: Doubleday & Company, Inc., 1969.

Seeman, Bernard, *Your Sight: Folklore, Fact, and Common Sense.* Boston: Little, Brown and Company, 1968.

Sutton, Maurice, *Cancer Explained.* New York: Hart Publishing Co., Inc., 1970.

Thirteen | Preventing and Eliminating Environmental Contamination

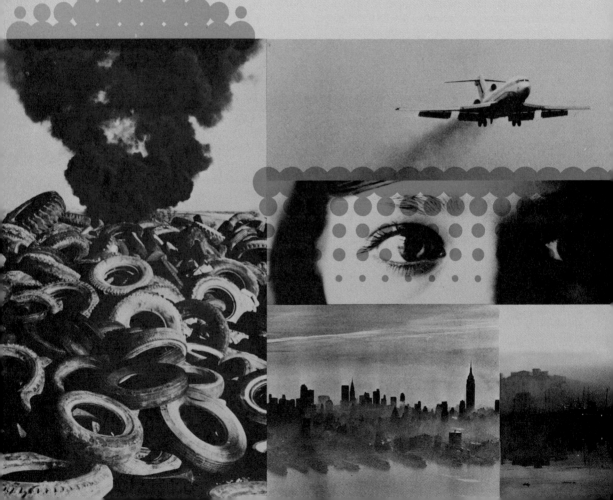

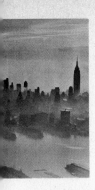

People have an amazing ability to adapt to new kinds of situations. Since the beginning of human existence, people have changed their environment to suit their purposes. Some of the changes have been for the better, but others have created serious environmental problems. For years, people have been able to adapt to these changes. Today, however, there is great concern about the effect of environment on health. Some of these environmental changes threaten people's ability to adapt. **There are ever-changing health hazards in the environment.** There is concern about whether people will be able to exist unless certain threats to health are controlled or prevented.

Two major requirements of life—the air people breathe and the water they drink and use—are in many ways a health threat. Other dangers to people's health have resulted from the use of radioactive materials and pesticides. Of great concern are the hazards that can result from an increasing amount of noise in the environment.

These concerns have become so great that in 1970 the Federal Government established the Environmental Protection Agency to oversee the environmental quality of life in the United States. This move consolidated into one agency the major federal programs dealing with air pollution, water pollution, solid waste disposal, pesticides regulation, and environmental radiation.

During the first year of its operation, major activities were developed to cope with water pollution problems, to implement the Clean Air Act of 1963 and the amendments of 1965 and 1970, and to ban the use of certain pesticides, including DDT.

In this chapter we shall explore these environmental hazards and their effects on health. We shall consider what is being done to lessen the hazards people have created. You will gain insight into how you may participate—even provide leadership —in future programs of control.

Air Pollution

The act you perform first and last in your life is to take a breath. Is the air you breathe free of harmful substances? No. The air you breathe has never been completely pure, and it is becoming less and less pure. If the air were purer, the length of time between your first and last breaths might be longer and more pleasant.

The Extent of the Problem

Air pollution is a public-health problem. It can cause acute symptoms of illness, aggravate symptoms of chronic disorders, and even kill.

Air pollution is also an economic problem. It can damage plants, clothing, and paint on houses and cars; it can destroy or stunt crops; and it can slow down transportation and make it more hazardous because of decreased visibility. In addition, automobile drivers and airplane pilots experience varied degrees of eye irritation and slower reflexes, creating still further transportation dangers.

Less dramatic, but also costly, are the smaller day-to-day economic effects of air pollution. You must wash and clean clothing more often, keep electric lights burning longer, and paint and wallpaper houses more frequently. It is estimated that expenses of this type are as much as $100 per person higher in cities with a major problem of pollution than in areas where the air is comparatively clean.

The problem of air pollution is worldwide. Hundreds of millions of people are affected.

The Causes of Air Pollution

Why is the air polluted? The answer is fairly simple. **Wherever there has been a substantial increase in the concentration of population and heavy industry, there has been an increase in air pollution.**

A great deal of pollution comes from the unburned gases emitted from automobile exhaust systems. The more cars there are on the road, the greater the potential of pollution. The more gasoline filling stations there are, the greater the possibility that increasing amounts of fumes will escape into the air as the gas is pumped.

The increasing burning of fuel oil and fuel gas releases large quantities of material into the atmosphere. In fact, any kind of burning, including the combustion of coal or trash, can discharge pollutants into the air. The growth of manufacturing, processing, and chemical industries also increases the possibility of airborne discharges.

Figure 13-1 • A clear day and a smoggy day in Los Angeles. What can be done to help eliminate air pollution?

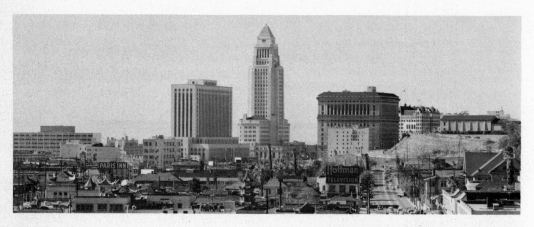

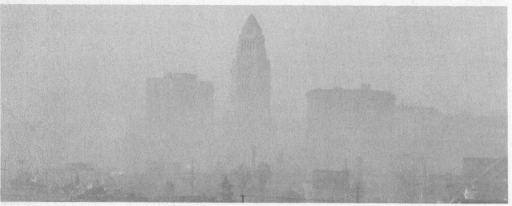

Estimated Nationwide Emissions
[In millions of tons per year]

Source	Carbon monoxide	Particulates	Sulfur oxides	Hydrocarbons	Nitrogen oxides	Total
Transportation	63.8	1.2	0.8	16.6	8.1	90.5
Fuel combustion in stationary sources	1.9	8.9	24.4	.7	10.0	45.9
Industrial processes	9.7	7.5	7.3	4.6	.2	29.3
Solid waste disposal	7.8	1.1	.1	1.6	.6	11.2
Miscellaneous [1]	16.9	9.6	.6	8.5	1.7	37.3
Total	100.1	28.3	33.2	32.0	20.6	214.2

[1] Primarily forest fires, agricultural burning, coal waste fires.

Figure 13-2 • Does your community have adequate smog controls for industry?

It is estimated that over 150 million tons of air contaminants are released into the atmosphere over the United States every year. Among the many types of air pollutants are smoke, gases, products of combustion (including those of cigarette and cigar smoking), pollens, radioactive matter, and dust. Figure 13-2 gives a breakdown of these pollutants. These air-polluting materials are the direct result of demands brought about by a rapidly expanding population.

Effects of Weather and Locality

It takes more than pollutants to cause health problems. Wind conditions (speed, direction, and turbulence), temperature, and geographical location of communities play an important role in determining how great the air pollution will be. Los Angeles, for example, is surrounded by mountains.

In addition, the air circulating around the area descends, and as it does so it becomes compressed and heated to form a warm, dense layer. This acts like a lid on a pot, preventing any upward escape of pollutants. Such a condition is known as a temperature inversion and may continue for several days. Narrow valleys may also be subject to similar inversion problems.

Inversions of varying degrees occur at all times. In the evening as the earth cools the air does not rise. The winds die down and the warm air above forms a lid. Pollutants accumulate until the sun rises and warms the air sufficiently to cause vertical movement. This does not usually occur until 10 A.M. or later. In spring and fall, very noticeable temperature inversions take place. In all these instances, when the pollutants become highly concentrated and are not dispersed by the movement of air, a "killing smog" may occur.

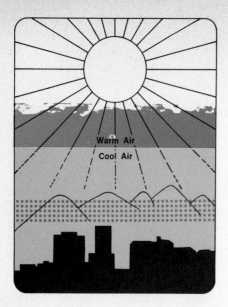

Figure 13-3 ● Warm air above the cooler air near the ground acts as a lid to hold pollution in the area.

The dangerous smog comes in two varieties. The type found in London, England, is more like a dirty fog. It is caused by pollutants from burning coal mixed with the moisture of fog. This produces a thick smog that interferes with respiration. The variety found in Los Angeles is influenced by the photochemical action of sunlight. The reaction causes the formation of ozone or oxidants from the atmospheric impurities. These products continue to react with organic pollutants to produce compounds that cause eye irritation, reduced visibility, crop damage, and other problems. This type of smog is more widespread than has been previously believed.

A different type of air pollution problem is related to pollen. Hay fever is a widespread disorder affecting many people in the United States. Research indicates that the pollen produced by ragweed is the principal offender. This plant is found all over the United States. It is controlled by spraying, which kills the plant before it has a chance to produce its seeds.

Health Hazards in the Air

There can no longer be any question as to whether or not air pollution is detrimental to health. A number of studies recently completed pinpoint air pollution as a complicating factor in a number of ailments, as well as in numerous deaths.

Air Pollution Episodes. There have been a number of episodes where loss of life has been attributed to air pollution. These have occurred in places as far apart as Belgium's Meuse Valley; Donora, Pennsylvania; London, England; New York City; and Tokyo, Japan.

In Donora, 20 deaths were directly attributed to air pollution, and thousands of persons were made ill within a short period of time.

One of the worst air-pollution disasters in history occurred in London in 1952. During one week, there were between 4,000 and 5,000 more deaths than would normally have been expected during a similar period. Some of those who died were elderly persons already suffering from respiratory or circulatory diseases. However, many young and healthy people were made seriously ill. A government report suggested that this high rate of illness and death was due to irritation of the respiratory tract caused by contaminants in the air that were present at that time. The contaminants probably came from the great amount of coal burned in inefficient open grates. Since 1952, London has had a number of additional major episodes of unusually high daily mortality, caused by air pollution.

Similar events have occurred in New York City, where many episodes of increased mortality due to air pollution have been noted. Tokyo, Japan has been one of the most hard-hit of cities in respect to air pollution. There is so much heavy industry concentrated around the city that heavy air pollution is almost always present. Like London and New York City, it has had many episodes where an increase in deaths attributed to air pollution has been noted.

In recent years, a number of air-pollution alerts have been called because of the high level of pollution in a large geographical area. Weather conditions have occurred that caused pollution to be trapped in stagnant air. In one episode, an area from the Great Lakes to the Gulf of Mexico and from the Mississippi River to the Atlantic Ocean was affected. Another episode involved the entire length of the Pacific Coast, extending inland to Denver, Colorado. Still another episode affected the Southwest area of the United States between California and the Great Plains.

All these episodes necessitated warnings to people and industries in the affected areas. Persons with respiratory diseases were asked to stay indoors. Those without respiratory diseases were asked to limit their physical activities. In many communities, industries were asked to shut down or cut back on their activities. Motorists were asked to reduce their driving.

The Effects on Health. Nobody can predict when and where the next killer smog will occur. With the increasing amount of pollutants in the air, it can come at any time.

Figure 13-4 ● Physical complaints reported by people affected by air pollution.

Physical Complaints of People Affected by Air Pollution

Symptoms reported by patients	Percentage of patients reporting
Cough	75.6%
Smarting of eyes	70.9%
Tearing of eyes	61.5%
Nasal discharge	52.0%
Dyspnea	44.5%
Sore throat	41.9%
Chest constriction	41.7%
Headache	41.2%
Choking	33.8%
Nausea	18.2%

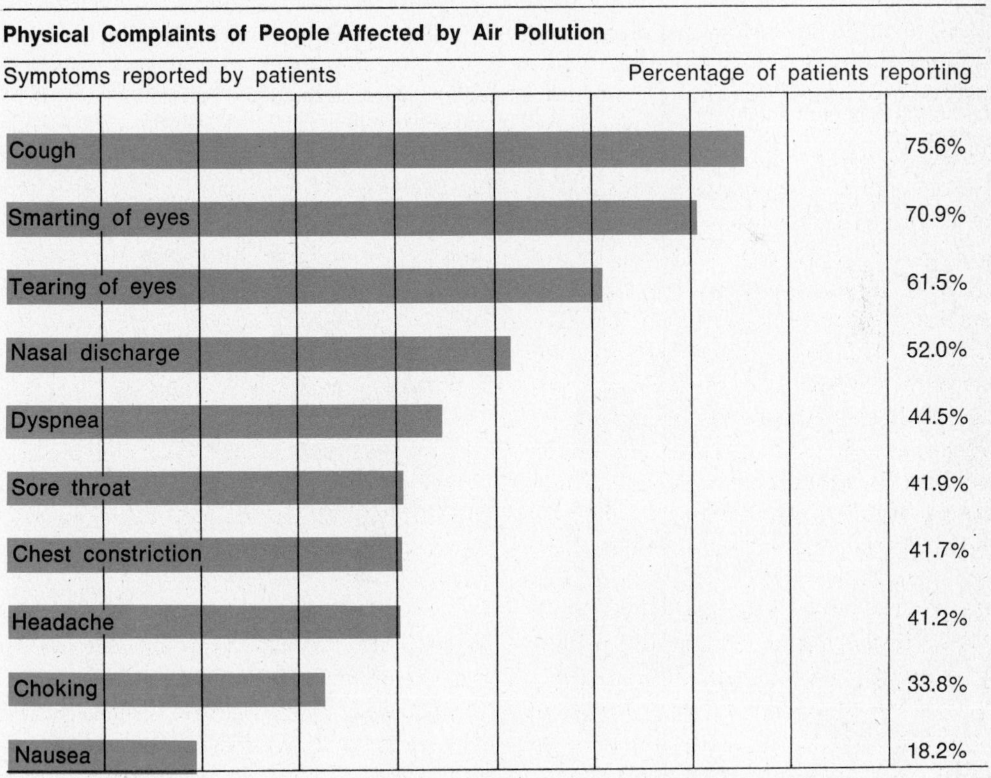

There is increasing evidence indicating that persons who have been severely affected by air pollution episodes are ill more often and die sooner than those not affected. For a number of years the U. S. Public Health Service Air Pollution Medical Program has conducted and sponsored studies of the effects of air pollution on health. The findings of these research projects suggest a strong relationship between illness and the amount and type of pollutants in the air. A survey of persons under medical care in Los Angeles, conducted by the Los Angeles County Medical Association in conjunction with the Tuberculosis and Respiratory Disease Association of Los Angeles County, disclosed that an estimated 10,000 patients had been advised by their physicians to move from that area because of air pollution.

Air pollution generally affects health by causing irritations. As a result, there may be damage to various membrane surfaces of the body, such as the eye and the respiratory tract. There may also be indirect effects on the heart. Investigations have shown a relationship between air pollution and allergies, cancer, and infectious diseases.

Thus far, research has revealed valuable information on the following health problems.

■ **Chronic Bronchitis.** In Great Britain, medical scientists have established a definite relationship between air pollution and chronic bronchitis. This disease is quite prevalent and serious there, being ranked third among causes of death and first among causes of economic loss due to illness. A particularly alarming characteristic of chronic bronchitis is that in many persons it seems to reach a stage where the effects are irreversible and premature death cannot be avoided. Although this condition is not nearly so

Figure 13-5 ● (Left) A cross section of a normal lung. (Right) A cross section showing the effects of emphysema. Note the large white spaces, indicating destruction of lung tissue.

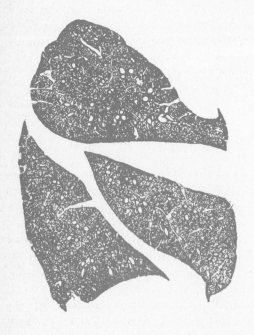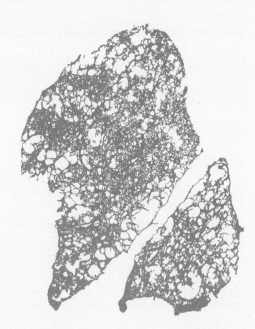

widespread in the United States, the number of cases has been steadily increasing in recent years. Many of the new cases have occurred in areas of high air pollution.

■ **Emphysema.** One of the most serious respiratory conditions in the United States is emphysema. In this disease, the air sacs of the lung lose their natural elasticity and become overinflated or enlarged. The lungs retain too much air, which cannot be exhaled. Over a period of time, breathing becomes increasingly difficult. The incidence of this condition is greatest in areas where air pollution exists. One medical researcher has demonstrated that emphysema patients show improvement in breathing when taken out of such an environment and placed in rooms where the air is filtered. There is evidence of a very definite rise in the number of cases of emphysema in the United States, and researchers believe this is due, at least in part, to air pollution.

■ **Lung Cancer.** Statistical studies indicate that where there is a high lung cancer rate there is also a high level of air pollution. Although medical scientists will not state positively that air pollution is a definite cause of lung cancer, they do see a strong relationship between air pollution and the increased number of cases. You have already learned that cigarette smoking is closely related to the development of lung cancer. Tobacco smoke is itself an air pollutant. Studies also have shown that where air pollution exists, the lung cancer rate is higher even among nonsmokers. For example, in Los Angeles County, members of a religious denomination which does not use tobacco have a higher rate of lung cancer than do members who live in relatively unpolluted areas.

■ **Other Cancers.** Studies also have shown a relationship between air pollution and mortality (death rate) from cancer of the stomach and esophagus. Large amounts of polluted air are swallowed. Persons exposed to the serious air pollution episodes in Donora and London complained of severe gastrointestinal symptoms. It appears, then, that the effects on the individual are not limited to the respiratory tract.

■ **Cardiovascular Disease.** The effects of air pollution on the heart and circulation are probably indirect. For example, when the exchange of air in the lungs becomes less efficient, the heart is forced to work harder to satisfy the body's demand for oxygen. In addition, studies have shown that there is a higher death rate from arteriosclerosis and other circulatory diseases in metropolitan areas where air pollution is most often a serious problem.

■ **Accidents.** Eye irritation caused by air pollution may result in accidents. The irritation brings about a severe watering of the eyes and a slowing of reflexes which interfere with driving ability. In addition, several air accidents have been blamed on poor visibility due to polluted air.

Controlling Air Pollution

Air pollution control activities have been sporadic and uneven in the past. In recent years, efforts to solve the problem have become more organized.

Local Community Activities. California initiated action against air pollution in 1947, when a law was adopted authorizing the creation of county air pollution control districts. As a result, Los Angeles County was able to pass a law banning the use of commercial, industrial, and backyard incinerators. This was done to reduce impurities in the air. In addition, a rule was adopted limiting the sulphur content of fuels burned during the months when air pollution is heaviest. When the pollutant exceeds the limit, an alert is announced and industry must switch to natural gas for fuel.

New York City has passed laws regulating the use of fuel burners and refuse incinerators in apartment buildings. The law limits the amount of sulphur in the fuel to be burned and requires that monitoring and recording devices be installed on the incinerators.

Some cities are curbing the use of surface transportation to help control air quality. These efforts include plans to close streets, limit the amount of parking area in mid-city, and even start rationing the amount of gasoline that can be purchased.

Still other cities, including Boston, San Francisco, Washington, D.C., Chicago, and Cleveland are developing rapid-transit systems to help get automobiles off the roads.

Many communities are becoming more concerned about contamination from power-generating sources. They are investigating new sources of power, such as nuclear reactors, as a possible way of reducing contamination.

State Efforts for Control. One of the greatest sources of air pollution is the automobile exhaust. In California, the State Legislature passed a bill in 1960 requiring most automobiles to be equipped with special exhaust devices. One device is used to eliminate crankcase (engine) emissions. Another device is designed to regulate emissions from the exhaust, or tailpipe. These devices are not in use throughout the United States.

However, this latter device still presents problems. To be efficient, an exhaust device must be capable of eliminating over 100 different kinds of exhaust gases. Thus,

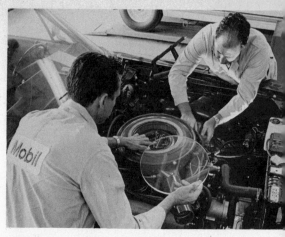

Figure 13-6 • Carburetor and exhaust smog control devices are now mandatory on automobiles. Proper maintenance is necessary if these devices are to be effective.

the original devices need to be improved so that more of the pollutants from the automobile exhaust can be eliminated. Regular maintenance is needed to keep the device functioning at the accepted level of efficiency.

A number of states have established automobile-inspection stations equipped with gauges to measure these emissions, as a means of enforcing the standards.

National Efforts for Control. In recent years the national attack on air pollution has become more intense. The Clean Air Act, passed in 1963 and amended in 1965 and 1970, provided money for air-pollution research. The act also made it possible to establish air quality standards. Amendments to the Act in 1970 required that by 1976 auto emissions of hydrocarbons, carbon monoxide, and oxides of nitrogen be reduced by over 90 percent. The Environmental Protection Agency has been given the responsibility of enforcing this legislation. This means that, in order to reach these levels, new devices will have to be added to the exhaust system of an automobile, or new engines will have to be designed and built.

Now that those who have direct responsibility for control of air pollution have coordinated their efforts, it remains for you and other citizens of your community to do your part. You can do this by cooperating with local air pollution officials, by supporting their programs, by following their directives, and by encouraging others to do the same.

Water Pollution

Water pollution presents a menace to our health and a threat to the economy, and contributes greatly to the ever-growing problem of water shortage since it reduces our supply of clean water.

The Extent of the Problem

- In the Southwest, salt brine is limiting water supplies and contaminating water, so that it cannot be used by agriculture and industry.

- In suburbs throughout the country, phosphates, a product of home laundries and dishwashers, have contributed to the growth of green mats of algae on the surface of rivers and streams.

- Many people think the water in their homes is free from bacteria or chemicals that can cause disease. Usually, this is true. However, in recent years some concern has been expressed as to the quality of water available for drinking. A Public Health Service survey indicated that 36 percent of home water supplies that were tested exceeded public-health limits. In addition, there have been a number of instances in which a variety of water sources have been polluted.

- In Santa Barbara, California, the Gulf of Mexico, and the San Francisco Bay, oil spills have occurred that have polluted the water and surrounding land areas.

- The Cuyahoga River in Cleveland was so polluted with industrial and municipal wastes that it caught fire.

- In every state, miles of streams are being lost to fishing each year and millions of fish and other aquatic life are being killed.

- In many cities water is becoming less pleasant to drink because of pollutants in the water supply.

- Because of pollution, many bathing beaches, picnic areas, and boating marinas are less safe and attractive for use.

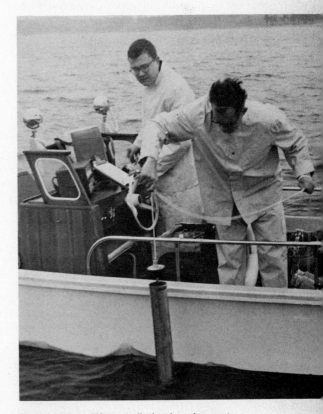

Figure 13-7 • Water pollution is a danger to health. A biologist takes a sample of water to determine the level of pollution.

Like air pollution, the water problem is directly related to population growth and industrialization. The population of the United States will reach approximately 260 million by 1980. Clearly, such increases in population will mean far greater demands on our already restricted water supplies. This is particularly true in cities. It is estimated that industrial uses of water will grow from the current 160 billion gallons of water per day to approximately 394 billion gallons per day in 1980.

The problem of pollution is further complicated by the increasing volume of waste materials to be disposed of. The current practice is to dump wastes into rivers, lakes, and oceans. Pollution is further complicated by hazardous new materials which are being produced, such as man-made fibers, detergents, weed killers, pesticides, and radioactive particles. These are reaching water sources in increasing quantities.

Solving the Problem

Water pollution can be controlled through enforcement of regulations designed to prevent contamination of our water supplies. The related water shortage problem can be solved by reclamation of used water and conversion of sea water to fresh.

The Federal Water Pollution Control Act permits legal action to be taken to protect the health of a community. In addition, funds are being made available to assist in the construction of waste disposal facilities. This will help eliminate the dumping of raw waste into the country's streams, rivers, and other waterways.

Great efforts are being made to solve the water shortage problem. An increasing number of persons are drinking "used" water. Along the Ohio River during certain months of the year water is used four times as it passes from Pittsburgh, Pennsylvania

Figure 13-8 • Note how the need for water in the United States has already overtaken the supply. Water pollution adds to this problem.

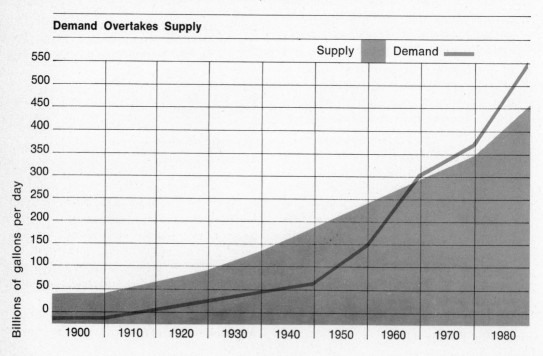

to Cairo, Mississippi. Scientists can make this water safe by filtration and chlorination.

People are also turning to the sea for their water. Desalination plants are already producing several million gallons of fresh water daily. In terms of our daily needs, this is a very small amount of water. In addition, it is quite expensive. Moreover, the expense increases if the desalted water has to be transported any great distance. With the current research taking place, it may be that giant nuclear plants will be used to convert sea water to fresh water. When this process is available, the cost will not be so great.

Radiation

Radioactivity is older than humans. Cosmic rays and mineral deposits have given off nuclear radiation for centuries. Little attention was paid to this process, since it was of no immediate practical concern. Now in this nuclear age of atomic industrial revolution, we must learn to keep exposure to radioactivity within safe limits.

The Extent of the Problem

Serious health problems may result from exposure to radiation. For many years problems arose mainly from using X rays and radium without adequate safeguards. Today, the greater use of these and new radioactive materials has increased the hazard. There has been a ninefold increase in X-ray exposure to the average individual since 1925. Approximately 160 million X-ray exposures are performed annually for medical-diagnostic purposes.

Radiation exposure also has resulted from the use of radioisotopes in medicine, industry, meteorology, agriculture, and space exploration. The greatest growth in the use of radioisotopes has been in medicine. Public-health authorities estimate that more than 500,000 patients each year are given radioisotope tracers for diagnosis of health conditions.

Our greatest potential contamination problem is presented by the nuclear power industry. There are at least 200 nuclear power reactors in operation in the United States today, with many more under construction or being planned. Although the importance of this source of power is unquestioned, its use will result in a greatly increased amount of radioactive waste material. The problem is proper disposal of this type of waste so that human beings are not exposed to its radioactivity.

Another source of environmental contamination is radioactive fallout from the testing of nuclear weapons. Despite the Test Ban Treaty, fallout from previous testing will continue for many years. Since not all nations have signed the Treaty, it is possible that there will be additional atmospheric testing with further contamination of air.

Health Hazards

The radiation hazard presents a unique problem to the medical scientist. Because of its many desirable uses, radiation cannot be eradicated. Instead, radiation must be contained and allowed to work for the benefit of humanity. Great care must be taken in its use. **The continued use of radiation or radioactive material presents numerous health hazards.**

Chronic Conditions. Excessive radiation has been linked with skin disorders, loss of hair, cancer, leukemia, birth defects, and genetic changes. In addition to these effects, some reports have indicated a relationship between excessive radiation and a shorter life expectancy.

Ill effects from radiation result when the cumulative exposure during your lifetime, from all sources, reaches a certain level. It is generally believed that this level is 15 roentgens (the standard unit of measurement). Most individuals always remain within safe limits. For example, you receive about 0.1 roentgens from a chest X-ray. Any reasonable number of X-rays taken during a lifetime, therefore, would not endanger your health.

There are other sources from which you can receive radiation. Because of the many safeguards, this total amount of accumulated radiation can be kept within safe limits.

Preventing health complications due to radiation involves keeping a check on the amount of radiation to which one is exposed. The Division of Radiological Health of the United States Public Health Service maintains a large number of sampling stations in many parts of the country to check daily on radioactive fallout. Samples of pasteurized milk from numerous sections of the country are also checked, because milk is the food item most often consumed and used as an indicator of isotope intake. In addition, diet studies are conducted in a number of boarding institutions across the country. Each institution provides one complete seven-day diet sample each month. The foods are then checked to determine the amount of radioisotopes present, if any. Water is also analyzed for radioactivity. Agencies at all levels of government conduct routine tests on a continuous basis.

Better control than ever before is also being exercised over dental and medical X-ray units. When you visit your doctor or dentist, notice the precautions taken.

Acute Effects of Radiation. If you are exposed to a high-level dose of radioactivity over a short period of time, you may suffer radiation sickness. The sickness may be slight, or it may result in death.

Radiation damages body cells by causing chemical changes. The amount of damage depends on the amount of radiation received, the duration of exposure, the amount of body exposed, and the age and general health of the person exposed.

The possibility of excessive exposure to radiation is relatively small. Excessive radiation is the kind that might be experienced in a nuclear attack. It is hoped that you will never have to protect yourself from such an attack. However, you should be aware of ways of minimizing exposure and providing emergency treatment.

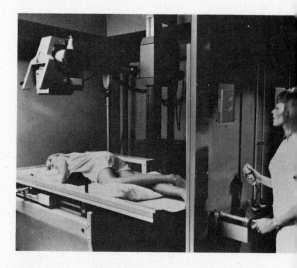

Figure 13-9 • Protective devices used in medicine and dentistry have greatly reduced radiation exposure.

Controlling Exposure

The degree of exposure is lessened and protection is achieved by shielding, distance, and time.

Shielding means placing some barrier between you and the falling radioactive debris. Because fallout has high penetrating power, the thicker the walls of your shelter, the better your protection. Being inside a well-constructed building is the next safest thing to being in an underground shelter.

Distance from the source or place of radiation is another important protection factor. Since fallout will drop to the ground, keeping your distance from the contaminated ground level would be beneficial. The middle floors of a tall building would be a good location in terms of protection. Here you would be away from any fallout accumulated on the ground and on the rooftop.

Time is an important factor since the danger of fallout decreases with radioactive decay. The decay is rapid in the first 24 hours after a nuclear explosion. It would be best, therefore, to stay shielded for the first 48 hours after an attack. Following this time, you could leave your protection for brief periods, but it would be several days before it would be safe to leave permanently.

Radiation Sickness. People exposed to high-level doses of radioactivity will probably suffer radiation sickness. Radiation damages body cells by causing chemical changes. The amount of damage depends on the amount of radiation to which the person is exposed and the duration of exposure. Most people suffering from moderate radiation sickness will recover.

The symptoms of radiation sickness are lack of appetite, nausea, vomiting, fatigue, drowsiness, weakness, sore mouth, headache, loss of hair, bleeding gums, diarrhea, and bleeding under the skin. Not all of these symptoms will appear in every person affected, and some will be noticeable only in cases of severe exposure.

Those with mild exposure probably will show only a few symptoms and will be able to continue their regular activities. But such victims should have more rest than usual.

With moderate exposure, the symptoms will appear about two hours after contamination. Generally, the victim will suffer—increasingly through the first day—upset stomach with nausea, vomiting, lack of appetite, drowsiness, and fatigue. The symptoms will generally disappear on the second day, and by the third day the person should feel normal. With proper rest, the victim can return to limited activity at this time.

Victims of severe exposure will suffer all the symptoms mentioned, but these symptoms will last longer. Some appetite and vigor will return in about three days, but fever, diarrhea, and soreness in the mouth will show up in the second week of illness. Ulcers or bleeding may appear in the mouth. Loss of hair will usually occur in the third week. Most patients with severe exposure will recover, though they might continue to have fever and mouth ulcers for seven or eight weeks. However, if the radiation is acquired within a short period of time, the person might continue to weaken and die.

Emergency Treatment. It is important to know the emergency treatment for radiation sickness. In the aftermath of a nuclear attack, physicians and nurses would be so busy with blast and flash casualties that they would have little or no time to treat fallout victims.

The best emergency procedure is simply to treat the symptoms of the individual. Keep the patient warm, quiet, and resting. Try to replace the fluids lost by those who are vomiting or have diarrhea. Give aspirin for headache. If the exposure is not too great, the symptoms will disappear in several days. As soon as feasible, the patient should be treated by a physician.

Pesticides

⚛ **The widespread use of chemicals in combating pests has created additional environmental health hazards.** These chemicals (pesticides) are widely used in agriculture and industry, and by various governmental agencies. In addition, most people use them in the home and garden to kill insects and rodents.

Value of Pesticides

Pesticides were developed to protect your health. Their earliest use was to control diseases such as malaria, yellow fever, typhus, and plague. Insects, rodents, or both, are involved in the transmission of these diseases. Millions of people are alive today because pesticides were developed to kill these carriers of disease.

Pesticides have also been valuable in protecting food. By destroying the pests that attack crops, agriculturists are able to provide us with a wider variety of food, higher in quality and lower in cost. In addition, pesticides have helped keep our food supply ample, thus reducing the incidence of such food-deficiency diseases as pellagra, scurvy, and rickets.

Hazards of Pesticides

Because pesticides are poisons, one potential danger is accidental ingestion either by swallowing or inhalation. This is of particular concern among those in agricultural occupations.

Public-health officials are also concerned about the possibility of long-term ill effects which could result from contamination of air, water, food, and soil by im-

Figure 13-10 • Pesticides are widely used in protecting the nation's food supply.

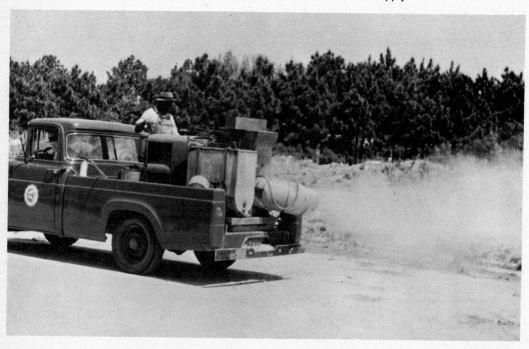

proper use of pesticides. This possibility is under constant study. Medical researchers study the gradual buildup of residues of pesticides in body tissues. Samples of food and water are routinely analyzed. If residues in a food go beyond a specified limit, that particular food product cannot be sold.

Of great concern to many persons is the potential danger of pesticides to marine life and wildlife. There are many examples in which the ecology was upset by the improper use of pesticides. In these instances, birds, fish, and other living things have been killed by the use of certain pesticides. As a result of the concern for the safety of people and other living creatures, some pesticides such as DDT can no longer be used in the United States. Federal laws require that all pesticides that are shipped interstate must be registered with the Environmental Protection Agency. If a hazard exists with one of these pesticidies, interstate shipment can be stopped.

Safe Use of Pesticides

Since pesticides are chemical poisons, they should be handled with extreme care and stored in a proper fashion. The following suggestions are important, whether you use these chemicals in the home or on the job.

■ Use a pesticide only when you are sure it is needed. Use the one best suited to your needs. The label on the product explains its proper uses.

■ Keep the pesticide in a plainly labeled container, preferably the one in which it was bought. Never transfer pesticides to unlabeled or mislabeled containers.

■ Store pesticides under lock and key, away from food items and out of reach of children, pets, and people who might not be able to read the label or understand their danger.

■ When handling, mixing, or applying pesticides, avoid inhaling dust and fumes and avoid getting the materials on the skin.

■ Do not spray or treat plants or animals or animal feeding areas with pesticides unless you are certain such treatment is safe for that use.

■ Check the label for the antidote before using the product, so that you know what to do quickly if there is an accident. In case of an accident, call a doctor or take the patient to a hospital immediately.

■ If you suspect you may have a special sensitivity to pesticides, you should consult an allergist and avoid any exposure to the offending agent.

■ Wash your hands thoroughly after using pesticides and before eating or smoking.

■ Dispose of used pesticide containers in a way that will not leave the leftover contents as a hazard to people, particularly children.

■ When mixing or using inflammable chemicals, be especially careful to avoid the fire hazards of smoking, defective wiring, and open flames.

■ Cover food and water containers when using pesticides around livestock or in pet areas.

■ When so directed by the label, wear protective clothing, such as goggles, gloves, aprons, respirators, and masks.

■ In applying pesticides to food plants and crops:
   a. Use the proper amount recommended for the purpose.
   b. Allow the full recommended time between applying the pesticide and harvesting the crop to avoid having a harmful amount of pesticide remaining on food to be eaten. Do not plant food crops near ornamental plants which are to be sprayed.

- Check sprayers before each use, to make sure that hose connections are tight and that valves do not leak.

- Do not spray into the wind.

- Change your clothing after each day's operations and bathe thoroughly. If the clothing or skin become contaminated, wash the skin and change to clean clothing.

- Work in a well-ventilated area, to avoid inhalation of fumes.

If an accident occurs and a pesticide is ingested, follow first-aid procedures for poisoning. The antidote for that particular poison will be indicated on the label of the container. Call a doctor or get the patient to a hospital immediately.

Noise

A form of pollution that you may overlook because it constantly surrounds you is noise. The ear is an amazing part of the body. It has the ability to hear without damage many different kinds of sound. However, there is increasing concern about the effect of noise on the health status of people.

Excessive exposure to noise can have both physical and psychological effects on an individual. Very often the first signs of the effect of excessive noise on an individual are discomfort, annoyance, headache, muscle tension, and irritability. A temporary loss of hearing is not uncommon. If the same kind of exposure continues over a long period of time, permanent hearing loss can result.

Noise is measured in terms of decibels (units of sound level or pressure) and frequencies (number of cycles or sound waves per second). Persons exposed to noise levels exceeding 85 decibels have been shown to have a slight shift in their hearing threshold. Over a period of time, this might lead to permanent hearing loss.

The difficulty of controlling excessive noise is complicated by the fact that the ears of some individuals are more easily injured by noise than those of other people. From a psychological point of view, the ability to withstand excessive noise also varies greatly. Consider how differently you and your parents react to the sound level of music or television.

In some industries, noise volume is being reduced to a safe level through the use of sound-absorbing walls or sound-conditioned machinery. In certain situations, workers may wear special ear protectors to prevent hearing loss.

More and more cities have drafted new building codes requiring better soundproofing of apartments, homes, and office buildings. Materials are available to reduce transmission of sound through walls. Fans, compressors, and other noisy equipment can be enclosed to reduce noise.

The Outlook

The future control of these environmental health problems will depend on continued research, new legislation, enforcement of laws, and the support of the general public in following recommended procedures. **Maintaining a healthful and safe environment is the responsibility of the individual, the family, and society.**

Specifically, some of the possibilities in the future include:

- More consideration of environmental contamination in urban planning

- Elimination of automobiles from the center of cities or the return of the electric automobile
- Planting of grass and trees between industrial and residential areas
- New ways of eliminating industrial wastes other than by dumping them into the air or the waterways
- Further advances in the reclamation and reuse of water, and the use of sea water.
- Reduction of the tremendous loss of stored water through evaporation by covering reservoirs with "chemical shields"
- Increased monitoring for pesticides and radioactive material in air, food, and water by government agencies
- Increased efforts by medical scientists to discover dangers to health from environmental contamination, perhaps even isolating some cause-and-effect relationships

Summary

The ability to alter the natural environment has created many health problems.

Accumulating evidence indicates that air pollution is associated with a variety of health problems. It has been established as a primary cause of one disease, chronic bronchitis. There is no doubt that it is an irritation that affects the eyes and the respiratory system.

Increasing evidence supports the theory that air pollution contributes to the high morbidity (incidence of disease) and death rates associated with cancer of the lung, trachea, stomach, and esophagus, as well as circulatory conditions. Finally, it is an important influence in causing accidents.

Everyone has a responsibility to participate in the fight against air pollution and the shortage of water. President Kennedy, in a message to Congress, expressed the nation's water goals as follows: ". . . to have sufficient water, sufficiently clean, at the right place and at the right time." Attainment of this objective will require the support and understanding of the entire population.

As the struggle against environmental contamination goes on, individuals will be called upon to do their part. Activities that you might be asked to engage in include refraining from burning leaves, supporting financial programs with your vote, or serving on committees attempting to solve these problems. Controls will depend upon the entire community working together.

In addition to air and water pollution, radioactive materials, pesticides, and noise add further environmental hazards that have widespread effects on man's health.

The extent of the problem has led to governmental controls at the national, state, and local levels. The success of these controls depends on the degree of cooperation each individual in the community gives to the programs developed.

in making health decisions . . .

Understand These Terms:

desalination
emphysema
inversions
morbidity
pesticides

pollutants
radioisotopes
shielding
water reclamation

Solve This Problem:

Ricky Martinez has become active in his school's Environmental Health Club. As a result of his activity and experiences, he thinks he wants to pursue a career in the environmental health field. What kind of work could he find after completing high school? After college? What educational background should he have for this work?

Try These Activities:

1. Borrow a decibel meter from the science class. Take readings at various sites in your school and in the surrounding community. Make a class chart illustrating your findings. Discuss your findings with your class.

2. Check to determine whether you have insecticides in your home. If you have, what are they? Where are they kept? What is the proper first aid for ingestion of each of them? Correct any deficiencies in their labeling or storage.

3. Prepare a written response to the statement "All pesticides should be banned because of the danger to all forms of life."

4. Prepare a report for your class showing the relationship between air pollution and each of the following:
   a. Human health
   b. Wildlife
   c. Production of meat and produce
   d. Upkeep of the home
   e. Maintaining an automobile

   Identify the most significant way in which people can contribute to solving this problem.

Interpret These Concepts:

1. Water pollution presents a menace to our health and a threat to the economy, and contributes greatly to the ever-growing problem of water shortage.

2. Wherever there has been a substantial increase in the concentration of population and heavy industry, there has also been an increase in air pollution.

3. There are ever-changing health hazards in the environment.

4 Maintaining a healthful and safe environment is the responsibility of the individual, the family, and society.

Explore These Readings:

Air Pollution Primer (pamphlet). New York: American Lung Association, 1971.

"The Big Cleanup: The Environmental Crisis '72," *Newsweek,* June 12, 1972.

Brennan, A. J. J., "Environmental Health: A Look at the Cost of Air Pollution," *The Journal of School Health,* Vol. XLIII (May, 1973), pp. 300–302.

Research and Monitoring: Cornerstone for Environmental Action (pamphlet). Washington, D. C.: United States Environmental Protection Agency, 1972.

Toward a New Environmental Ethic (pamphlet). Washington, D. C.: United States Environmental Protection Agency, 1971.

Fourteen Living Safely

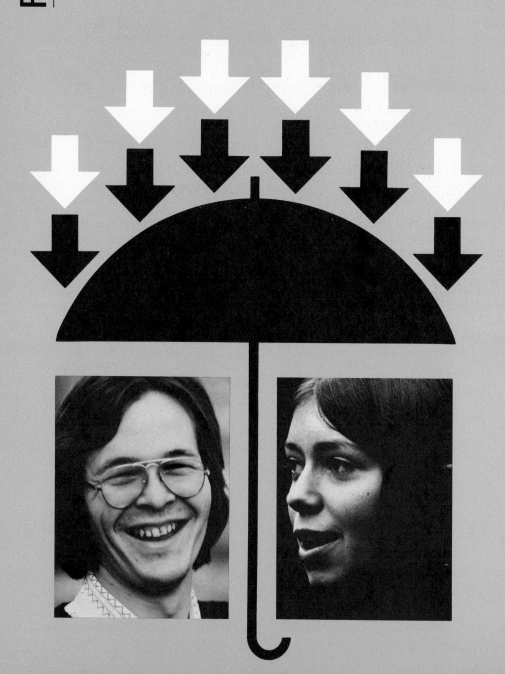

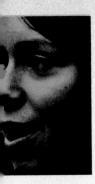

The loss of human resources is an important health problem in the United States. One of the more dramatic illustrations of such loss is the number of accidental deaths and injuries which occur each year. Accidents are ranked as the fourth most common cause of death in this country. As new medical developments combat chronic health conditions and reduce them, it is possible that accidents will have an even higher ranking in the future.

In recent years more than 115,000 persons have been killed annually by accidents. In addition, each year more than 11,000,000 persons suffer disabling injuries which restrict their usual activities for at least a full day beyond the accident. The number of accidents in which there is no personal injury or in which the injury involves less than a day of restricted activity is almost too great to calculate with reasonable accuracy.

The economic implications of accidents are staggering. Each year the loss exceeds 29 billion dollars. It includes medical and hospital fees, wage losses, insurance claims, property damage in motor vehicle accidents, property damage by fire, and production lost due to accidents which take place on the job.

Accidents also have many social implications. When the head of the family is involved in an accident, it might mean a readjustment in the lives of all the other family members. Because of a loss in the family income, the family standard of living may be lowered drastically. Injuries that result in a permanent handicap can cause serious problems of readjustment, retraining, and job replacement. All these services involve expenses for the family of the injured person or for public agencies.

What Is An Accident?

An accident is usually thought of as an unplanned act or event resulting in injury or death to persons or in damage to property. It would be better thought of as an unplanned act that *usually* results in injury or death or in damage to property. The latter definition takes into account that many accidents occur *without* injury and damage.

The key to an accident is that it was unintended or that an unplanned occurrence in a series of events triggered it. Living safely depends upon controlling both the behavior of individuals and factors in the environment so that the unintended events can't take place.

Accident Patterns

Much study and research are necessary to determine the factors affecting an accident. The following information should help you develop a perspective of the total problem.

Age-Group Variation

The types of accidental deaths and injuries vary greatly among different age groups. For people under 36 years of age, accidents are the leading cause of death. Among young people between 15 and 24 years of age, accidents claim more lives than all other causes combined, and nearly seven times more than the next leading cause.

Rates of accidental injury reach their peak among young people, with more than three out of ten injured each year. This is primarily due to the great number of motor-vehicle injuries and to injuries associated with work. The accidents may reflect the inexperience of the young people.

Accidents and Other Causes of Death in the 15–24 Age Group [1]

Cause	Number of Deaths			Death Rates [2]		
	Total	Male	Female	Total	Male	Female
All Causes	**41,140**	**29,953**	**11,187**	**124.4**	**183.5**	**66.8**
Accidents	23,012	18,480	4,532	69.6	113.2	27.1
Motor-vehicle	*16,543*	*12,911*	*3,632*	*50.0*	*79.1*	*21.7*
Homicide	3,357	2,688	669	10.1	16.5	4.0
Cancer	2,731	1,637	1,094	8.3	10.0	6.5
Suicide	2,357	1,789	568	7.1	11.0	3.4
Heart Disease	946	545	401	2.9	3.3	2.4
Pneumonia	851	492	359	2.6	3.0	2.1

[1] Source: National Center for Health Statistics.   [2] Deaths per 100,000 population.

Work injuries reach their peak in persons between 25 and 44 years of age. All other injuries have a higher incidence among those under 24 than among those over 24.

Rates of accidental death in the over-65 age group are about three times as high as those of any other age group. Older persons have more difficulty in adapting to some aspects of the changing environment. They have trouble particularly in adapting to fast-moving traffic.

Sex Variation

The accident death rate of males is greater than that of females in all age groups except the very old. Men either take greater risks or they are more susceptible to accidents. The rate of accidents among men for all ages combined is more than twice the rate of accidents for women.

The ratio of deaths between males and females in the 15–24 age group is shown in the chart on page 238. Actually four out of five accident victims in this age group are males.

Geographic Variation

There is a great variation in incidence of accidental deaths and injuries from state to state and from region to region in the United States. States west of the Mississippi River and the southeastern Gulf States have higher accident death rates than other areas in the country.

There is no single reason for these different patterns. Part of the reason may be the difference in age distribution among the populations of these states and regions. Varying types of occupation—agricultural versus industrial—may also account for some of these differences.

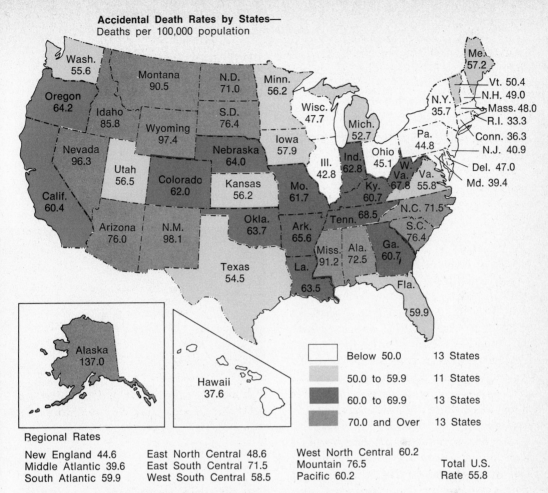

Accidental Death Rates by States—
Deaths per 100,000 population

Wash.	55.6
Montana	90.5
N.D.	71.0
Minn.	56.2
Me.	57.2
Oregon	64.2
Idaho	85.8
Wisc.	47.7
Vt.	50.4
N.H.	49.0
N.Y.	35.7
Mass.	48.0
S.D.	76.4
Wyoming	97.4
Mich.	52.7
R.I.	33.3
Nevada	96.3
Iowa	57.9
Pa.	44.8
Conn.	36.3
Nebraska	64.0
Ohio	45.1
N.J.	40.9
Utah	56.5
Ill.	42.8
Ind.	62.8
Del.	47.0
Calif.	60.4
Colorado	62.0
Kansas	56.2
Mo.	61.7
W. Va.	67.8
Va.	55.8
Md.	39.4
Ky.	60.7
Arizona	76.0
N.M.	98.1
Okla.	63.7
Ark.	65.6
Tenn.	68.5
N.C.	71.5
S.C.	76.4
Texas	54.5
La.	63.5
Miss.	91.2
Ala.	72.5
Ga.	60.7
Fla.	59.9
Alaska	137.0
Hawaii	37.6

Below 50.0 — 13 States
50.0 to 59.9 — 11 States
60.0 to 69.9 — 13 States
70.0 and Over — 13 States

Regional Rates

New England 44.6
Middle Atlantic 39.6
South Atlantic 59.9

East North Central 48.6
East South Central 71.5
West South Central 58.5

West North Central 60.2
Mountain 76.5
Pacific 60.2

Total U.S.
Rate 55.8

Figure 14-1 ● Accident death rates by states. How does your state rank?

Seasonal Variation

Accidental deaths reach their peak during the months of June, July, and August. This peak results from an increase in the number of deaths from drowning. The winter peak is in December and results from increases in motor-vehicle accidents, falls, fires, and explosions. The varying types of weather conditions seem to have an influence on the number and types of accidents that will occur.

Environmental Variation

The potential for accidents exists everywhere in our environment. Almost half of accidental deaths occur on the highways as a result of motor-vehicle accidents. Just under one fourth occur in the home; the remainder occur in places of work, places of recreation, and other public places. The percentage of home accidents has been increasing slightly in recent years; the others are decreasing slightly or staying constant.

Human Factors that Influence Accidents

Accidents occur at different rates and have different causes in different groups of the population. When characteristics of the population group that has the greatest risk for a given type of accident can be considered and identified, specific control procedures can be developed.

Age

The frequency of accidents, especially motor-vehicle accidents, is high among young people. Youth is the time when sensory perception, speed of reaction, and motor skills are at their highest. An analysis of accidents reveals that other qualities associated with youth may contribute to these higher accident rates. These qualities are inexperience, lack of judgment, and willingness to take risks. Preventive measures must therefore take these qualities into consideration.

In people of advanced age, the speed of reaction and motor skills decrease. As a result, older persons are not so efficient as younger people in carrying out a sequence of responses within a short period of time. As people grow older, their ability to organize incoming stimuli and to react decreases. The slower responses of the aged must also be considered if accidents are to be reduced.

Accident-Proneness

Recently efforts have been made to identify some individuals as "accident-prone." This term usually refers to the person who, because of inherent and persistent behavior tendencies, has accidents repeatedly.

Accident Proneness

Individual Adjustment

Emotions

Alcohol

Human Factors that Influence Accidents

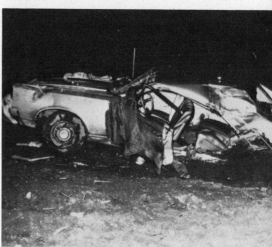

Physical Defects and Disorders

Fatigue

Drugs and Medicine

Age

Figure 14-2 ● Human factors that influence accidents. How can you control these risks of accidental injury?

Information to support this concept of accident proneness is quite limited. In fact, there is some doubt that there exists an identifiable type which could be labeled an accident-prone personality. Even if the concept of accident proneness were accepted, it would explain only a few of the cases involving a high frequency of accidents. Some people are accident-repeaters on the basis of chance alone or because they are frequently exposed to risk.

Individual and Social Adjustment

Researchers are interested in the number of accidents to the same person as a result of poor adjustment in meeting the demands of daily life. **The individual who constantly makes mistakes in meeting the personal and social obligations of life has a greater likelihood of making mistakes in situations that can lead to accidents.**

In this regard, the role of personal traits and attitudes has been under close study. One study of no-accident and high-accident drivers among military personnel indicates the two groups differ markedly in their personal traits and attitudes. Their risk-taking behavior is influenced by their attitudes toward speed, traffic regulations, competing traffic, and the actions of other drivers.

Fatigue

Research indicates that alertness, efficiency, skill, and judgment are temporarily decreased by fatigue. As a result, accidents are more likely to occur when people are fatigued.

Many studies have shown that a variety of accidents take place more frequently in the late morning and the late afternoon. These findings provide a good argument in favor of rest periods.

Fatigue is related to how long people have engaged in a particular activity. It is also related to the amount and quality of previous rest, as well as the kind of previous activity. As fatigue develops, efficiency becomes impaired. Individuals think they are doing as well as formerly, yet they are performing less skillfully, no longer recognizing or appreciating their errors.

Emotions

Much more research is needed on the relationship of emotions and accidents. It seems reasonable to assume such a relationship does exist.

When persons are emotionally upset or preoccupied, they pay less attention to what they are doing and to their surroundings. Under such conditions, they may misinterpret a situation and therefore make the wrong response, which may contribute to an accident.

Alcohol

Many substances taken for their supposedly stimulating effect or for the relief of pain may endanger safety. The effects of alcohol on human behavior have been studied extensively. It has been found that the risk of an accident when the driver has even a low level of alcohol in the blood is very great.

Alcohol affects the speed of reaction and the motor skills. It contributes to lack of judgment. This may cause a wrong response and result in an accident.

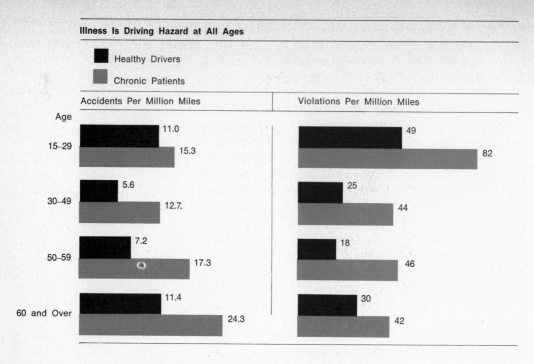

Illness Is Driving Hazard at All Ages

■ Healthy Drivers
■ Chronic Patients

	Accidents Per Million Miles	Violations Per Million Miles

Age

15–29
- Healthy Drivers: 11.0
- Chronic Patients: 15.3
- Healthy Drivers: 49
- Chronic Patients: 82

30–49
- Healthy Drivers: 5.6
- Chronic Patients: 12.7
- Healthy Drivers: 25
- Chronic Patients: 44

50–59
- Healthy Drivers: 7.2
- Chronic Patients: 17.3
- Healthy Drivers: 18
- Chronic Patients: 46

60 and Over
- Healthy Drivers: 11.4
- Chronic Patients: 24.3
- Healthy Drivers: 30
- Chronic Patients: 42

Figure 14-3 • Good health reduces your risks from accidents while driving.

Drugs and Medication

Many drugs prescribed by a physician or purchased over the counter have side effects that contribute to accidents. Unless individuals are properly instructed, they may not realize that drugs they are taking may have a sedative effect for as long as 24 hours. A drug may alter vision and equilibrium and create periods of drowsiness. In addition, certain drugs may produce a dangerous attitude of overconfidence. As a result, people may do things they would not ordinarily do.

You need to know your reactions to various drugs and medications. Take proper precautions when under their influence. This will help you avoid accidents. Avoid driving when you are taking a new medication that may have side effects of which you are not aware.

Physical Defects and Diseases

Many physical defects and diseases result in reduced alertness and perception, faulty coordination and balance, and even loss of consciousness. Individuals suffering from such ailments as epilepsy, diabetes, and multiple sclerosis, as well as amputees, run a higher risk of accidents than healthy persons do. These accidents may take place at home, at work, in school, during recreation, and on the highway.

Special measures are often required to help protect the afflicted individual and the unsuspecting public. A number of states have regulations regarding fitness to drive. In these states, "special-risk" drivers may be licensed as long as they are under continuing medical surveillance.

Many industries try to employ eligible physically handicapped persons when it can be done without undue risk to the individual and the employer. Special equipment is often installed so that these people may work without increasing the risk of accidents for themselves or others.

Home Safety

Most people consider the home a place of safety and security. Unfortunately, statistics contradict this impression. One-third of all nonfatal injuries from accidents and almost one-fourth of all fatal injuries from accidents occur in and around the home. The National Safety Council estimates that one person in 50 was disabled one or more days by injuries received in home accidents during a recent year. One-fourth of these injuries resulted in some permanent impairment.[3]

Many kinds of home accidents that occur today were unheard of a few years ago. Many modern appliances and power tools have caused injury and death when carelessly and improperly used. New drugs, household and garden sprays, paints, cleaning agents, and other chemical products have caused sickness and death when not used according to instructions.

Prevention of home accidents requires constant alertness. Be especially alert to conditions that might cause accidents.

---

[3] National Safety Council, *Accident Facts.* Chicago: National Safety Council, 1972.

Figure 14-4 ● Is your home a safe place in which to live?

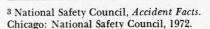

Remove Home Fire Hazards

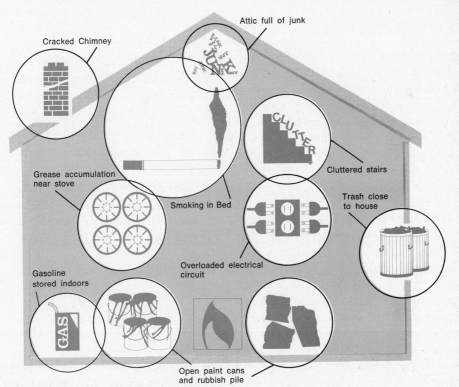

Cracked Chimney

Attic full of junk

CLUTTER

Cluttered stairs

Grease accumulation near stove

Smoking in Bed

Trash close to house

Gasoline stored indoors

Overloaded electrical circuit

Open paint cans and rubbish pile

Accidents Among Children

Nearly two-thirds of the fatal accidents to children under five years of age occur at home. Home injuries account for nearly 60 percent of all injuries to children. The high home-accident rate for this very young age group comes from their lack of experience, knowledge, and skill. The very young fail to recognize that many situations actually involve danger.

Falls cause the greatest number of injuries in this age group. However, when causes of accidental death are examined, those listed most frequently are suffocation, choking on objects caught in the windpipe, fires, and poisonings.

Children in the 5–14 age bracket have frequent accidents with guns. This is particularly true among boys. After the age of 14, vehicle accidents involving bicycles, motorcycles, and automobiles show a definite increase.

To prevent accidents to the very young, it is extremely important for parents, to "safety-condition" the environment. This means removing all possible hazards from the home. As children grow older, they must learn to take responsibility for themselves. Parents, however, should recognize that teaching safety is one of their responsibilities. The best teaching method is setting the proper example.

Accidents Among Older Persons

Old people are highly susceptible to home accidents. Nearly half of the fatal home accidents are to persons 65 years of age and older. Many of the factors associated with advancing age—poorer vision and hearing, common diseases associated with the aging process, and reduced speed of reaction and motor skills—contribute to accidents.

Preventing accidents to the very old requires an approach similar to that for the young, "safety-conditioning" the environment. In addition, older persons must be helped to realize their physical limitations and their decreased ability to carry on their former activities.

Your Responsibility

When you become a parent, you will have many responsibilities in protecting your children and teaching them to avoid accidents. More important, you will be teaching them how to behave in a safe manner.

However, there are many things you can do now. You can take the lead in your household to make sure the environment is safe. Some aspects of home safety that you should try to check regularly are:

- Are stairways and hallways well lighted?
- Are fuses the right strength?
- Are medicines properly labeled and stored out of reach of children?
- Are poisonous substances stored in their original containers and away from food?
- Are poisonous substances and prescription drugs properly disposed of after they have served their purpose?
- Do you have adequate ventilation when you use household cleaning substances and insecticides?
- Are oily rags and inflammable liquids properly stored?
- Are glass doors in your home made of safety glass?
- Are the glass doors marked by decals or other easily seen devices?
- Are power tools in proper working order? Are they stored in the right place?

- If you have a gun in the home, is it stored properly? What training in firearm safety have the household members had?

- Are gas heaters and stoves properly vented?

Home safety is everyone's responsibility. You can help your family eliminate or reduce hazards in and around the house. More important, you can help them develop sound attitudes that will enable them to live safely.

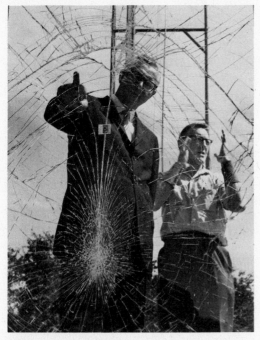

Figure 14-5 ● Scientists testing the safety features of plate glass.

Traffic Safety

The motor vehicle is both a blessing and a problem. Approximately 2 million persons are injured each year and more than 50,000 killed as a result of motor-vehicle accidents. The total number of persons killed and injured in motor-vehicle accidents constitutes almost half of the number killed and injured in all accidents per year.

An increasing number of traffic accidents are caused by motorcycles. Each year, the deaths due to motorcycle accidents increase, and one reason for great concern is that the age group most affected is between 17 and 25 years old.

A motorcycle accident is potentially much more dangerous than an automobile accident. Many of the safety features of the automobile cannot be built into the motorcycle. As a result, the behavior of the driver is of prime importance. The protective clothing worn and the judgment and skill of the driver can reduce the number of accidents, and also reduce the seriousness of the accidents.

If you are thinking of riding a motorcycle, you should be familiar with the following "Tips for Safer Cycling."[4]

- Train before you drive. Even if you can drive a car, you must learn starting, gear shifting, balance, braking, and the other operations unique for motorcycles.

- Protect your head. Always wear a helmet with goggles or face shield, whether you are a passenger or the driver.

- Keep yourself covered. Never ride with bare arms or legs. Experienced cyclists wear heavy footgear and durable types of clothing to protect themselves against cuts and scrapes.

- Keep in the left half of your lane. Then a car behind you must change lanes to pass. This is the safe procedure for both of you.

- Stop before a U-turn. Before making a U-turn, come to a full stop and look in all directions to make sure no one is coming. Then take a second look before making the turn.

---

[4] Harris E. Dark, "Your Youngster and the Motorcycle," *Today's Health,* vol. 45 (May 1967), p. 23.

- Think ahead. Allow enough space to brake safely in an emergency. At 50 miles per hour you need about 175 feet to stop. A car needs 243—so beware of the car behind you.

- Brake from back to front. Rear brake first is the rule. Then ease down gently on the front. Brake smoothly on slippery surfaces. Brake before entering curves, not after.

- Know your surfaces. You're on a two-wheeled vehicle that can suddenly skid out of control on oil spots, ice, water, wet leaves, sand, or gravel.

- Think small—you are. Remember, you can't always be seen by car drivers—especially in rear-view mirrors.

- Get "pass protection." Wait for a clear road ahead and allow plenty of margin between you and the car you pass—especially as you swing back into the right lane.

Many of the tips suggested for safe cycling can also be applied to other types of vehicles. Keep this in mind as you consider the additional factors that can influence traffic accidents. The only way to be safe is to practice safety measures at all times.

Figure 14-6 ● The driver is the most important factor in preventing accidents. What are your responsibilities when you are behind the wheel?

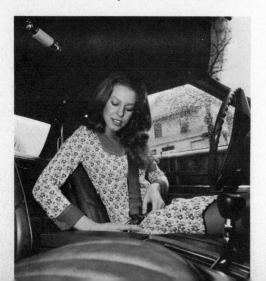

With the American family becoming more and more dependent on the use of automobiles, it is a national tragedy that so much suffering is also created in this use. For your age group, accidents are the leading cause of death, and traffic accidents are a major part of the total problem.

There are several factors that influence traffic accidents.

The Driver

The behavior of the driver is the most important single factor in preventing accidents. The driver is the one who makes judgments regarding the control of the vehicle. No matter how safe the vehicle or the road, the vehicle must be operated properly to avoid accidents.

As a driver, you have the responsibility of understanding and applying sound principles of traffic efficiency and safety. You must recognize the need for laws and regulations and abide by them. **You must accept personal responsibility for the conservation of life and health on the highways.**

The Vehicle

The condition of the motor vehicle itself is an important consideration. Too few drivers maintain their vehicles in a completely safe operating condition. Some states have automobile inspection laws to require drivers to maintain safe vehicles.

Recently, interest in the safety of the vehicle itself has reached a new high. Congressional inquiries have resulted in national regulations requiring the construction of safer vehicles. More and more attention is being paid to such items as brakes,

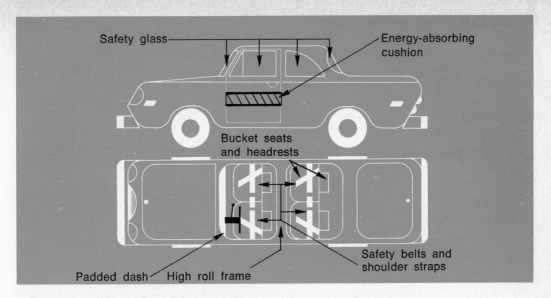

Figure 14-7 • An example of a safe automobile design. Included are: (1) high roll frame; (2) bucket seats close to the midline of the car; (3) contour of seats, headrests, and shoulder belts added to protect against impact from the side; and (4) doors with deep, energy-absorbing cushions and flexible glass. What other suggestions can you make for a safe car?

lights, steering, and tires. In addition, more emphasis is being placed upon seat belts, recessed steering-wheel posts, padded dashboards, and doors that do not open on impact.

Research has demonstrated that lap type seat belts or shoulder harnesses, when properly used, reduce injuries and save lives. They keep you from being thrown against the dashboard or out of the vehicle. Unfortunately, even when the vehicles come equipped with seat belts, not everybody uses them. To ensure your own safety when traveling in an automobile, use a seat belt or shoulder harness.

Another recent innovation that should help to reduce injury in auto accidents is to equip the car with an air bag. The air bag automatically inflates when accidents occur, to protect front-seat passengers and drivers. It is anticipated that the air bag, along with lap seat belts and shoulder harnesses, should significantly reduce accidental deaths and injury in auto accidents.

Alcohol

A major cause of traffic accidents is the use of alcohol by drivers. Even one drink affects the driving ability of many persons. Drinking has been indicated to be a factor in at least half of the fatal auto accidents, according to special studies. In more than half of such accidents, the drivers were between the ages of 20 and 34 years.

Speed

Speed is a contributing factor in a number of fatal traffic accidents. In many of these instances, the driver was violating the speed law. This does not necessarily mean that the driver was going faster than the posted limit. It can mean that the driver was going faster than was safe, whether it was 25 or 50 miles per hour, or even faster.

The severity of traffic accidents is related to speed. More injuries occur in accidents that take place at higher speeds.

Driving too slowly also contributes to the traffic hazard. This tends to encourage other drivers to proceed around the slowly moving vehicle, thereby increasing the risk of an accident.

Traffic accidents occur more frequently at night than during the daytime. At night the problem of reduced visibility and headlight glare is added to fatigue and drowsiness. The situation is further complicated by driving at speeds which are inappropriate for the conditions of visibility and alertness.

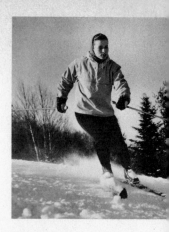

Roads

Unfortunately, many of the roads in use today were not constructed to serve the amount of traffic they currently carry. This problem is of great concern to the local, state, and national governments. Great sums of money are being spent on planning better driving conditions and correcting faulty conditions. There is special interest in constructing roads that would be less hazardous under conditions of rain, snow, and ice.

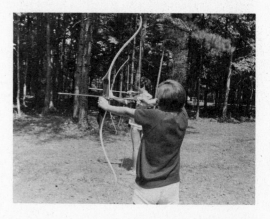

Recreational Safety

The tremendous increase in outdoor recreation emphasizes the need to have fun safely. **Developing skills, staying within the limits of your ability, and avoiding hazardous conditions can add to your enjoyment of recreational activity.**

Safe Boating

Not too many years ago, boating was engaged in only by the wealthy. Today, more than 40 million persons take part in some type of boating recreation. Unfortunately, there are many accidents because of failure to practice commonsense rules of boat handling.

If you are interested in boating, learn how to handle a boat properly. Make sure the boat is in good repair. In addition, become familiar with the rules and regulations that must be followed on the water. Obey these rules at all times. This is just as important as following rules and regulations for operating a motor vehicle. You should also become familiar with and use all the safety equipment available on boats.

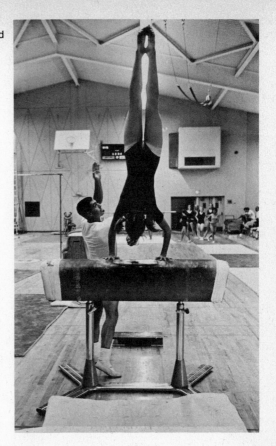

Figure 14-8 ● Increase your enjoyment from recreational activities by taking recommended safety precautions.

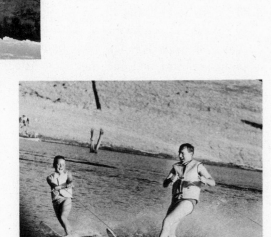

Swimming Safety

More and more people are enjoying swimming activities today. Public swimming pools, streams, rivers, lakes, and the oceans are being increasingly used for a variety of water sports. In addition, private swimming pools have added to the number of persons who swim daily.

New water and swimming activities are becoming popular. More and more people are water skiing, skin and scuba diving, and surfing. To reduce the risk of accidents in all of these activities, it is important for you to develop skill, to use proper equipment, and to know and obey safety rules. Above all, while enjoying the water you should be alert to the potential danger of water activities.

Firearm Safety

Hunting, target shooting, and other forms of recreation in which firearms are used require instruction, education, and constant safe practices and procedures. The potential danger in these activities is widely recognized. Even so, many needless deaths occur.

More firearm accidents can be avoided if you repeat the following precautions so that they become automatic:

- Keep a gun unloaded when it is not in use.
- Always keep a gun pointed away from people.
- Keep the "safety" on when the gun is not pointed at a target.

Safety in Competitive Sports

Injury due to competitive sports can be avoided if the following precautions are taken:

- Compulsory physical examinations will eliminate those who are physically unfit for certain types of athletic competition. These individuals can be counseled to go into other types of activity.

- Conditioning programs are of extreme importance in preventing injuries which might result from muscular weakness, fatigue, and lack of endurance.

- Protective equipment should be worn when indicated. Good protective equipment is now available for most contact sports. It is important that such equipment be properly fitted and used.

- Whatever the game, the rules for playing it must be followed. Rules help reduce injury.

Medical Self-Help

You should be prepared to meet emergency health needs when professional medical care is not available. It should be understood that such **emergency assistance is only temporary aid to the sick and injured until such time as a physician's services can be obtained.**

The Division of Emergency Health Services of the Public Health Service, Department of Health, Education, and Welfare, and the Office of Civil Defense, Department of Defense have prepared a medical self-help guide to help you meet emergency health needs. The following selected emergency care procedures are adapted from this guide, *Family Emergency Health Care.* In each procedure things to do and, in some cases, things not to do are presented.

Artificial Respiration

What to Do

Mouth-to-Mouth Method

1. Place the person who has stopped breathing in a prone position, face up.
2. Clear the mouth and throat completely to ensure an open airway to the lungs.
3. Tilt the head back so that the chin points upward and lift the lower jaw from beneath and behind so that it juts out.
4. Start artificial respiration immediately. The most important lifesaving action is to get air into the person's lungs through either the mouth or the nose. Open your mouth wide and place it tightly over the person's mouth. Pinch the nose shut. Or close the victim's mouth and place your mouth over the victim's nose. With an infant or small child, place your mouth over both the nose and mouth, making an airproof seal.

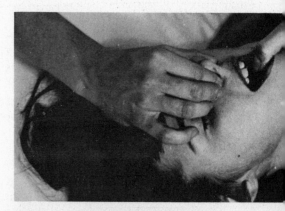

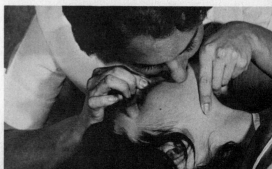

5. Blow into the mouth or nose, continuing to hold the unconscious person's lower jaw so that it juts out, to keep the air passage open.

6. Remove your mouth from the patient's mouth. Turn your head to the side and listen for the return of outflowing air coming from the patient's lungs. If you hear it, you will know that an exchange of air has occurred.

7. You can then continue your breathing for the patient. Blow vigorously into the mouth or nose 12 times a minute for an adult and about 20 times a minute for an infant.

8. If you are not getting an exchange of air, turn the person on the side and strike the person several times between the shoulder blades. This will help to dislodge any obstruction in the air passage.

9. Normal breathing may start any time. If it does not you should continue the artificial respiration until you are positive life is gone.

The Chest Pressure-Arm Lift (Silvester) Method [5]

If there is foreign matter visible in the mouth, wipe it out quickly with your fingers or a cloth wrapped around your fingers.

1. Place the victim in a face-up position and put something under the shoulders to raise them and allow the head to drop backward.

2. Kneel at the victim's head, grasp the arms at the wrists, cross them, and press them over the lower chest. This should cause air to flow out.

3. Immediately release this pressure and pull the arms outward and upward over the head and backward as far as possible. This should cause air to rush in.

4. Repeat this cycle about 12 times per minute, checking the mouth frequently for obstructions.

When the victim is in a face-up position, there is always danger of aspiration of vomitus, blood, or blood clots. This hazard can be reduced by keeping the head extended and turned to one side. If possible, the head should be a little lower than the trunk. If a second rescuer is available, have that person hold the victim's head so that the jaw is jutting out. The helper should be alert to detect the presence of any stomach contents in the mouth and keep the mouth as clean as possible at all times. This procedure is very important.

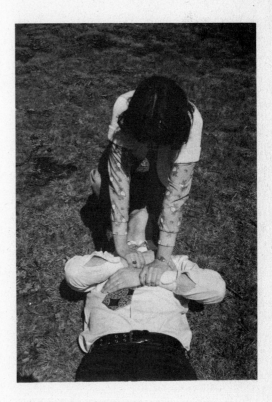

[5] Material on this method is from *First Aid Textbook,* copyright © 1933, 1937, 1945, 1957 by The American National Red Cross. Adapted from this source by permission.

Bleeding and Bandaging

What to Do

1. Apply a dressing or pad directly over the wound.
2. Apply direct even pressure. Use your bare hand, if necessary, when the bleeding is serious and a dressing is not immediately available.
3. Do not disturb the dressing.
4. Continue pressure by applying a bandage.
5. Secure the bandage in place. Check to be sure the bandage is not tight and cutting off circulation.
6. Elevate the limb above heart level, except where there is a possible broken bone.
7. Treat the patient for shock.
8. If blood soaks through the dressing, do not remove it but apply more dressings.
9. Do not use a tourniquet unless it is impossible to stop excessive bleeding by any other method.

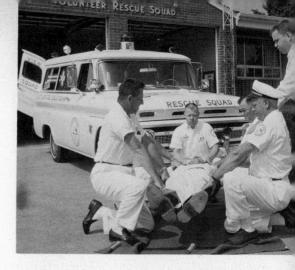

3. Give complete emergency treatment before moving the injured person.
4. Be gentle in moving the patient. Have enough help to assure safe moving.
5. Always carry a stretcher to an injured person, not the person to the stretcher.
6. Always use a stretcher for seriously injured persons and also for transporting the injured over a long distance.
7. Be sure the injured person will not slip or fall from the stretcher while being carried.
8. Always use a two-man carry in preference to a one-man carry, if a hand carry is used.

Transportation of the Injured

What to Do

1. Before transporting any sick or injured person:
   a. Stop all bleeding.
   b. Be sure the patient is breathing.
   c. Splint the fractures.
   d. Treat for shock.
   e. Complete all other lifesaving methods.
2. Determine carefully the type and seriousness of the injuries and the condition of the injured person.

Shock

What to Do

1. Keep the patient lying down.
2. Keep the head lower than the legs and hips, if there is no evidence of chest or head injury.
3. Have the head and shoulders slightly raised, if it is a chest or head injury or if there is difficulty in breathing.

4. Keep the patient from chilling.

5. Encourage the patient to drink if the patient is conscious.

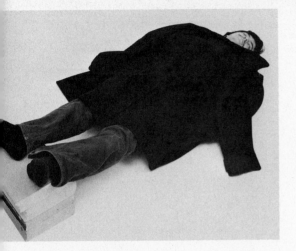

What Not to Do

1. Never attempt to give fluids to an unconscious person.

2. Never use alcoholic beverages as a stimulant. Shock may cause death if not properly treated.

Burns

What to Do

1. Treat the patient for shock.

2. Relieve pain.

3. Prevent infection from starting.

4. Cover the burned area with a dry sterile or clean cloth.

5. Encourage the intake of fluids to replace the fluids lost from the body.

6. Give the patient a salt and soda solution to drink (one teaspoonful of salt and one-half teaspoonful of soda to a quart of water).

What Not to Do

1. Do not pull clothing off the burned area.

2. Do not remove pieces of cloth that stick to the burn.

3. Do not try to clean the burn.

4. Do not break the blisters.

5. Do not use grease, ointment, petroleum jelly, or any type of medication on severe burns.

6. Do not use iodine or any other antiseptic on burns.

7. Do not change dressings that were initially applied until absolutely necessary. The dressings may be left in place five to seven days.

Poisoning

What to Do

1. Administer first aid immediately: minutes count. The aim is to dilute and remove the poison, and to help the body fight the poison. If possible, neutralize the poison by giving an antidote. However, there are but few effective antidotes and they are not generally available.

2. Quickly administer water in large amounts—four glassfuls or more for adults. Do not attempt to give fluids to an unconscious person.

3. Call a physician or your local Poison Control Center. If indicated by them, try to remove the poison from the patient's stomach immediately by inducing vomiting (except in those cases described below).

4. If you can find the package from which the poison came, you may find its antidote on the label. If available, use the antidote as directed.

First Aid for Poisoning

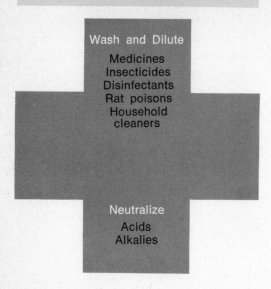

Wash and Dilute

Medicines
Insecticides
Disinfectants
Rat poisons
Household
cleaners

Neutralize

Acids
Alkalies

5. Unless the poison was a sedative (such as an overdose of sleeping tablets), have the patient lie down after vomiting several times. Keep the patient warm and quiet.

6. However, if the poison was a sedative, keep the patient awake by talking and encouraging the patient to walk about. Give the patient several cups of black coffee every two hours until the condition improves.

Special Procedures for Special Poisons

Acids: Dilute quickly with a glass of water and then give milk of magnesia. Several glassfuls may be given, but do not induce vomiting. Then give milk, olive oil, or egg white to protect the membranes of the digestive tract.

Alkalis: Give a glass of water quickly, then vinegar or lemon juice in the diluting fluid to neutralize the alkali. Follow this with milk, olive oil, or egg white. Do not induce vomiting.

Unconsciousness

What to Do

1. A person who is feverish and flushed, and has a strong, slow pulse should lie down with the head slightly raised above the level of the body. Apply cold wet cloths to the head. If breathing stops, start artificial respiration.

2. A person who has lost color, is cold and clammy to the touch, and has a weak pulse should lie down with the head slightly lower than the rest of the body. If available, hold aromatic spirits of ammonia under the nose (except where a head injury is suspected). If breathing stops, start artificial respiration.

3. A person who has a bluish face, weak pulse, and irregular breathing should lie down and be kept warm. If breathing stops, start artificial respiration.

What Not to Do

1. Do not give the patient a stimulant, food or drink.

2. Do not move the patient, except to move out of danger.

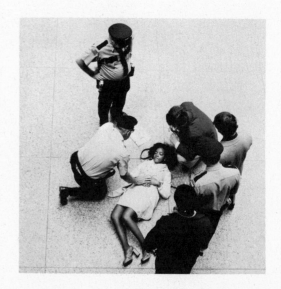

One Final Word

These selected medical self-help suggestions are not intended as a substitute for professional medical care. They are intended only to help maintain health and alleviate suffering during any period of disaster or emergency when professional care and normal services are not available. After giving aid, be sure to take the individual to a hospital or call a doctor.

What You Can Do

To live safely you must be able to adjust to new situations day after day and year after year. You must be able to adapt to your physical surroundings and to the people around you. Make a conscious effort to acquire personal traits that will enable you to lead a safe, productive, and enjoyable life:

- **Knowledge.** Develop a knowledge of the particular hazards in various life situations and of the preventive action to take to avoid these hazards.
- **Practice.** Follow accepted safety practices. Constantly evaluate what you are doing.
- **Skill.** Develop the skills required for the activities in which you wish to engage. Once you have developed these skills, maintain them by constant practice.
- **Attitudes.** Develop desirable attitudes, such as alertness, observation, caution, thoughtfulness, regard for the safety of others, respect for rules, patience, and pride in behaving safely.

Summary

The annual loss of human resources because of accidental death or injury has both social and economic implications.

There are a number of human factors affecting the occurrence of an accident. These include age, accident proneness, degree of respect for others, fatigue, emotions, alcohol, drugs and other medications, and physical defects and disease.

The home is usually considered a place of safety. Unfortunately, a significant number of injuries and deaths due to accidents take place in and around the home.

The motor vehicle, while important to people, injures millions of persons each year. Increased interest and participation in outdoor recreation has resulted in more accidents associated with boating, water sports, firearms, and competitive sports.

To live safely, you must be able to adapt to new situations to prevent accidents. This means you should acquire traits that will enable you to live a safe, productive, and enjoyable life. When emergency situations arise, you should be prepared to meet these emergencies and act promptly to reduce serious damage to health.

in making health decisions . . .

Understand These Terms:

accident
accident proneness
antidote
medical self-help
medical surveillance

"safety-conditioning" the
  environment
shock
suffocation

Solve This Problem:

Thomas Crawford is a high-school graduate who took many classes in industrial arts when he was in school. He has been working in an industrial manufacturing plant during the year since his graduation. He has become interested in industrial safety. What type of job opportunities might be available to him? What preparation would he need for them? What special skills would he need to develop? After you have answered these questions, refer to Chapter 16 for more information.

Try These Activities:

1. Survey your home for safety hazards. Based upon this survey, develop a plan for making your home a safer place in which to live. Include the role of all family members for maintaining safety.

2. What are the special skills needed and safety precautions that should be followed in your favorite recreational activity? Select an activity that you might want to learn. What special skills are necessary and what safety precautions are associated with it?

3. Analyze an accident to understand its causes and how it might have been prevented. Choose any accident you are familiar with and follow these steps:
   a. Learn all you can about the safety factors of the agent (the car, equipment, or tool that was involved in the accident).
   b. Study the actions of the host (the victim involved in the accident).
   c. Analyze the environment (the physical conditions surrounding the accident, such as weather, time of day, road conditions if it is an automobile accident, etc.).

   Now give your opinion of what caused the accident. What precautions, if followed, would have prevented the accident?

Interpret These Concepts:

1. The individual who constantly makes mistakes in meeting the personal and social obligations of life has a greater likelihood of making mistakes in situations that can lead to accidents.

2. Developing skills, staying within the limits of your ability, and avoiding hazardous conditions can add to your enjoyment of recreational activity.

3 The potential for accidents exists everywhere in our environment.

4 Emergency assistance is only temporary aid to the sick and injured until such time as a physician's services can be obtained.

Explore These Readings:

Accident Facts. Chicago: National Safety Council, annual.

Hafen, Brent Q., Alton L. Thygerson, and R. Peterson, eds., *First Aid: Contemporary Practices and Principles.* Minneapolis: Burgess Publishing Co., 1972.

Kelly, John, "Avoid the 50 Most Common Winter Accidents," *Family Health,* Vol. IV (December, 1972), pp. 15–16.

"Product Hazards: What Can Be Done About Them," *Consumer Reports,* September 1970, pp. 559–564.

Thygerson, Alton L., *Safety: Principles, Instruction, and Readings.* Englewood Cliffs, N. J.: Prentice-Hall, Inc., 1972.

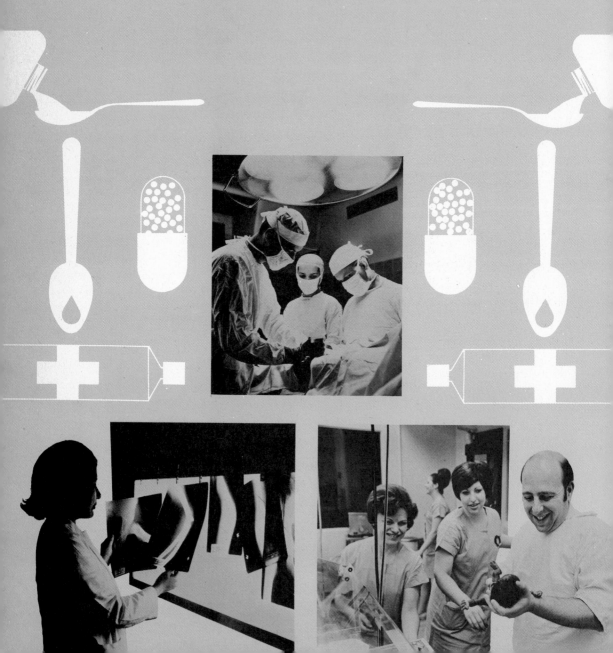

Fifteen

Selecting Medical Products and Services

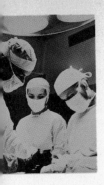

During your lifetime, we have had available to us more and better medical care than at any other time in history. This improvement in medical care is linked with dramatic advances in medical science, along with better methods of sanitation, increased levels of nutrition, and higher standards of medical practice.

Still, there has been a growing awareness in the United States by a large section of the population, including the President, that we are facing a crisis in our health-care system. The crisis is the result of a variety of factors which include the high cost of medical care and the fact that medical care is not available to all citizens. There is much speculation as to what type of reform will take place to meet our changing health-care needs. Some of these plans, including public and private health-insurance plans, will be discussed later in this chapter.

In the meantime, it is necessary to take advantage of those products and services which are available today. You should have some knowledge about health and hospitalization insurance programs. You need to understand the differences among the various practitioners identified by the title "Doctor." It is important that you understand what quacks are and what methods they use. You should also have some insight into the differences between "ethical" and "proprietary" drugs.

Ethical drugs are dispensed by prescription only. They are advertised only in professional journals read by the medical profession. Proprietary drugs (formerly called patent medicines) are sold in pharmacies, supermarkets, and other stores without prescription, and are advertised to the public via newspapers, magazines, radio, television, outdoor advertising, and promotional mail.

Selecting Health Products

Oliver Wendell Holmes, the physician and author, once suggested that if all the medicine in the world were thrown into the sea, it would be so much better for humanity, and so much worse for the fish. This might have been true in the era of patent medicines, but it certainly is not true today. It is estimated that three million people are alive today in the United States only because of the medications developed during recent years. **When properly prescribed by a physician, modern tested medications are a great boon to humanity.**

Self-Medication

You have probably heard the saying "He who treats himself has a fool for a patient and an even greater fool for a physician." Old as this saying is, it is still true. Self-medication may indeed be dangerous.

At least one-third of the people in the United States do not consult a physician even for an annual medical checkup. Usually this does not indicate good health, but rather that these people are trying to care for their ailments themselves.

Certainly there are a number of nonprescription medicines that you can use safely by properly following the directions printed on the label. You probably have a number of these in your medicine chest—aspirin, for one. That same medicine chest probably contains many items that are potentially hazardous. These items include high-potency pain relievers, tranquilizers, antihistamines, amphetamines (energizers), liver pills, stomach pills, and vitamins, among others. The indiscriminate use of any of these products may be harmful.

What may the presence of these nonprescription items indicate? Have you treated yourself for conditions that should have been diagnosed and treated by a physician?

There are two real dangers in self-treatment. First, it is possible that you will cover up symptoms of a more serious disorder than the one you recognize and treat. Second, although you may correctly diagnose your ailment, there is the chance that you will treat it inadequately with nonprescription drugs. Conditions such as persistent headaches, coughs, and stomach cramps should be called to the attention of your physician. **When any symptom persists, you should see a physician to get the proper diagnosis and treatment.**

The tremendous volume of advertising of proprietary drugs has helped create many of the problems associated with self-medication. Research by the medical profession and the Federal Food and Drug Administration has contradicted the claims made by many advertisements. The studies concerning the relative merits of highly advertised aspirin products are a good illustration of this issue. A comparison of five brands of aspirin showed that the highly advertised brands, which were usually higher in price, were no more effective than the unadvertised brands. Cough and cold remedies are other products that are often misrepresented in advertising. Recently, 16 different manufacturers of cold products were named by the Federal Trade Commission for improper advertising.

If you want to be an intelligent consumer, you should evaluate advertising appeals, such as "There is no better product on the market than ours." This may be true —but there may be a dozen others just as good. Compare labels, where standards are listed, and compare prices. Careful attention to advertising claims will help you make a better choice. Figure 15-2 will help you understand what to look for on a label.

Figure 15-1 • Americans spend about two billion dollars a year on nonprescription drugs. Which of these drugs are really necessary?

Contents of the $2-Billion Medicine Chest

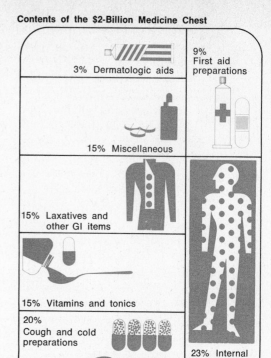

3% Dermatologic aids

9% First aid preparations

15% Miscellaneous

15% Laxatives and other GI items

15% Vitamins and tonics

20% Cough and cold preparations

23% Internal analgesics and other CNS* drugs

* Central Nervous System

The Modern Prescription Drugs

Ethical (prescribed) medicines have been very effective in treating illness. However, some problems have arisen in connection with their use. To care for your health and have confidence in the medication prescribed by your doctor, you should know the nature of modern drugs and some of the problems connected with their use.

Many of the drugs marketed today have been developed from new ingredients. Approximately 90 percent of the ingredients now in use were not known prior to 1950. In addition, many modern drugs are used for only two to five years and are then replaced by still newer drugs.

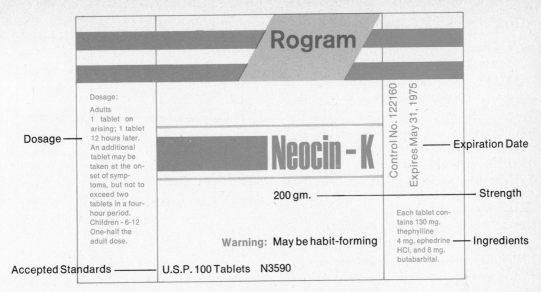

Dosage

Dosage:
Adults
1 tablet on
arising; 1 tablet
12 hours later.
An additional
tablet may be
taken at the on-
set of symp-
toms, but not to
exceed two
tablets in a four-
hour period.
Children - 6-12
One-half the
adult dose.

Rogram

Neocin - K

Control No. 122160
Expires May 31, 1975

Expiration Date

200 gm.

Strength

Each tablet con-
tains 130 mg.
thephylline
4 mg. ephedrine
HCl, and 8 mg.
butabarbital.

Ingredients

Warning: May be habit-forming

Accepted Standards

U.S.P. 100 Tablets   N3590

Figure 15-2 • Important information to check in purchasing a medical product.

It is extremely important that new drugs be adequately tested before they are made available for human consumption. **Nearly all drugs have some side effects.** Some side effects are of a minor nature, while others pose serious problems. It is the responsibility of the Federal Food and Drug Administration (a division of the Department of Health, Education, and Welfare) to carry out the proper testing of drugs to protect your health. Until recent years, the Food and Drug Administration was handicapped in providing this protection because the laws governing drug safety were not adequate.

The Importance of Safeguards. The importance of safeguards in permitting the use of new drugs was illustrated dramatically in the early 1960's, when a tranquilizer called thalidomide came into wide use in several countries. Originally used in Germany as a "harmless soother" for fretful babies, it came to be prescribed in some countries as a sleeping pill for women in the early stages of pregnancy.

Unfortunately, not enough research had been done on its possible side effects on human beings. An alert research physician in the Federal Food and Drug Administration, Dr. Frances O. Kelsey, while testing the drug before releasing it as safe for use in the United States, developed serious doubts as to its "harmlessness" and withheld approval. This prevented the drug from being distributed in the United States.

In the meantime, in various countries there appeared case after case of infants without fully developed arms and legs, born to women who had used the drug. It appears that the drug had a tendency to prevent proper development of the fetus. The growing number of "thalidomide babies" caused serious international concern.

This concern helped bring about new legislation in the United States concerning the release of new drugs. The Kefauver-Harris Law, also known as the Drug Amendments Act of 1962, requires that a drug manufacturer test his product and prove not only that it is safe but also that it is effective for the purpose for which it is intended. This law gives the FDA authority to withdraw a drug from the market if it does not meet these standards. Such regulations protect the consumer from dangerous or worthless drugs.

Demands of Patients. Another problem arising from the use of modern drugs is the patient's expectations. Many people feel neglected if their doctor does not write a prescription when they are ill. They may even become angry. As a result, they put pressure on the physician to prescribe something. Some physicians will appease such patients by writing a prescription. This is usually done to avoid an emotional problem, rather than to cure a physical disease. Thus many unneeded prescriptions are written every year.

Figure 15-3 • Before drugs are released for human consumption, they undergo rigorous tests.

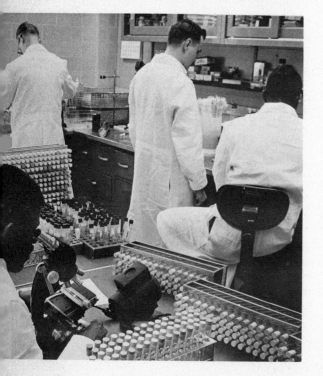

You should develop confidence in your physician and not demand a prescription your physician considers unnecessary. Physicians are able to make the proper decisions for your treatment. You are purchasing their services because they are qualified to make medical decisions. Allow them to do so.

High Cost of Drugs. Still another problem resulting from the use of modern drugs is cost. It has been estimated that American consumers spend more than a billion dollars a year unnecessarily for prescription drugs. There is a price markup of 200 percent on some highly advertised products. To counteract this, officials in New York City passed legislation requiring pharmacies to post prices of certain prescription drugs. Such action helps the consumer become a selective buyer.

Dangers of Indiscriminate Use of Drugs. Leftover drugs are a potential health hazard. Once a prescribed drug has been used for a specific ailment, it should never be reused at some other time without consulting a physician.

Improper use of an antibiotic, for example, may cause one to develop a tolerance for that drug, so that it becomes ineffective in combating illness.

In some instances, reused drugs may be hazardous because they have increased in potency. In other instances, the drug may be contaminated.

How to Select Health Products Safely

Great care must be exercised in the selection of health products. When you are selecting health products, be sure to remember the following rules:

■ Disregard high-powered advertising.

- Study the label for ingredients and directions for use.
- Follow the recommendations of your physician.

You can have the advantages of modern drugs without spending a great deal of money, if you use good judgment. Follow your physician's instructions carefully and be discriminating in your use of nonprescription drugs.

Selecting Health Services

Selecting competent physicians and dentists and utilizing adequate services requires some knowledge on your part. Your life may at one time or another rest in the hands of those you choose.

How to Choose a Doctor

It is a good idea to have a personal physician who can take care of most of your ailments. Such a person will help you get the services of a competent specialist when you need one. This is much better than selecting a specialist on your own.

If you or your parents are in the position of having to find a doctor, the following recommendations should be helpful to you:

- Ask people you trust and respect to give you the name of a doctor. If you are new to a community and do not know anyone, ask the secretary of the local medical society to supply the names of several physicians who practice in your immediate neighborhood.
- Look up the doctor's professional background in the American Medical Direc-

tory, which is available in most public libraries. This directory will provide you with information regarding each doctor's medical training, specialty, medical society memberships, and any teaching affiliations the doctor may have.

- If there is an emergency and you cannot reach your doctor or you are in a strange community, telephone the medical emergency call service. If this service is not available, get help from the telephone operator, the local hospital, or the police.

Help the physician you choose by giving all the information that will be needed. Follow the physician's advice. If you are in doubt about what you are supposed to do, ask your doctor for clarification. If you are not satisfied with the services you receive, choose another doctor. **You should have a doctor who takes an interest in you and in whom you have complete confidence.**

Figure 15-4 • *The American Medical Directory* is a valuable resource for information on the medical qualifications of physicians. Check the meaning of the code numbers listed after the doctor's name.

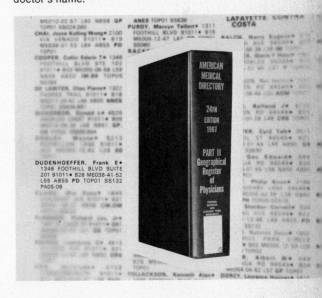

Medical practice has changed greatly during the past few decades. The change has been necessary to meet the ever-increasing volume of patients and to keep abreast of scientific and technological advances. Because of these advances, there has been a trend in medicine toward more and more specialization. When you consider the new discoveries in diagnostic equipment, drugs, and treatments, it becomes clear why specialization has advanced. The specialties are described in Figure 15-5.

The "old family doctor" seems to be disappearing. The general practitioner is being replaced by either the specialist in general practice or by the diagnostician or internist (specialist in internal medicine). This is a person who is skilled in diagnosing illness. Experience has shown that the internist can handle most of the problems patients present. When the internist recognizes an illness requiring the attention of another specialist, an appropriate referral can be made. Consulting this type of physician is much better than selecting specialists on your own. Such an individual will be more likely to treat you as a total person and be concerned with your total health. The specialist is more likely to be concerned with one specific part of the body.

Other Practitioners

You have thus far considered the M. D. (medical doctor). There are several other groups of practitioners, with whose preparation and training you should be familiar, as well as with the services they render.

Doctor of Dental Surgery (D.D.S.)

The art and science of oral health is the concern of the dentist. Professional training qualifies the dentist to treat the diseases of the teeth, jaws, and gums. In addition, the dentist is concerned with promoting oral health as a part of total health.

While not all dental schools require four years of college as a prerequisite to admission, many applicants to these schools do hold bachelor's degrees.

There are now approximately 50 dental schools in the United States. These schools provide training in the fundamental sciences, as well as in dental science and procedures, and also provide practical experience in clinics. They also offer opportunities for research and for postgraduate work.

There are specialists in dentistry who have undergone training similar to that of medical specialists. Some of these specialists are included in the following list.

- **Orthodontist**—concerned with the diagnosis and treatment of irregularities and poor alignment of the teeth
- **Periodontist**—specializing in the prevention and treatment of diseases of the supporting tissues of the teeth
- **Prosthodontist**—concerned with providing artificial replacements for missing natural teeth and/or supporting structures
- **Endodontist**—specializing in the diagnosis and treatment of diseases of the pulp chamber and pulp canals
- **Oral Pathologist**—concerned with the study of disease processes of the hard and soft tissues of the oral cavity.
- **Oral Surgeon**—specializing in surgery dealing with diseases, injuries, and defects of the mouth, the jaws, and associated structures
- **Pedodontist**—concerned with the prevention, detection, and treatment of dental disorders of children

Before an individual can practice dentistry in a state, state board examinations must be completed successfully.

Optometrist (O.D.)

Optometrists (O.D.) are trained to measure visual acuity, to fit glasses, and to give instruction regarding practices that will help preserve vision. They are concerned with visual development in the growing child and the prevention, as well as correction, of visual problems. Although optometrists do not treat diseases of the eye, they are trained to detect these problems. If they detect a disease, they then refer the individual to an ophthalmologist who specializes in the treatment of such diseases. All states now require optometrists to be licensed to practice optometry. To be eligible to take a state examination, an individual must be a graduate in optometry from an accredited school or college of optometry.

All the accredited colleges of optometry in the United States require a six-year curriculum which includes two years of pre-optometry education at an accredited college and four years at a school of optometry.

Opticians complete the team of optical specialists. They are skilled in grinding lenses according to the prescription written by the optometrist or ophthalmologist. They are generally not qualified to examine eyes.

Doctor of Osteopathy (D.O.)

Osteopathy is the healing art in which the trained practitioner is most nearly like the M.D. Osteopathic physicians use generally accepted physical, medical, and surgical methods of diagnosis and therapy. However, they place much more emphasis on body mechanics and manipulation of the bone structure as a means of detecting and correcting ill health.

The preparation of the osteopathic physician includes at least three years of college plus four years at an osteopathic college and one year of internship. Three-fourths of all osteopathic physicians complete a four-year college program before beginning their medical preparation. The student can also prepare for one of the osteopathic specialties by serving terms of residency and special practice.

The D.O. is licensed to practice in all 50 states and the District of Columbia. Forty-one states and the District of Columbia grant the D.O. unlimited practice rights.

Recently there has been increased recognition of osteopathy as a healing art. This was aided by a decision in California to grant the M.D. degree to osteopaths who met the preparation standards for the degree. This action may start a trend toward combining medicine and osteopathy throughout the country.

Doctor of Podiatry (Pod.D.) or Chiropody (D.S.C.)

Podiatry, or chiropody as it was formerly known, is the prevention and treatment of disorders of the feet. Care is given by medical, mechanical, and surgical means. Podiatrists also treat skin ailments such as athlete's foot, papillomas (benign growths on the skin such as warts and moles), and diabetic and varicose ulcers. They advise patients on preventive measures in foot health such as proper exercise and care of the feet and, when appropriate, they prescribe corrective shoes.

Medical Specialists

Specialists in these fields supplement the work of the family physician

Figure 15-5 • Medical specialists your doctor may recommend.

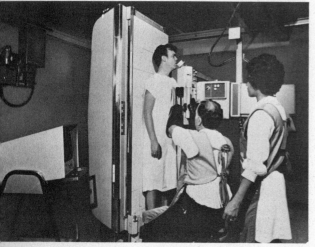

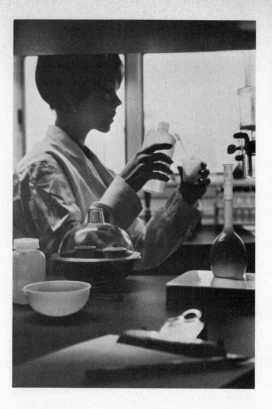

Internal Medicine

The internist diagnoses and treats diseases of the inner organs. Other specialists in internal medicine include cardiologists (heart), allergists, gastroenterologists, etc.

Pathology

A pathologist uses laboratory tests to diagnose and aid in the treatment of disease.

Orthopedic Surgery

The orthopedic surgeon is concerned with the corrective treatment of diseases and deformities of bones, muscles, and joints.

Anesthesiology

The anesthesiologist gives local and general anesthetics.

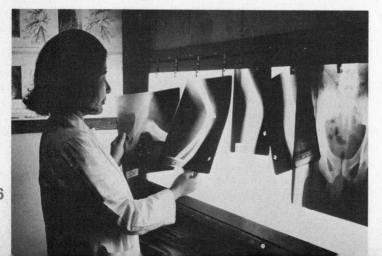

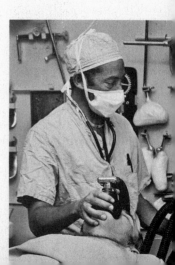

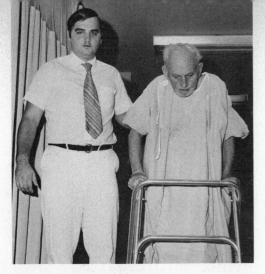

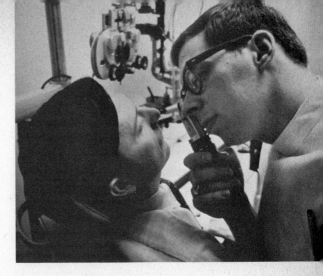

Physical Medicine and Rehabilitation

This specialist deals with the diagnosis and treatment of disease and disability through physical means (electricity, radiation, heat, cold).

Ophthalmology

The ophthalmologist examines and treats the human eye to maintain and improve sight.

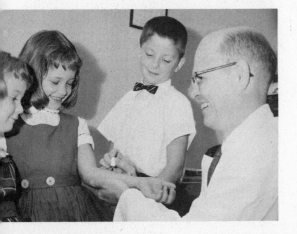

Pediatrics

The pediatrician specializes in preventing and treating diseases in children and adolescents.

Dermatology and Syphilology

The dermatologist and syphilologist deals with diseases of the skin (including hair and nails) and syphilis.

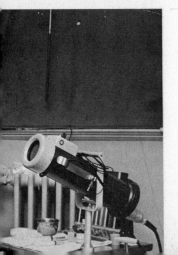

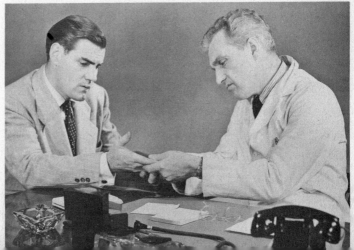

Preventive Medicine

Doctors in this field work to prevent the occurrence of disease through scientific methods such as vaccination, etc.

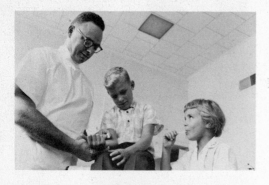

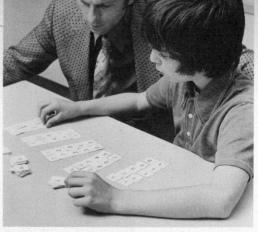

Psychiatry and Neurology

The psychiatrist specializes in the treatment of emotional and mental disorders. The neurologist specializes in organic disorders of the nervous system.

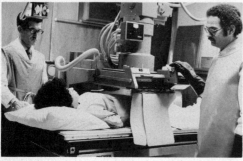

Radiology

The radiologist uses X rays for diagnostic and therapeutic treatment and gives radium treatments. Radiology includes nuclear medicine.

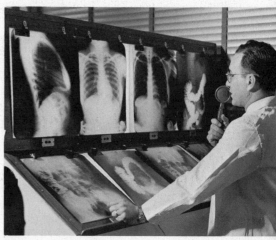

Proctology

The proctologist deals with the diseases of the anus, rectum, and sigmoid colon.

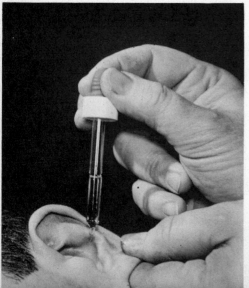

Otorhinolaryngology

This specialist is concerned with the ear, throat, windpipe, upper trachea (larynx), and the nose.

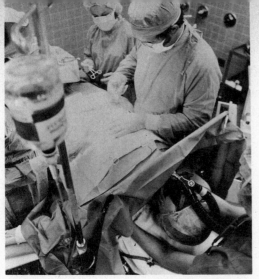

Surgery

The surgeon diagnoses and treats diseases and injuries and performs operations when they are needed.

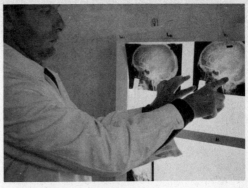

Neurological Surgery

The neurological surgeon performs surgery of the brain and nervous system.

Obstetrics and Gynecology

The obstetrician cares for women before, during, and after childbirth. The gynecologist specializes in women's diseases in general.

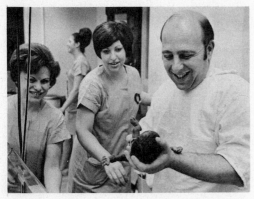

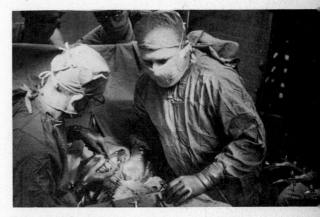

Plastic Surgery

A plastic surgeon repairs or builds up lost or injured tissue, restores parts, and repairs deformities.

Thoracic Surgery

The thoracic surgeon diagnoses and treats diseases of the chest and performs surgery in this area.

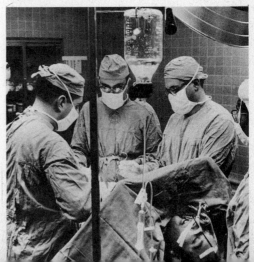

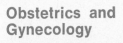

269

All schools of podiatry require a minimum of two years of college work for entrance to their four-year course. The course requires a total of 4,276 clock hours of instruction in the classroom, laboratory, and clinic.

All states require podiatrists to pass an examination before they are licensed to practice. Some states also require a clinical internship after the individual has completed four years of study.

The podiatrist is trained to detect general symptoms of disease that occur in the feet. These may include such problems as heart disease, diabetes, and kidney disorders. In such situations, the podiatrist refers the individual to the family physician for treatment.

Doctor of Chiropractic (D.C.)

Chiropractic is a nonmedical approach to healing. It is based on the belief that the nervous system controls all other systems of the body, and that disease is caused by improper or abnormal nerve function; therefore, the treatment of illness is the proper alignment of the body structures to relieve pinching of the spinal nerves. The primary function of the chiropractor is to manipulate and adjust body structures such as the spinal column, to correct the condition.

Other approaches used by the chiropractor include nutritional guidance and emotional counseling.

Doctors of chiropractic do not have the same educational standards as osteopaths and medical doctors. However, their standards are being raised. All schools of chiropractic require high school graduation as an entrance requirement. A recent trend is to require two years of college as a prerequisite for admission.

The training programs in the schools of chiropractic vary. Chiropractors are licensed to practice in all but four states. Before being allowed to take the state licensing examination, a chiropractor must have from two to four years of professional training.

The chiropractor is not qualified by training or experience to detect or treat infectious diseases or conditions such as heart disease and cancer. These require the skills of the medical doctor or the osteopath.

Quackery

You are constantly being confronted with all sorts of claims about products to use for your health. These promise a cure for every disease under the sun. Unfortunately, many people are misled by catchy slogans and attractively packaged products. They waste their money and, in many instances, they endanger their health by wasting valuable time before going to a qualified physician.

To be an intelligent consumer, you should be aware of the unethical practices of individuals whose only aim is to lighten your wallet.

Figure 15-6 ● Many worthless devices are peddled by quacks as cures for arthritis and cancer.

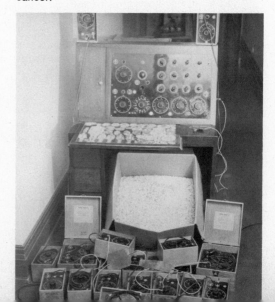

Quackery may be defined as the use of discredited, unproven, or disproved methods in the diagnosis and treatment of health problems. It is the practice of making false or misleading claims for any food, drug, device, or service, or the pretense of medical skill by a person not qualified to practice medicine.

Many organizations are working to eradicate quackery. To be successful, these organizations need your help, because the quack looks to you for profit.

Who Is a Quack?

A quack is an incompetent person. A quack pretends to have medical knowledge and skill but does not possess them. Getting money is the sole motive. Because of this, the quack makes promises that cannot be kept.

How Does the Quack Operate?

The quack very often advertises services or products. When questioned about the form of treatment used, the quack is quite secretive. The quack will not submit the product for public analysis, or the method for professional evaluation.

One of the quack's favorite approaches is to cite testimonials from people who supposedly have been cured by the services or product.

Very often, the quack selects for a target those who are suffering from painful and long-lasting diseases which medical science has difficulty combating. Quacks do their greatest damage to victims of arthritis and cancer. They are also extremely active among those with nutritional problems, especially obesity. It is estimated that Americans spend well over 300 million dollars a year on worthless treatments and products.

Arthritis "Cures"

Approximately 12 million persons in the United States have arthritis in one form or another. The Arthritis and Rheumatism Foundation estimates that every day about 700 new victims are diagnosed as having this disease.

Unfortunately, there is no cure for this disease. The arthritis patient can usually be helped somewhat by the medical profession, but the relief is often temporary. This leaves the door open for the quack and the claims for a surefire cure. For example, the Federal Food and Drug Administration recently seized a quantity of sea water that was being sold for three dollars a pint. It was being advertised as a cure for arthritis and other ailments. Many sufferers of arthritis had been enticed by the false claims.

Another product dispensed by arthritis quacks is the "glorified aspirin tablet." This is nothing more than regular aspirin combined with some valueless ingredient such as dehydrated alfalfa leaf. The charge for such a preparation can be 25 times that of ordinary aspirin.

Electronic devices are also advertised as "cures" for arthritis. The intelligent consumer realizes that such devices are useless. But people suffering great pain often seize upon any product or device that offers hope of relief.

Cancer "Cures"

The cancer quack is particularly dangerous because a person might be delayed from getting proper treatment. Early detection is the key to the proper treatment of cancer. The longer a cancer is permitted to develop unchecked, the greater the likelihood that it will reach a point where medical science cannot be of any help. The person who buys services from a quack is postponing proper treatment and risking death.

One of the most famous cases involving a "cure" for cancer was the Hoxsey treatment. This employed a combination of potassium iodide, licorice, red clover blossoms, several types of roots, and buckhorn powder. Over a period of approximately 30 years, thousands of people paid millions of dollars for the product. The federal courts stopped the sale of the product in 1956, when medical authorities were able to prove it was completely ineffective in curing cancer.

Investigation into a woman's death from chemical burns uncovered another cancer quack in San Diego, California. It was revealed that the burns were caused by a salve she had been using "to cure cancer." The quack who sold her the salve was arrested and convicted. A study of the quack's files disclosed that persons "diagnosed" as having internal cancer were given a light-colored salve. Those "diagnosed" as having external cancer received a dark-colored salve. Naturally, everyone who came to this quack was "diagnosed" as having some form of cancer, no matter what the symptoms were. The cost for the "cure" ran as high as $600.

Many drugs have been widely publicized in well-written articles in many of the major newspapers and magazines. Even though the drugs have not proven to be of value, many people are led to believe that they are effective cancer cures by the mere fact that they have been publicized. The public must learn to discount material unsupported by scientific proof, and free itself of the common belief that whatever appears in print must be true.

Consumer Protection

There are laws and governmental agencies to protect the consumer. In recent years concentrated efforts have been made to combat quackery.

The basic law used to combat quackery is the Federal Food, Drug, and Cosmetic Law of 1938. It is administered by the Food and Drug Administration. The intent of this law is "to insure that foods are safe, pure, and wholesome, and made under sanitary conditions; drugs and therapeutic devices are safe and effective for their intended uses; all of these products are honestly and informatively labeled and packaged." New amendments have been added to strengthen this law.

What You Can Do

Laws, however, are not enough. An informed and intelligent public is needed. **If the consumer would not purchase worthless services and products, the quack would be forced to go out of business.** Learn how to evaluate claims for health products and services. Know the earmarks of the quack.

The American Medical Association has suggested this rule of thumb for spotting a quack.
Beware:

■ If a "medical expert" uses a special or "secret" machine or formula claiming to cure disease

■ If a quick cure is guaranteed

■ If advertisements are used or if case histories and testimonials are used to promote the cure

■ If the "expert" claims that opposition by medical men is unfair persecution because they are afraid of competition

■ If the "expert" tells you that surgery, X-rays, or drugs will cause more harm than good

If you have a health problem, or think you have a problem, see a qualified physician. Don't be misled. Report frauds or suspected frauds to the proper authorities.

Medical Care

The costs of medical care seem to be high. Yet the consumers of medical care continually demand more health protection and higher-quality care. This is normal, since medical care is no longer considered a privilege, but rather a right.

Because of this feeling, many authorities are predicting that a form of national health insurance for all citizens is forthcoming in the United States. All advanced countries in the world, with the exception of the United States, have some type of national health-insurance program for the majority of their citizens.

Figure 15-7 ● How the medical care dollar is spent in the United States.

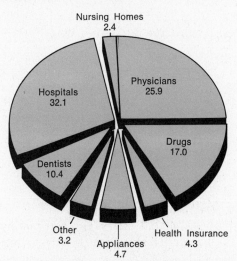

At the present time, your needs in medical care are probably taken care of by your parents. However, soon you will be faced with making your own decisions on how to provide for your medical care. Part of this decision may well include taking part in political decisions that would provide a national insurance program in this country. To do this intelligently, you should know about the current costs of medical care and the various health-insurance programs now available to the people.

The Cost of Medical Care

The people of the United States spend over 6 percent of the national annual income on medical care. This amounts to billions of dollars—a great deal of money indeed. But when you consider the benefits received, you will agree that it is money well spent. Countries where there is a national health-insurance program have been able to keep their costs to 4 to 5 percent of their national income and still provide excellent medical care.

Figure 15-7 shows how the medical-care dollar is being spent in the United States. You will notice that hospital costs take the greatest share of the dollar. These costs have steadily increased over the past several years. The Health Information Foundation predicts that hospitals will continue to take an increasing percentage of the medical-care dollar.

A major reason for this rise is the expansion in the range and volume of services provided for the patient. Better diagnostic tests and more intensive treatment are constantly being made available. More personnel are employed by hospitals to provide the increasing service. Nursing assistants, physical therapists, X-ray technicians, and laboratory technicians are just a few of the experts needed in the modern hospital.

Another major cost of medical care is health insurance. This has become the primary means of paying medical and hospital bills today. Approximately 80 percent of the people in the United States are now covered by health insurance.

Selecting Health Insurance

Health insurance is designed to protect individuals and families from the unpredictable costs of medical care. The programs are such that protection can be purchased individually or in group plans.

Ideally, sufficient insurance should be purchased to cover medical expenses that cannot normally be handled by the family budget. Consideration should be given to possible hospital expenses, surgical expenses, and regular medical expenses, including physicians' services and prescription drugs.

Major-Medical Health Insurance

This type of insurance was popularly called "catastrophic coverage" when it was first issued in 1949. It is most often purchased as a group plan. Major-medical insurance is written on the premise that the average family budget can meet relatively small medical expenses (between $50 and $500). Therefore, the insurance policy contains a deductible clause similar to that in an automobile insurance policy. This clause provides that the person insured pays the first $50 or $100. The insurance company then pays all or a percentage of the balance, up to a specified maximum. There is generally a limitation on the amount to be paid or on the time allowed for one illness or one accident. A limit of $10,000 or three years is common.

Coverage under this type of plan is usually quite broad. It generally takes care of hospital fees, physicians' services, laboratory services, and prescription fees. Some

Figure 15-8 ● The percentage of people covered under various voluntary health insurance programs.

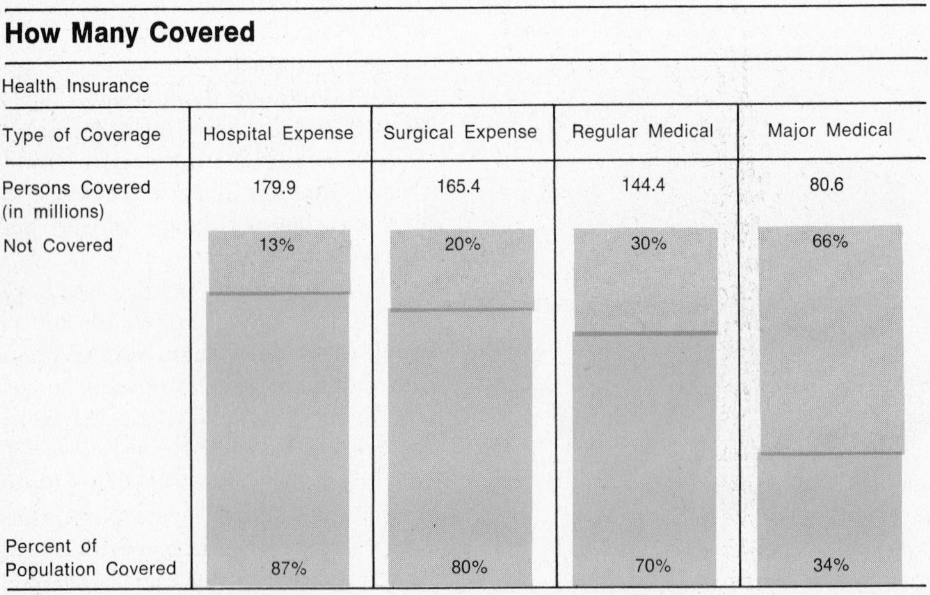

How Many Covered

Health Insurance

Type of Coverage	Hospital Expense	Surgical Expense	Regular Medical	Major Medical
Persons Covered (in millions)	179.9	165.4	144.4	80.6
Not Covered	13%	20%	30%	66%
Percent of Population Covered	87%	80%	70%	34%

policies also cover home-nursing care, dental care, eye care, and treatment for mental illness.

When you are ready to select a major-medical insurance policy, consider the following suggestions:

■ Get broad coverage. Do not buy policies that list only specific diseases.

■ Have the insurance limit high enough to meet any emergency and check on the limitation for any one illness or accident.

■ Be sure that all your dependents are covered.

■ Buy policies that are renewable and non-cancellable.

■ If you are considering a group policy, make sure it can be converted to an individual policy whenever desired.

Hospital Insurance

Hospital insurance developed out of the hospitals' need to be assured of payment for their services. This type of insurance is purchased by more Americans than any other coverage. It is protection against that part of the medical care that costs the most.

Because these types of insurance plan vary so much regarding cost and coverage, you should compare them carefully before you sign up. Buy the insurance that gives the most benefits for what you pay. Avoid buying what you don't need.

Surgical-Expense Insurance

This kind of insurance protection developed from the surgeons' need to be assured of payment for their services. Most plans provide payment of a percentage of the fees charged by the surgeons.

Many plans are based on ability-to-pay approach. In these plans, people with incomes under $7,500 per year have almost all of their surgical services paid by the insurance company. As incomes rise, the insurance policy covers a smaller and smaller percentage of the surgical service.

Medical Insurance

Through this type of insurance coverage, you are enabled to pay for physician services. Originally, it was developed to pay for hospital visits made by doctors to patients. Today many companies also include in their coverage office and home calls.

A limit is imposed on the number of calls during any one year. In addition, a limit is placed on the amount of the doctor's fee to be paid by the insurance company. Another limitation is that coverage for office and home calls starts only after the third or fourth visit for the same illness or injury.

Other Insurance Plans

There are many plans being developed to provide more comprehensive prepaid health protection. These plans include coverage for dental care, prescription drugs, eye care, and psychiatric care.

Dental insurance has been available for some time, but its growth has been slow. In recent years this type of coverage has received much support from labor unions and business and industry. More and more labor contracts include dental insurance as a part of the fringe benefits for workers.

In Wisconsin a prepaid prescription-drug plan has been initiated. It is a family plan that requires an enrollment fee and an annual prepaid premium, and has a $25 deductible clause. All prescription drugs deemed necessary for the treatment of the patient are covered, after the first $25.

Insurance policies that will cover short-term outpatient psychiatric treatment are being studied in New York. This is an attempt to provide more care outside a mental institution for those with emotional problems. If this approach is successful, future health-insurance programs may well include similar provisions.

Any insurance plan you purchase as protection against short-term illness or disability should be as comprehensive as possible. A prepayment plan in which the monthly payment is deducted from the paycheck seems to work best.

Medicare

A health-insurance plan which provides many of the services described in the preceding section is now being provided by the federal Social Security program.

Medicare provides medical and hospital services for more than 20 million persons over 65 years of age. Also covered in this program are the blind, the disabled, and children in need of medical care, whose parents cannot afford this care. Medicare provides basic hospital and medical insurance. The hospital insurance covers:

■ Sixty days of hospital care for any one period of illness (with a small deductible —paid by the patient), plus an optional

Figure 15-9 ● Provisions of the federal Medicare law.

Basic Coverage Under Social Security
(To be financed by increased Social Security taxes)

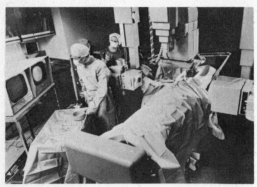

Hospital Care

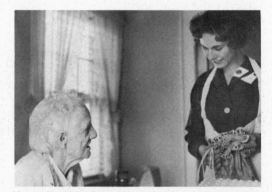

Home Nursing Care

Nursing Home Care

Outpatient Service

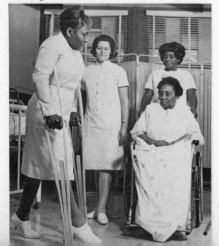

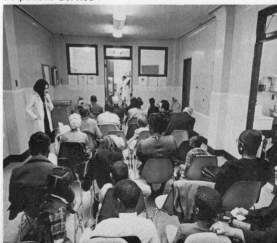

30 additional days of hospitalization (with the patient paying a small amount)

■ A "lifetime reserve" of 60 additional hospital days. The patient may use any of these if he requires more than 90 days of hospital care in any benefit period, but each day used permanently reduces the total number of days left. All covered hospital services are paid for, except a small amount a day, paid by the patient.

■ Up to 100 medically prescribed home visits by nurses, physical therapists, or other health workers

The medical-insurance coverage of Medicare is available to persons over 65 years of age who are willing to pay a small monthly premium. In addition, the individual covered must pay the first $50 of any medical expense. Medicare then pays 80 percent of the balance. This insurance plan covers the physician's consultation, surgery, home and office calls, and diagnostic services.

The Medicare plan allows patients to choose any doctor they desire. The law prohibits the government from attempting to control or supervise medical practice.

The purpose of the plan is to provide a certain portion of the population with a means of paying for needed medical care before they get sick. During the years when a person works, if covered by Social Security, a specified portion of the salary is deducted for future Medicare benefits.

Additional Coverage Under Voluntary Insurance (To be financed by monthly premiums and federal funds)

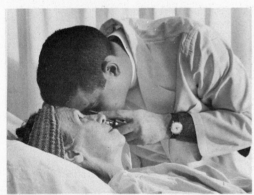

Physicians' Care
Mental Hospital Care

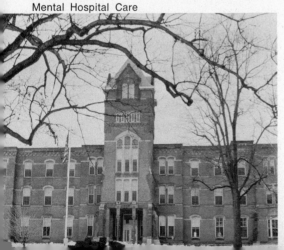

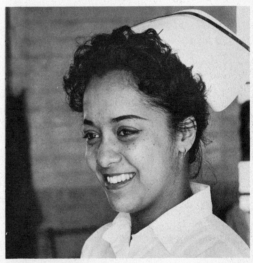

Home Nursing Care
Health Services

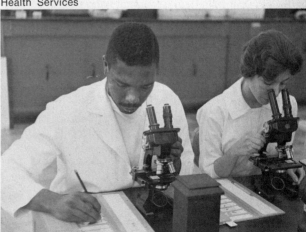

Summary

More and better medical care than at any other time in history is available today. It is your responsibility to take advantage of this excellent care by carefully selecting health products, health services, and health insurance. In selecting health products, you should disregard high-powered advertising. Read, compare, and evaluate what is written on the labels of health products. Follow the recommendations of your physician. Above all, do not diagnose persistent symptoms or treat them yourself with proprietary drugs.

When you select health services, do not hesitate to inquire into the professional background of physicians. You should clearly understand the many medical specialties and the differences among the various healing arts.

Quackery is a dangerous and serious problem. Do not be misled by promises that cannot be kept. Avail yourself of the services of qualified physicians and avoid quacks.

The best way to protect yourself against unpredictable costs for medical care is to purchase prepaid health insurance. Select a plan that will provide the most comprehensive coverage at a cost you can afford.

in making health decisions . . .

Understand These Terms:

diagnostician

ethical drugs

Food and Drug Administration

health insurance

Medicare

proprietary drugs

quackery

self-medication

specialist

testimonials

Solve This Problem:

Joan Ramsey has always wanted to be a doctor. She has taken the college preparatory courses in high school and has earned excellent grades in these courses. She was planning to take a premed course at the state university, but has been somewhat discouraged by stories that medical schools are full and difficult to get into. What should Joan do? Whom should she talk with? What other careers might she consider if she can't get admitted to medical school?

Try These Activities:

1. Write a short description of several advertisements on medications seen on television. Tell how the effects of the medications have been distorted in the ads.

2. Study your family's health-insurance policy. Evaluate it on the basis of the discussion on health insurance in this chapter. How well does it meet the suggested requirements for sound insurance? How could it be improved?

3. Prepare a brief report on how each of the following agencies help protect the public against quackery:
   a. The American Medical Association
   b. The American Dental Association
   c. The Better Business Bureau
   d. The Pure Food and Drug Administration

Interpret These Concepts:

1. When properly prescribed by a physician, modern tested medications are a great boon to mankind.

2. You should have a doctor who takes an interest in you and in whom you have complete confidence.

3. When any symptom persists, you should see a physician to get the proper diagnosis and treatment.

4. You can have the advantages of modern drugs without spending a great deal of money, if you use good judgment.

Explore These Readings:

Burns, Eveline, "A Critical Review of National Health Insurance Proposals," *Health Services Reports,* Vol. 86 (February, 1971), pp. 111–120.

Facts About Quacks (booklet). Chicago: American Medical Association, 1971.

"Prepaid Group Practice That Works: Kaiser-Permanente Organization," *Forbes,* 111:29 (March 15, 1973).

"Price of Life: Federal Support Under Medicare," *Time,* Jan. 1, 1973.

Read the Label (booklet), Food and Drug Administration Publication No. 73-1005. Washington, D.C.: U.S. Department of Health, Education, and Welfare, 1972.

Sixteen

Finding
Health
Careers

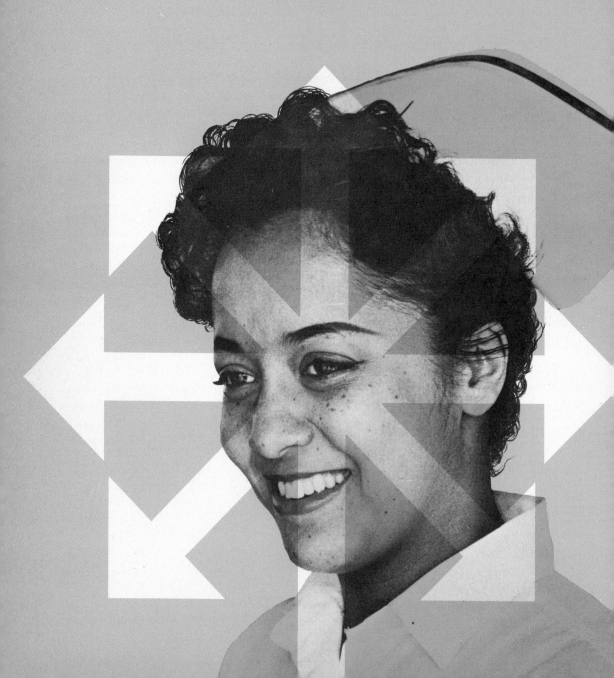

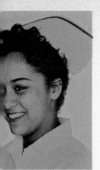

There is a shortage of workers in health occupations in the United States and throughout the world. This shortage has been created by programs for expanded health care of the populations of the world, and by the technological discoveries in the health field which create new jobs.

The serious shortage of workers in the health occupations has been of growing concern to the Department of Labor for the past several years. **Large numbers of health personnel are required to meet the health needs of our society.** The Department of Labor has estimated that there is a need for half a million more workers in this field. This estimate projects the need for 10,000 new health workers each month for a period into the 1980's.

If action is not taken, the shortage will become greater because of the increasing population and the heightened demand for services. Greater efforts will be required to enlist, educate, and train additional workers for the health team. All of this puts you into an enviable position if you are interested in pursuing a health career. The pages that follow will describe some of the specific opportunities available to you.

Nature of Health Careers

A variety of opportunities exist for health careers. Of all the occupational opportunities that await you, the health field probably has the greatest variety of positions from which to choose. In the medical-care field, for example, for each physician there are approximately 12 other health workers. The same type of situation exists in dental services, public-health services, and other allied health fields.

Another important factor is that people can advance in the health occupations. Some high school graduates obtain jobs in medical offices, hospitals, or clinics, and then go on to more formal education to accompany their on-the-job training. Courses are available to help people move ahead in many health careers. Many people develop special interest and return to college to complete degrees and qualify for higher-level positions.

If you are interested in serving other people, it would be well for you to look into a health career. All health careers have as their basis the objective of maintaining the health of the peoples of the world. People need to feel that their work is meaningful, not merely monotonous and regimented. If you find your work satisfying and gratifying, you will be a happier person, not only at work, but in all your personal relationships. A health career might provide such fulfillment for you.

Some Health Careers

If you are interested in a health career, the best thing to do is to talk with someone who can provide you with reliable information. Start with your family doctor, the personnel director of a hospital, and your high school vocational counselor. Ask them where else you might get additional information about health careers. Your school counselor, for example, might have the government publication *The Health Careers Guidebook,* which has a description of more than 200 health careers.

Varying amounts of education and experience are required for health careers. Some careers require only a high school education. There are many that require a high school diploma and a short period of technical training—some of which can be

Figure 16-1 • This chart shows the estimated average of health-related jobs opening each year to 1980.

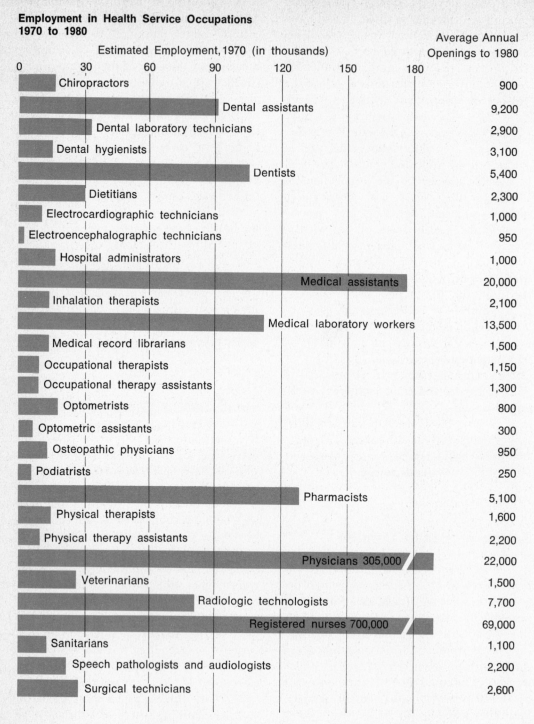

Employment in Health Service Occupations 1970 to 1980

Estimated Employment, 1970 (in thousands)

Average Annual Openings to 1980

Occupation	Average Annual Openings to 1980
Chiropractors	900
Dental assistants	9,200
Dental laboratory technicians	2,900
Dental hygienists	3,100
Dentists	5,400
Dietitians	2,300
Electrocardiographic technicians	1,000
Electroencephalographic technicians	950
Hospital administrators	1,000
Medical assistants	20,000
Inhalation therapists	2,100
Medical laboratory workers	13,500
Medical record librarians	1,500
Occupational therapists	1,150
Occupational therapy assistants	1,300
Optometrists	800
Optometric assistants	300
Osteopathic physicians	950
Podiatrists	250
Pharmacists	5,100
Physical therapists	1,600
Physical therapy assistants	2,200
Physicians 305,000	22,000
Veterinarians	1,500
Radiologic technologists	7,700
Registered nurses 700,000	69,000
Sanitarians	1,100
Speech pathologists and audiologists	2,200
Surgical technicians	2,600

acquired on the job. Still other opportunities exist for those with a two-year community college preparation. In addition, higher-level positions exist for those who complete college and postcollege degrees. An attempt has been made to standardize terminology in relation to level of training for health careers. It is as follows:

Technologist or therapist—college degree or above

Technician or assistant—two years of college or other formal training beyond high school

Aide—specialized training of less than two years beyond high school, or on-the-job training

Perhaps you will find a health career of interest to you among those discussed in the following pages.

Entry-Level Health Careers

The entry-level health careers are those that require the least amount of formal education or other preparation. They provide a young person with an access to a career from which he might move ahead. Some of these entry-level health jobs are described in the pages that follow.

■ **Certified Laboratory Assistant.** The certified laboratory assistant usually works under the supervision of a medical technologist performing the simpler laboratory tests and procedures. Graduation from an accredited high school, preferably with ability and interest in science and mathematics, is required for admission to a school approved by professional groups. The preparation includes a 12-month course of practical and technical training. Graduates who pass the exami-

nation given by the Board of Registry of the professional association may place the letters CLA (ASCP) after their names.

■ **Dental Assistant.** The dental assistant's primary function, that of assisting the dentist at the chairside, includes preparing the patient for treatment, keeping the operating field clear, mixing filling materials, and passing instruments. Other duties involve exposing and processing X-ray films, sterilizing instruments, assisting with laboratory work, ordering supplies, and handling the office records and accounts.

All dental schools now routinely train dental students in the effective utilization of chairside assistants. The utilization of assistants has progressively increased until today more than four of every five dentists in private practice employ at least one dental assistant.

Traditionally, dental assistants have been trained on the job by their dentist-employers. However, the number of institutions offering accredited training programs for assistants is increasing.

■ **Dental Laboratory Technician.** Dental laboratory technicians are highly skilled workers who perform many tasks involved in the construction of complete and partial dentures, fixed bridgework, crowns, and other such dental restorations and appliances. Dentists are relieved of many time-consuming procedures by utilizing the skills of technicians who perform such tasks as waxing, investing, casting, soldering, finishing, and polishing. Technicians do not have direct contact with patients, but perform their work in accordance with instructions received from the dentist.

Dental laboratory technicians may be employed in a dental office and work directly for a dentist. Most technicians, however, are employed in commercial dental laboratories which serve the majority of the nation's dentists.

Most dental laboratory technicians have received their training on the job in commercial laboratories or dental offices. Relatively few formal educational programs for technicians are available at the present time.

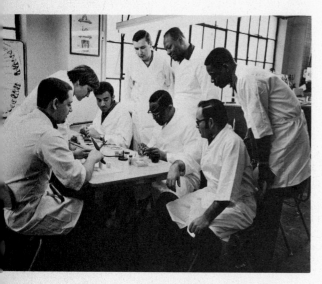

Figure 16-2 ● Dental laboratory technicians receive much of their training on the job.

■ **Electrocardiograph Technician.** Electrocardiography involves recording the changes of electrical potential occurring during the heartbeat by use of an electrocardiograph (ECG or EKG) machine. It is used in diagnosing abnormalities in heart action or recording the progress of patients with heart conditions, as well as providing follow-up for those patients receiving cardiotoxic medications. The electrocardiograph technician operates the machine and gives the recorded tracings to physicians who are qualified in cardiology for analysis and interpretation. They perform in a laboratory or at the patient's bedside if the patient cannot be moved. The technician attaches electrodes to various parts of the patient's body and moves the chest electrodes to successive positions across the patient's chest, obtaining several different tracings of the heart action by the ECG machine.

No specialized formal education is required for this job. However, high school graduation with courses in the physical sciences and some college work are desirable. On-the-job training in a hospital usually lasts from three to six months, under the supervision of an experienced technician or cardiologist.

■ **Electroencephalograph Technician.** Electroencephalography involves detecting, measuring, and recording brain waves by the use of an electroencephalograph (EEG) machine. It is of great importance in the diagnostic evaluation and treatment of patients with various types of brain disease or trauma. The electroencephalograph technician is trained to use the machine to record brain waves. These tracings are interpreted by a physician, usually a neurologist with training in electroencephalography.

The EEG technician may take on-the-job training in a hospital EEG department, generally serving an apprenticeship lasting three to six months, with some programs lasting six to twelve months. This practical experience may be supplemented by lectures on nueroanatomy, neurophysiology, and electronics. A minimum background of high school science courses and an aptitude for working with complicated electrical equipment, together with a desire to handle patients with a variety of diseases, are needed. Formal training programs are being developed in a number of universities and hospitals. For some of these programs a minimum of two years of college preparation is required prior to admission.

■ **Food-Service Workers.** The entry-level positions in food services in hospitals and health-related institutions include *dietetic technicians* and *dietetic aides.* The dietetic technician assists the dietitian and functions as the middle-management person in the department. The dietetic aide supervises employees and food-service areas. Food-service workers have a wide range of jobs, including food receiving, storage, preparation, cooking, and serving.

Post-high-school programs to prepare dietetic technicians and aides are offered by more than 200 vocational schools, technical institutes, and community colleges. Most of the preparation is in on-the-job training or in a supervised practical educational experience.

■ **Nursing Aide or Orderly.** A nursing aide or orderly works under the supervision of a professional nurse. An aide may bathe patients, assist in feeding them, distribute food trays, deliver messages, escort patients to other departments, and perform other duties that are necessary for patient care. Aides and orderlies who work in mental hospitals are called *psychiatric aides.* Nursing aides and orderlies are trained on the job in hospitals, nursing homes, and other patient-care facilities. Training takes approximately three months.

■ **Secretarial and Office Services.** These services are usually provided for medical personnel by *receptionists, secretaries,* and *office assistants.* Professional offices and admitting offices of hospitals and related institutions usually employ one or more persons to perform many and varied duties, such as scheduling appointments, receiving patients, recording case histories, ushering the patient into the consultation or examination room, setting out the necessary instruments, and perhaps assisting the doctor by passing instruments or performing other functions. There are also clerical duties involving correspondence, payments, monthly statements, supplies, insurance forms, and reports. The person who prepares the examination room and hands instruments and materials to the doctor as directed is frequently called an office assistant or aide, rather than a secretary. The receptionist's office procedures are closely related to those of the secretary. However, secretarial duties play a more important role in the secretary's job, which often requires a knowledge of medical or dental terms.

High school graduation is the minimum educational requirement for secretarial and office services. Training in office procedures and skill in typing, shorthand, and bookkeeping improve opportunities for employment. Courses in biology, chemistry, health education, and medical (or dental) terminology, as well as ethics and personal relations, are desirable as part of the education of medical (and dental) secretaries. Formal programs are available in an increasing number of community colleges and in technical and vocational schools, and are supplemented by training and experience on the job.

■ **Surgical Aide and Other Aides.** Hospital assistants or aides are identified according to the service in which they work. For example, surgical aides work as members of the surgical team under the direction and continuous supervision of the physician and/or nurse. They assist in the care of patients in the operating room, delivery room, or emergency room, and perform tasks associated with maintaining aseptic conditions essential for patient care. The surgical-technical aide also helps set up the operating room with surgical instruments and equipment needed for each operation; assists in the care, preparation, and maintenance of sterile and nonsterile supplies and equipment; and assists in the handling and sterilization of instruments and equipment.

Most surgical aides are high-school graduates who have received at least three to six months of in-service training, primarily in hospitals. A few vocational schools and community colleges, in conjunction with cooperating hospitals, now offer a program of one year or longer duration, leading to a certificate.

■ **Vocational Nurse.** The entry level in nursing is that of vocational nurse. The vocational nurse provides nursing care and treatment of patients under the supervision of a physician or a registered nurse. The care and treatment might include giving routine medications and taking and recording temperatures, pulse, respiration, and blood pressure. They may also assist with the supervision of nursing aides and orderlies. The majority of practical nurses work in hospitals, clinics, homes for the aged, and nursing homes. Licensure of practical nurses is provided for by law in the 50 states and the District of Columbia. For licensure as a licensed practical nurse (L.P.N.) or licensed vocational nurse (L.V.N. in California and Texas), an applicant must graduate from a state-approved school of practical nursing and pass a state board examination.

Requirements for admission to a practical-nursing school program vary. In most states the applicants are required to have completed at least two years of high school; a few states require a high-school diploma. The program is usually 12 to 18 months and may be obtained in trade, technical, or vocational schools operated by public school systems or in private schools controlled by hospitals, health agencies, or colleges.

■ **Ward Clerk.** Ward clerks are sometimes floor clerks or stations clerks. They act as receptionists and are responsible for much of the paper work done at a nursing station. The position requires typing ability and accuracy in spelling and arithmetic. Ward clerks are trained on the job in approximately one to two months.

Intermediate-Level Health Careers

There are many health careers that require some formal college education, but not a bachelor's degree. You can prepare for most of these careers in a community (two-year) college. Because these careers require more preparation, they usually pay more than the entry-level jobs and often involve responsibility of supervising some other workers. Examples of some of these careers are described below.

■ **Biomedical Engineering Technician.** This health worker is responsible for constructing, adapting, operating, and maintaining medical devices and instrument systems. These technicians may enter from many diverse fields to use their special skills in this occupation. Persons with special training in plastics, for example, work on repair and replacement materials and the development of artificial organs. Courses in biomedical engineering technology are being developed by some technical institutes as a two-year program and also to supplement on-the-job training of biomedical engineering aides.

■ **Clinical Laboratory Technician.** There are three health careers in clinical laboratories at the intermediate level. They are the cytotechnologist technician, the histologic technician, and medical laboratory technician. *Cytotechnologists* specialize in screening slides in the search for abnormalities that are warning signs of cancer. Minimum prerequisites include two years of college with 12 semester hours in science, eight of which are in biology. The cytotechnology course provides for six months of education, plus six months of full-time experience in an acceptable cytology laboratory. *Histologic technicians* are employed in pathology laboratories. These histologic technicians specialize in cutting and staining body tissues for microscopic examination. The Board of Registry of Medical Technologists gives limited certification, following examination, to persons with a high-school diploma plus one year of supervised training in a clinical pathology laboratory or in a community college. In addition, there are training courses in some hospitals. *Medical laboratory technician* is a new intermediate level of laboratory personnel. These technicians usually work under the supervision of a medical technologist, performing at a level between the medical technologist and the certified laboratory assistant following successful completion of an examination. Requirements for registration are an associate degree from an accredited junior or community college including supervised clinical experience in an acceptable laboratory. Certified laboratory assistants and graduates of 12-month military laboratory programs and persons with five years' laboratory experience may take the certifying examination, if they have an associate degree or demonstrate comparable academic standing.

■ **Dental Hygienist.** Dental hygienists are the only dental workers who, like den-

tists, are required in each state to obtain a license to practice. The hygienist, working under the direction of a dentist, performs prophylaxis (scaling and polishing of the teeth), exposes and processes dental radiographs, applies fluoride solution to children's teeth, instructs individual patients in toothbrushing techniques and proper diet as related to the teeth, and performs other duties in conformity with the training and licensing standards. The great majority of dental hygienists provide services to patients, working primarily in private dental offices, but also in public and private schools, public and private clinics, hospitals, and other institutions. Some hygienists, however, are engaged in other activities, such as determining dental treatment needs of schoolchildren, reporting these findings to parents, and giving dental-health talks in classrooms.

Figure 16-3 ● Many colleges and community colleges now offer two-year career programs for dental hygienists.

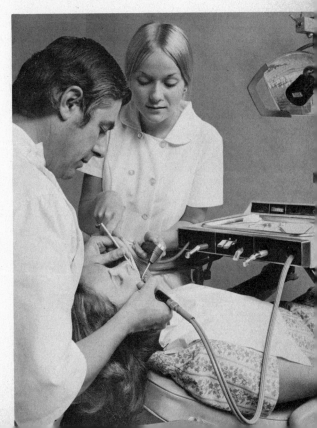

Dental hygienists receive at least two years of education at the college level. The dental-hygiene curriculum, which includes basic sciences, dental sciences, and liberal arts, is usually open to high school graduates. However, in 1969, about one institution out of every six required some college training for admission to this program. Originally, dental-hygiene programs were provided primarily by schools of dentistry, but increasing numbers of colleges and technical schools are now offering this training. Two types of college training are available to the hygiene student. The two-year associate degree or certificate program qualifies a hygienist for clinical practice. The level of training required for leadership positions in teaching and public health is provided by the four-year bachelor's-degree program in dental hygiene. Hygienists completing the latter program qualify for graduate training leading to the master's degree in related fields.

■ **Environmental Technician.** As environmental-protection facilities and services have increased in number and complexity, the need for increasing numbers of trained technicians and aides has become more apparent. Environmental technicians assist professional personnel in carrying out the various elements of prevention, control, and service programs including inspections, surveys, investigations, and evaluations to determine compliance with laws and regulations. They obtain appropriate samples of air, food, and water, and assist in performing tests to determine the quality of these samples. They operate or assist in operating water purification and waste-water treatment plants and systems, and solid wastes collection and disposal facilities. The minimum educational requirement for

the environmental technician is an associate degree in environmental health, environmental science, radiologic technology, or related areas of specialization. A number of community colleges or technical institutes offer technical training in these areas.

■ **Inhalation-Therapy Technician.** Inhalation-therapy technicians use, under medical supervision, a wide variety of therapeutic skills, procedures, techniques, medical gases, drugs and medications, and equipment to restore normal functioning of the respiratory system. They also use various testing techniques to assist in diagnoses, monitoring, treatment, and research. The majority of inhalation-therapy technicians work under the direct supervision of the anesthesiology department or the pulmonary department of hospitals. An increasing number are being employed in clinics and doctors' offices. Others work for firms that provide emergency oxygen service for clinics or for municipal organizations. Courses of study provide no less than 12 months for those preparing to become certified technicians and no less than two years of college for those preparing to become registered therapists. The courses are open to high school graduates and graduates of nursing schools.

■ **Medical-Record Technician.** The medical-record technician assists the medical-record librarian and performs the technical tasks associated with the maintenance and use of medical records. Associate degree programs in community colleges require two years of study, and hospital-based programs nine to ten months. Instruction is given in medical terminology, anatomy, physiology, and medical-record procedures. A correspondence course is open to persons who are employed in medical-record work and who are high school graduates as another avenue to becoming a medical-record technician. Those who satisfactorily complete the 25-lesson course are eligible to apply for the national accreditation examination, as are those who graduate from approved schools.

■ **Medical Assistant.** These workers assist the physician, usually within the professional office or the hospital. The duties may include preparing patients for the doctor's examination, sterilizing gloves, preparing the examination room, performing simple laboratory tests and X-ray procedures, and assisting with or carrying out treatments prescribed by the physician. Certification examinations for medical assistants can be prepared for in special vocational schools or in an increasing number of community colleges.

■ **Orthotist and Prosthetist.** On the basis of a physician's prescription, the *prosthetist* makes and fits artificial limbs, while the *orthotist* makes and fits orthopedic braces. After the appliance has been fitted to the patient and checked by the physician, the physical therapist and occupational therapist train the patient in the use and care of his new device with the assistance of those who made them. The individual who designs and fits these appliances may be certified in both prosthetics and orthotics. Persons are employed in privately owned facilities or laboratories, rehabilitation centers, or hospitals, or by a government agency. Applicants for the examination to qualify for these careers are required to possess at least an Associate of Arts degree from a community college.

■ **Radiologic Technician.** Radiologic technology involves the use of radiant energy in the field of medicine to assist the doctor in diagnosis and treatment of disease. The primary function of radiologic tech-

nicians is to operate X-ray equipment under the direction of a physician who is usually a radiologist (specialist in the use of X-ray). For diagnostic purposes, the technologist prepares the patient for radiographic examination, positions the patient between the X-ray tube and film, selects the proper exposure, and records an image of a part of the body as prescribed by a physician. For therapeutic purposes, the technologist operates special X-ray equipment and assists in the preparation of radium or other radioactive materials for controlled application by the physician.

The three specialties within the field include the diagnostic X-ray technology, nuclear-medicine technology using radioactive isotopes, and radiation-therapy technology using radiation-producing devices.

Programs are conducted by hospitals and medical schools and by community colleges with hospital affiliation. The courses are open to high school graduates, although a few require one or two years of college or graduation from a school of nursing. The length of the training varies from a minimum of two years in a hospital radiology department or a community college offering an associate degree, to a four-year university course leading to a bachelor's degree.

Figure 16-4 ● The radiologic technician performs a valuable function in diagnosing and treating people.

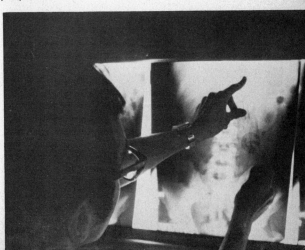

■ **Registered Nurse.** Individuals in this profession may function in a variety of positions within different employment settings. They render nursing care to patients or perform specialized duties in hospitals, infirmaries, nursing homes, sanatoriums, clinics, doctors' offices, industrial plants, schools, or in patients' homes through a public-health department or other service agency. They also serve as teachers of nursing. Registered nurses are responsible for the nature and quality of all nursing care that patients receive. They are also responsible for carrying out the physicians' instructions and for supervising practical nurses and other nonprofessional personnel who perform routine care and treatment of patients.

Figure 16-5 ● A career as a registered nurse offers women and men an opportunity for responsible and rewarding service to others.

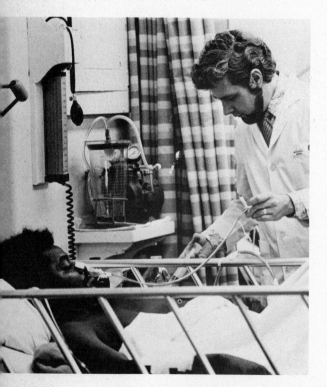

A license to practice nursing is required in all states and the District of Columbia. For licensure as a registered nurse (R.N.), an applicant must have graduated from a school of nursing approved by the state board for nursing and have passed a state board examination. Graduation from high school is required for admission to all schools of nursing. There are three types of initial programs of nursing education which prepare persons for licensure as R.N.'s. Diploma programs are conducted by hospital schools, and usually require three years of training; associate-degree programs usually located in community colleges are approximately two years in length; baccalaureate programs usually require four years of study in a college or university, although a few require five years. Nurses who would like to go into administration or education must complete postgraduate work. Many earn master's degrees and Ph.D. degrees.

■ **Therapists.** *Occupational therapy technician* and *physical therapy assistants* work under the direction of occupational and physical therapists, respectively. They help to carry out programs of rehabilitating patients in hospitals and other health-care facilities. Two-year programs of training have been developed in hospitals, health agencies, vocational and adult education schools, and community colleges.

■ **Vision Specialists.** Several categories of health personnel are involved in providing services for the relief of visual complaints. At the intermediate level these include the dispensing opticians, the optical technicians, and the orthoptists. *Dispensing opticians* make, fit, supply, and adjust eyeglasses according to prescriptions written by opthalmologists or optometrists to correct a patient's optical defects. They do not examine eyes or prescribe treatment. Mechanical grinding and polishing of the lenses and assembling in a frame are done by *optical technicians,* who follow the work order prepared by the dispensing optician. An apprenticeship of one to four years is required to practice opticianry in most licensing states. Six states also specify high school graduation. Qualifications for initial licensure usually include successful completion of written, oral, and practical examinations. An alternate method of entering this occupation is through completion of a one- or two-year formal program in ophthalmic-dispensing optical technology in a community college or in a military or technical school.

A special category of ophthalmic assistants is the *orthoptist.* Orthoptists work under the direction of the ophthalmologist in the specialized field of diagnosis and treatment of eye muscle and fusion anomalies. They work with children and adults who need training in coordinating the use of the two eyes. The orthoptist teaches patients certain exercises that help to overcome the handicap of crossed eyes or, in other patients, to train eyes that are not working well as a pair to work together efficiently. An orthoptist must have two years of college and 15 months of training in an accredited training center.

Health Careers for College Graduates

There are a considerable number of health careers that require a bachelor's degree from a college or university as preparation. People who complete their education and get a few years of experience in these ca-

reers can generally get further preparation to move into even higher-level positions. Some of the health-career opportunities for college graduates are described in the following pages.

■ **Biomedical Engineer.** Biomedical engineering involves the application of the principles and practices of engineering science to biomedical research and health care. It serves and supports life-science research and diagnosis, therapy, and prevention of human disease and disorder. Typical activities in this field include the development of new instruments and systems for use in research, patient care, and delivery of health services. Included as well are the invention and perfection of orthotic and prosthetic devices, the application of physical systems analysis, computer technology, and engineering methods to problems of living. This work is being conducted in academic institutions, hospitals, federal and private research laboratories, and a variety of manufacturing and service industries. The minimum educational requirement for biomedical engineers is a bachelor's degree in engineering with some training and experience in the biomedical sciences. Virtually every engineering school in the country offers formal curricula to prepare persons to work in the field.

■ **Clinical Laboratory Technologist (Medical Technologist).** These health professionals perform chemical, microscopic, bacteriologic, and other tests under the supervision of a physician or medical scientist. Some serve as laboratory supervisors or assist in the training of student medical technologists and other laboratory personnel. Presently, the minimum educational requirement for such medical technologists is four years of college including one year in a medical-technology educational program.

■ **Communication Specialist.** Science writers, health information specialists, and technical writers are responsible for making authoritative health information available to the public in an understandable and appealing form. Some are also involved with making professional, scientific, and technical information accessible to the health specialists themselves. *Science writers* are journalists who specialize in health or other scientific subjects. They write for newspapers, magazines, radio, television, or for scientific or professional publications to acquaint the public with developments in the fields of science, including medicine. Science writers are employed by newspapers, serve as editors or writers on magazines and in publishing houses, or have staff positions as information specialists in scientific and health organizations. Some are freelance writers working on their own time. *Health-information specialists* are employed by health organizations to inform the public of achievements as well as programs of the organization. To accomplish this, they make use of leaflets and other publications, newspapers, magazines, radio, television, exhibits, direct mail, and motion pictures.

Technical writers and science writers deal with the same general subject matter, but each focuses mainly on a particular group of readers. The technical writer's specialty is writing about scientific and technical developments primarily for professional persons in the field. Since the material is written for this group and is technical in nature, the emphasis is on specifics written in great detail. The minimum education requirement for a communication specialist is a bachelor's degree, usually in English or journalism, with some supplementary science courses.

■ **Dietitian.** Dietitians are specialists, professionals responsible for the nutritional care of individuals and groups. They may specialize in one or more of four recognized areas of specialization: administration, nutritional care, research, and education. Their work includes applying principles of nutrition and management in planning and directing food-service programs in hospitals and related medical-care facilities, educational institutions, and other public and private institutions. In addition, they provide guidance and instruction to individuals and groups in applying principles of nutrition to eating habits and the selection of foods, and may be engaged in research related to dietetics. For qualification as a professional dietitian, the American Dietetics Association recommends the completion of an approved dietetic internship of three years of qualifying experience, following a bachelor's degree in dietetics. Some dietitians take graduate courses leading to a master's or doctor's degree.

■ **Environmental-Control Specialist.** The nation's growth and productivity have resulted in many complex environmental problems that seriously challenge our health and well-being. Included are problems related to the contamination of air, water, soil, and food; occupational and community stresses; noise, temperature, and vibration; inadequate housing and work environments; highway and home hazards; and radiation and other hazards.

Environmental control represents a diverse area of work; thus it draws heavily on well-established disciplines. These include chemistry, physics, and biology of many specialties, hydrology, meteorology, oceanography, engineering, sanitation, ecology, medicine in several specialties, law, mathematics, statistics, political science, economics, and social work. Efforts in controlling environment are carried out by many professionals, including environmental engineers, sanitarians, and program specialists.

Environmental engineers apply engineering and scientific principles and practices to the prevention, control, and management of environmental factors that may influence our physical, mental, and social health and well-being. They are engaged in the broad area of public works with major responsibilities for such environmental practices as public water supply, community waste disposal pollution control, and housing control activities.

Sanitarians apply their knowledge of the principles of the physical, biological, and social sciences to the improvement, control, and management of the environment. Sanitarians safeguard the cleanliness and safety of the food people eat, the liquids they drink, and the air they breathe. They inspect food-manufacturing and processing plants, dairies, water supplies, supermarkets, restaurants, and other places for health hazards. They seek compliance with local regulations and with state and federal laws relating to public health. They also plan and conduct sanitation programs, administer environmental health programs, and promote the enactment of health regulations and laws.

Program specialists work in industrial hygiene, radiation protection, and air-pollution control. Basic industrial-hygiene activities include the recognition, evaluation, and control of those environmental factors which have an adverse effect on the health and efficiency of workers in places of employment or among citizens of the community. *Industrial-hygiene personnel* examine the work environment for identification and determination of hazardous concentrations of dusts, fumes, gases, or vapors; for determination of unhealthful conditions, such as excessive noise and inadequate ventilation; for collection of samples for chemical analysis; and for recommendations for the control of hazardous conditions.

Radiation-protection personnel at the professional level include health physicists, engineers, chemists, biologists, and other scientific and technical specialists with particular training in the health aspects of radiation. The radiation-exposure problems with which they are concerned are associated with the use of electronic products, such as X-ray machines, particle accelerators, microwave ovens, and color television; radioactive materials; and nuclear reactors; as well as with environmental radioactive contamination. Their work is conducted principally in industrial, medical, research, or educational institutions that use radiation sources, and in health agencies that have responsibility for protection of the public health.

Air-pollution-control personnel include engineers, chemists, meteorologists, statisticians, physicists, biologists, sanitarians, technicians, inspectors, and a variety of other professionals. The principal activities that comprise air-pollution-control programs are the measurement of chemical pollutants, determination of the effects of air pollution on living things, control of air pollution, and development and enforcement of air-quality standards.

The minimum educational requirement for environmental engineers, sanitarians, and certain other environmental disciplines is the baccalaureate degree. However, in a number of other instances, postbaccalaureate education is required for disciplinary qualification or for program specialization. In several careers the qualifying professional degree is the doctorate.

■ **Food Technologist.** Food technologists apply science and engineering to the production, processing, packaging, distribution, preparation, and utilization of foods. Their scientific knowledge and special skills are employed to solve technological problems connected with the development of new products, processes, or equipment; selection of raw materials; fundamental changes in the composition or physical condition of food for industrial processing, or the nutritional value and suitability of such foods for human consumption. A bachelor's degree in food science or in a related science such as chemistry, biochemistry, biology, bacteriology, or in engineering is the minimum educational requirement for entrance into the field.

■ **Food and Drug Inspector.** The Food and Drug Administration of the U.S. Department of Health, Education, and Welfare has broad responsibilities for food and drug protective services and employs inspectors and analysts who are concerned with the purity and safety of food, drugs, and cosmetics, and with the effectiveness of drugs. The *food and drug inspector* tries to provide protection before the product reaches the consumer by checking the processes involved from raw material to delivery, including the conditions under which it is manufactured and the package labeling. The inspector is usually a college graduate with a science major.

■ **Health Statistician (Biostatistician).** These specialists are primarily concerned with the use of statistical theory, techniques, and methods to determine useful measurements or meaningful relationships of quantified information on a par-

ticular subject relating to health or disease. They help in identifying and measuring health problems as a basis for planning and evaluating progress of programs and also in the scientific study of the causes, processes, and cures of disease. Another major function of the health statistician is to devise special studies and analyses for use in planning and evaluating health services. A bachelor's degree with courses in statistics, mathematics, biological sciences, social sciences, and physical sciences is the usual requirement for beginning positions as *health statisticians.* Advanced training in statistics and public health leading to a master's or doctor's degree is desirable.

■ **Medical-Record Librarian.** Medical-record librarians are responsible for designing health-information systems; planning, organizing, directing, and controlling medical-record services; developing, analyzing, and evaluating medical records and indexes; cooperating with the medical staff in developing methods for evaluation of patient care; and cooperating with medical and administrative staff in research projects utilizing health-care information. The minimum educational requirement for professional registration as a medical record librarian is a baccalaureate degree in medical-record science.

■ **Therapist.** The health careers in therapy include occupational therapist, physical therapist, corrective therapist, educational therapist, music therapist, recreation therapist, and home economist in rehabilitation.

Occupational therapy is the art and science of using purposeful activity in the promotion and maintenance of health, the prevention of disability, and as treatment in the rehabilitation of persons with physical or emotional dysfunction. *The occupational therapist,* as a vital member of the rehabilitation team, determines the objectives of the treatment program according to the individual needs of each patient. The required preparation includes a bachelor's degree in occupational therapy and approximately six months of supervised clinical practice.

Physical therapy is concerned with the restoration of function and the prevention of disability following disease, injury, or loss of a body part. The goal is to help patients reach their maximum performance and to assume their due places in society while learning to live within the limits of their capabilities. The therapeutic properties of exercise, heat, cold, electricity, ultrasound, and massage are used to achieve this goal. Upon referral by a physician, the physical therapist evaluates the patient and plans the program which will be most effective. *Physical therapists* must complete a bachelor's degree and four months of clinical educational experience.

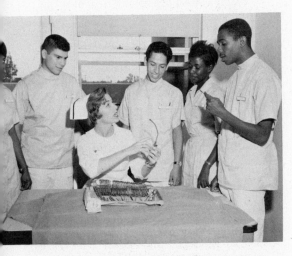

Figure 16-6 • Junior college students receiving instruction in one of the allied health professions. Have you considered a vocation in the health field?

Corrective therapy is the treatment of patients by medically prescribed physical exercises and activities designed to strengthen and coordinate functions and to prevent muscular deconditioning resulting from long convalescence or inactivity due to illness. *Corrective therapist* is the usual title used by those persons who work in hospitals, nursing homes, and rehabilitation centers, while those employed in educational institutions are known as *adapted physical educators.* The minimum educational requirement is a baccalaureate in physical education from an accredited school followed by a period of clinical training.

Education therapy is the utilization of academic teaching designed to develop the mental and physical capacities of hospitalized patients. The *educational therapist* administers medical treatment through the use of educational activities and materials that are of significance to the patient. The educational therapist is a college graduate who has majored in education or physical education. In addition, two to seven months of clinical training is required.

The professional application of the art of music for therapeutic purposes is relatively new and has a wider application in the treatment of mental illness than in physical illness. The *music therapist* uses instrumental or vocal music to bring about changes in behavior that can serve as a basis for improved mental and physical health. To do this, the trained music therapist follows the specific treatment aims prescribed by a physician. For employment as a qualified music therapist, the college graduate with a degree in music must complete a six-month internship.

Therapeutic recreation is a specialized service within the rehabilitation process, with therapeutic implications for the disabled, handicapped, and aged person. The elements of service commonly offered by the *recreation therapist* include activity programming (music, drama, sports and games, arts and crafts, camping, nature activities, hobbies, and social clubs) and recreation counseling. A bachelor's degree in recreation is the qualifying preparation for this career.

Within the framework of the family, *home economists in rehabilitation* apply their unique knowledge and skills in the areas of food and nutrition, textiles and clothing, housing and household equipment, family economics, home management, and family and child development to the needs of handicapped people and their families. Home economists in rehabilitation are college graduates with a degree in home economics followed or accompanied by in-service or graduate training in the education of the handicapped.

Health Careers Requiring Graduate Education

The health professions requiring the most preparation and experience are described on the following pages. They all include formal education in addition to the regular four-year college degree. Naturally, these are the better-paying health careers, and ones in which the worker has the most responsibility.

■ **Clinical-Laboratory Scientist.** Most of these scientists are employed in clinical laboratories directed by pathologists or other physicians, or an (allied) medical scientist or specialist. Others direct their own laboratories or work in independent laboratories. They have graduate degrees in chemistry, microbiology, or other biological sciences. An academic degree in a specific science followed by a period of work experience in a laboratory is the usual course of entry into this field.

■ **Health Educator.** Health education is the process through which individuals acquire knowledge and behavior consistent with the achievement of optimum individual and community health. The practitioners of health education are public health educators and school health educators. The *public-health educators* or *community-health educators* have major interests in educating all segments of the community and are concerned with those forces which create or change behavior. Their talents may also be directed toward planning and providing educational opportunities for other health personnel. The minimum educational requirement for public health educators is the baccalaureate degree in a program of community health education in an accredited institution. Many positions require a master's degree in public health.

School health educators are mainly concerned with classroom teaching and other influences which the school exerts on health knowledge, behavior, attitudes and practices. Within a school district, they may coordinate the work of all groups in the community which are interested in the health of the school child and furnish leadership in developing and maintaining a sound, well-balanced health program. School health educators must meet the regular certification standards for teachers in their state. They are required to have at least four years of college education leading to a bachelor's degree, with a background in the biological, physical, and social sciences as well as in the field of health education. A master's degree in the field of health education is being increasingly required.

■ **Hospital Administrator.** The hospital administrator acts as planner, organizer, educator, and adviser coordinating the operation of the entire institution—from ensuring that ample resources, facilities, equipment, and services are available, to providing continuing education programs for hospital staff and supportive personnel. Diplomat and liaison to the community, the administrator also extends the hospital's cooperation and leadership in combating disease and solving local health problems. Graduate programs leading to a master's degree in hospital administration consist of one or two years of academic study, and may include a period of up to one year of "administrative residence" in a hospital or other health-related facility or organization.

■ **Medical Illustrator.** Medical illustrators work with physicians, research scientists, medical educators, authors, and others to record graphically the facts and progress in the health field. They serve a vital role in dispensing scientific information through publications, exhibits, television, and other communications media. For the most part, medical artists work for hospitals, clinics, medical schools, public and private research institutes, large pharmaceutical firms, and medical publishing houses. Medical illustrators may also work on a free-lance basis, and some combine free-lancing with a part-time salaried position in a hospital or other medical institution.

Five medical facilities offer courses in medical illustration of not less than 20 months or two academic years. The entrance requirements usually include four to six years of undergraduate and graduate study with extensive course work in the biological sciences, art, and other related subjects.

■ **Medical Librarian.** Medical librarians are employed in health-care institutions, educational institutions, departments of public health, drug firms, insurance companies, and general biomedical-research institutions. They work with physicians and other health and research workers, as well as with students and instructors preparing for careers in health fields. The basic requirement for certification as a medical librarian is a master's degree from an accredited school of library science offering a course in medical bibliography. This five-year program may be followed by an internship or other specialized training.

■ **Nutritionist.** Nutritionists are specialists in human nutrition concerned with the maintenance and improvement of health throughout the life cycle. They may be responsible for nutrition components of health and medical-care services and their work includes planning and conducting programs concerned with food and nutrition, examining the processes through which food is utilized by the body, and analyzing food to determine its composition in terms of essential ingredients or nutrients. Nutritionists may engage in services to groups or individuals in administration, in teaching and/or research. They work in health and welfare agencies, agricultural agencies, hospitals and clinics, food industries, and educational facilities both governmental and non-governmental. Preparation for nutritionist positions usually requires academic training at both the undergraduate and graduate levels.

■ **Pharmacist.** Pharmacy is the health profession which is concerned with the preparation and distribution of medicinal products and entails a comprehensive knowledge of the physical nature, chemical composition, pharmacological action, and therapeutic use of the substances being employed. The pharmacist practices in community pharmacies, hospitals, extended-care facilities, and nursing homes. Others are employed in academic, industrial, governmental, and professional association settings. In addition to the traditional services of compounding, dispensing, and distributing drug products, pharmacist's services are becoming patient-oriented and clinical in approach. Clinical pharmacy is practiced in the community pharmacy by maintaining a patient-medication record and advising and counseling patients on their medications. In the hospital, the clinical pharmacist serves as the drug-information specialist to members of the hospital staff.

A minimum of five years of study after graduation from high school is required for a bachelor of science in pharmacy (B.S.) or a bachelor of pharmacy (B. Pharm) degree from a college of pharmacy. Most schools of pharmacy require one or two years of preprofessional college education. Students who do advanced study in one of the specialized areas of pharmacy may qualify for the master of science or doctor of philosophy degree.

■ **Research Scientist.** Science is basic to all activities in the health field. Scientists with an academic background in one of the basic scientific disciplines or in the application of mathematics to these disciplines engage in research to provide new knowledge and deeper insights in every health profession. The biological sciences provide the basic supply for medical research. However, modern medical research is also drawing heavily on scientists trained in an increasing diversity of fields of study within the sciences. Most research scientists are en-

gaged in medical research in universities and research institutes. Industry and government also employ these health professionals.

A doctoral degree in the basic sciences is the preparation usually required for these positions.

■ **Rehabilitation Counselor.** Rehabilitation counselors are concerned with evaluating the vocational potential of people. They try to match the abilities of patients with a suitable job when the time comes for starting work—either in their former position or in the one for which job training or retraining becomes a part of rehabilitation. Some counselors specialize in services for the blind, deaf, mentally ill, mentally retarded, or other specific groups. They not only provide counseling, but engage in community activities to interest employers in hiring qualified handicapped persons and others in the benefits of rehabilitation.

The minimum educational requirement for employment as a rehabilitation counselor is generally a bachelor's degree, preferably with a major in counseling psychology, social work, or education. Specialized graduate education is open to college graduates who have had some education or experience in rehabilitation counseling or in such related fields as those above. Two years usually is required to complete the master's degree in the fields of study preferred for rehabilitation counseling.

■ **Speech Pathologist and Audiologist.** Speech pathologists and audiologists are primarily concerned with disorders in the production, reception, and perception of speech and language. They help to identify persons who have such disorders and to determine the severity of specific disorders through interviews and special tests. They facilitate optimal

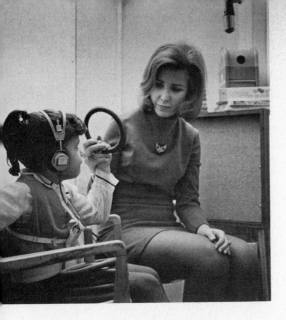

Figure 16-7 • Speech pathologists and audiologists work in schools and clinics.

treatment through speech, hearing, and language remedial or conservational procedures, counseling, and guidance. They work in the public schools and in special clinics. Both specialists require academic training at the master's degree level and one year of experience in the field, and must pass a national examination.

■ **Social Scientist.** Several of the social sciences have specialists concerned with the solution of health problems. *Cultural or social anthropologists* study cultural factors related to personality, mental illness, and psychological development and stress. Thus they are considered as part of the health-manpower resources.

Sociologists as part of the health field identify social factors influencing the occurrence of disease, the behavior of patients and the organization of the health professions.

Health economists appraise health as an economic asset and analyze ways in which the provision of health-care products and services affects the health of individuals.

About one-third of all *psychologists* are engaged in health activities. Clinical psychologists are engaged primarily in the diagnosis and treatment of mental illness in hospitals, clinics, and private practice. They also consult with community mental health programs and school systems. Counseling psychologists work in schools, industry and community agencies. They help individuals understand themselves so that they can deal with their own problems.

Social workers in hospitals and clinics work directly with patients and their families in helping them to cope with problems related to severe or long term illness, recovery, and rehabilitation.

The preparation of social scientists who work in health-related programs includes either a master's or doctoral degree in their field of study.

■ **Veterinarian.** Veterinarians treat sick and injured animals, give advice regarding the care and breeding of animals, and help prevent the outbreak and spread of diseases among them by physical examination, tests, and vaccinations. Veterinarians employed in the regulatory and public-health aspects of veterinary medicine assist in the provision of safe meat and dairy products. They also help to shield the human population from over 100 animal diseases.

The minimum time required to earn the Doctor of Veterinary Medicine degree (D.V.M.) is six years beyond high school. This period consists of at least two years of general college plus four years of professional training in an approved school of veterinary medicine. For some positions in public health, research, laboratory animal medicine, or teaching, the master's or Ph.D. degree in a field such as pathology, public health, or microbiology is required, in addition to the D.V.M.

Summary

Today, there are a considerable number of opportunities for people who would like a health career. Such job openings are expected to last until into the 1980's. There are over 200 health occupations from which to choose. Jobs are available for persons with high school preparation as well as at all levels of the college-education ladder. Many health careers can be prepared for in special vocational schools.

You should select a career that is meaningful to you. It should be one that you will enjoy and that will offer the employment advancement to meet your personal goals.

in making health decisions . . .

Understand These Terms:

audiologist
biomedical
dietetics
orthopedic
pathology

sanitarian
statistician
technician
technologist
therapist

Solve This Problem:

You have been elected leader of a student committee responsible for planning a one-day health personnel career conference during your school's annual Career Roundup Week. The following questions need to be resolved in preparation for your first committee meeting:

1. What health-related career representatives should be invited to speak at the conference?

2. What specific items should speakers be asked to include in their presentations?

3. How can you insure presentations that are equally appropriate for girls and for boys?

4. What are some conference follow-up activities that you may wish to suggest to your planning committee?

Try These Activities:

1. Ask your school or family physician for an opinion regarding the nature and degree of health-personnel needs ten years from now.

2. Make a list of health-related careers that deal primarily with things (machines and/or equipment) rather than with people. Compare this list with a list that contains careers that deal primarily with people. Why is it important to have interested and capable people in each group?

3. List the procedures you would follow in exploring the many offers of scholarships and work-study programs available through governmental agencies, hospitals, and colleges.

Interpret These Concepts:

1. Large numbers of health personnel are required to meet the health needs of our society.
2. A variety of opportunities exist for health careers.
3. Various amounts of education or experience are required for health careers.

Explore These Readings:

Gartner, Alan, "Health Systems and New Careers," *Health Services Reports,* Vol. 88 (February, 1973), pp. 124–130.

"Job Spurt Likely in Health Fields," *The New York Times,* Aug. 20, 1972, p. 17.

Koch, M. S. and Charles Hollander, "The Health Sciences Careers Program," *Health Services Reports,* Vol. 87 (November, 1972), pp. 787–802.

Montgomery, Erwin, "Health Helpers in Erie County, N. Y.," *Health Services Reports,* Vol. 86 (October, 1971), pp. 879–887.

New Careers Bibliography. Washington, D. C.: National Institute for New Careers, 1970.

Seventeen

Solving Future Health Problems

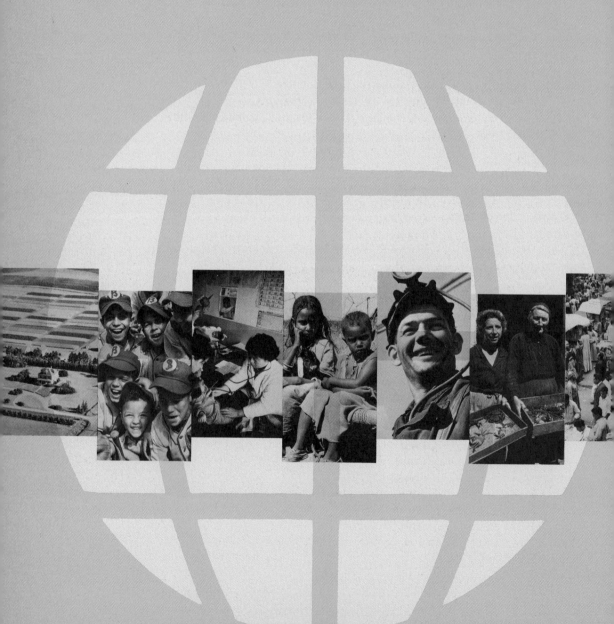

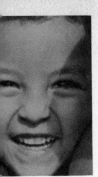

Many health scientists predict that within the next 50 years (very probably during your lifetime) we will see almost miraculous advances in the field of medical technology. For example, scientific results of current medical research indicate a strong possibility for the eventual development of procedures and techniques that would result in: a life expectancy of 100 years or more; tissue growth to replace missing limbs and damaged organs; extensive use of mechanical and artificial organs; the control of cancer; and the correction of genetic defects that result in health problems. These problems are not simple or independent. They are interrelated and require comprehensive planning for their solutions.

It is generally agreed, however, that a valid solution to future health problems must involve more than advanced medical technology. Some of the related problems receiving study and attention throughout the world include the need to improve and/or increase: health-care delivery systems; environmental controls; health-personnel resources; and personal responsibility for acquisition of health knowledge and practice of positive health behavior.

An Appraisal of Needs

It is important that you keep abreast of new developments in health care and relate them to your personal life. This can be done by intelligent reading, by consultation with your physician, and by active involvement in community health problems. As is true of any other aspect of education, health education should never end.

Organization for Health

It is no longer possible to think of certain health problems as affecting only a particular city, county, state, or country. **Health problems affect people without regard to political boundaries.** Air pollution, for example, does not end at the city line.

In the future you may see the organization of health services in connection with specific problems. Agencies will be developed to function across political lines. In this way, overlapping and duplication of services will be eliminated.

Comprehensive Personal Health Services

Comprehensive personal health services of high quality are needed for everyone in every community. Health services still are not available to everyone in every part of the United States. For example, a number of areas have no physicians, hospitals, or other services considered so important today. Individuals and agencies responsible for health services will need to combine programs gradually to provide comprehensive services that will be equally available and accessible to all.

The Personal Physician

Where possible, individuals should have their own personal physician. Through the physician, comprehensive personal health services can be made available. The physician will direct the individual to whatever services are needed, if specialists are required.

Because the number of physicians is limited, more and more health-care functions will be delegated to paramedical personnel (technicians and other trained or professional persons supplementing the work of the physician). Increasingly, the physician will become a coordinator of health services. To carry out this role, it will be necessary for the physician to become aware of all the health services and resources of the community, in order to mobilize them for treatment of the patient.

Control of the Environment

Ecology is a dynamic process; it is also a relationship-centered process. In short, ecology is the result of an organism's impact upon its environment, and the reciprocal impact of the environment upon the organism. The health implications of such a relationship are obvious.

Air, water, and land are not unlimited. You have learned that the environment is being contaminated at a rate that is rapidly approaching saturation. The health of the public is in danger.

Improving the quality of the environment will require more money and more laws and regulations. For example, a nationwide, continuous, automated air-sampling network will be necessary.

Additional research will be required to determine the immediate and long-range effects of pollutants on human beings, plants, and animals. Special education programs will be necessary to teach the consumer how to avoid the misuse of physical, biological, and chemical products.

Urban Design

Planning for a healthy environment will become an essential consideration in urban design. By the end of this century, nearly three-fourths of the population of the United States will be urban dwellers. The effect of so many people living so close together will require careful study.

Additional research is needed on the effect of population density and urban conditions on the physical, emotional, mental, and social health of people. Legislation protecting the public from hazardous, noisy, and unaesthetic environments will be developed as part of the health program.

Space must be provided for recreational and cultural activities. Comprehensive health and welfare services will need to be properly distributed so that they are available and accessible to everyone.

Voluntary Citizen Participation

Everyone has a responsibility for health. One reason the United States has been able to improve the level of personal and community health has been the participation of individuals and voluntary groups.

Volunteers play an important role in solving community health problems. More of this type of activity will be needed in the future.

Education for Health

Education for health is basic to all health programs. School districts will have to assume more responsibility for educating students in the area of health.

By stimulating each individual to be more concerned for maintaining personal health and to participate in community health activities, health education programs will help solve many of the problems that face the world now and in the future.

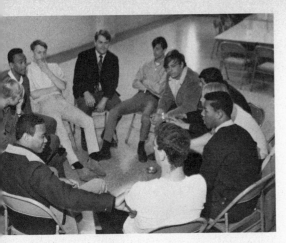

Figure 17-1 • Education is one of the keys to the protection of tomorrow's citizens.

In addition, the community has a responsibility for developing educational programs for those who have left school. **Health education should not end with graduation, but should be continued throughout life.**

New Technology

Scientific developments occur so rapidly that it is difficult to keep up with them. There is a time lag between discovery and application. Even so, we are already deriving benefits from the development of electronics, from the practial peacetime application of nuclear energy, and from the exploration of space.

Electronic Developments

One of the exciting electronic developments now being utilized for the betterment of man is the computer. Computers are widely used in the field of medicine and their use will be tremendously expanded in the future.

Research is being conducted on the use of the computer as an aid in diagnosing illness. The computer is fed information on a person's medical history, along with present symptoms of illness. Through proper programming, the computer can then be required to supply the physician with a list of possible ailments or diseases that might be present. These suggestions can then be further investigated by means of selected diagnostic laboratory tests. If such an approach can be devised, the diagnosis time can be substantially shortened. In addition, many unnecessary diagnostic tests might be eliminated. Perhaps even more important, diagnosis could become more accurate.

Another interesting possibility of computerization is the development of a lifelong health history for every citizen of the United States. All your health information could be stored in a central data-storage area. You would then carry a card with a medical number and a coded medical summary. Any doctor to whom you would go would then have access to your complete medical history. By inserting your card in the health history retrieval system, your complete medical history would be printed out.

Figure 17-2 • Computers and other electrical devices will find an increasing number of uses in health care.

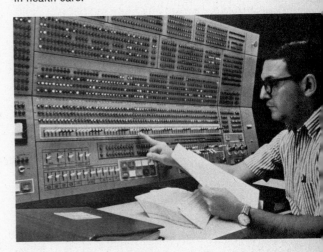

Advantages of such a system can be clearly seen. However, not everyone is completely happy about this approach. Some individuals feel that this is simply another step toward reducing human beings to mere numbers on cards. These people feel that the development of a personal relationship with the physician will be hindered by the use of the computer in this manner. If issues of this nature can be resolved, the technical knowledge to develop such a system is now available, and the program could be operational in the 1970's.

Additional uses for the computer are constantly being devised. In the future there will be greater use of these instruments in monitoring basic physiological processes of hospital patients. This will assist the physician and the nurse in rendering medical treatment.

Perpetual inventories of drugs and other medical supplies will be controlled by computers. This will reduce waste and spoilage.

In addition to the computer, new electronic developments will continue to add to doctors' equipment. Some that have already been developed are: tiny radio-pills that relay information from various organs of the body; telemetered diagnostic devices that eliminate the need for wires; small sensory devices for measuring body temperature and other physiological functions; "pacemakers" to control the heartbeat; and electrical stimulation of the brain as a means of diagnosis and treatment.

Nuclear Energy for Health

The discovery of nuclear energy has already advanced medical knowledge tremendously. It is predicted that even greater results will occur in the future.

More than three-fourths of the radioactive isotopes produced in the world are used in medicine, mainly for diagnostic purposes. For example, some thyroid conditions are diagnosed by means of radioactive iodine, which the patient is required to swallow in the form of a small capsule. A special instrument then measures the amount of the radioactive iodine taken up by the thyroid gland. This gives the physician some insight into how well the gland is functioning.

The dose requirements of the radioisotopes are not much higher than for an X ray, and some are considerably less. Thus they can be used with safety. This combination of radioactive material and radiation-detection devices has been improved to such a point that various parts of the body can now be monitored, including the brain, lungs, heart, liver, spleen, pancreas, kidneys, and skeleton.

Many hospitals are adding departments of nuclear medicine to carry on such activities and to make use of new discoveries.

Figure 17-3 • Radioactive materials will continue to be useful in the detection and treatment of disease.

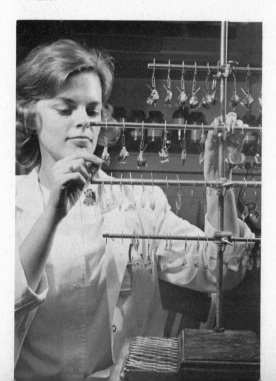

Space and Health

Constant advances in the conquest of space have led to many medical findings. The health aspects of space travel itself and the findings from space technology that are applicable on earth will probably be useful in solving health problems.

Astronauts have had to deal with problems such as weightlessness, high levels of radiation, pressure changes, wide temperature changes, nutrition, elimination of body wastes, and emotional stress. Some of these problems have been effectively overcome. The information gained from the space program has already been put to use in various industries that face problems similar to those of the astronauts.

In addition, two space-age devices are currently being used to aid amputees and paraplegics (people with paralysis of the legs and lower part of the body). The device developed for moving about on the moon (the Moonwalker) has been adapted to an eight-legged walker for paraplegics and amputees. The walker can move over sand and rough fields, and even climb slopes and curbs. The second device, a simulator, is being used to create the effect of weightlessness. In the simulator, paraplegics can be taught to fall safely. This is particularly helpful when the handicapped person is learning to use artificial limbs.

One of the more spectacular medical advances resulting from space research is the increase in knowledge concerning cryogenics (the science of extreme cold). To lift spacecraft from the ground, space scientists had to develop special fuels which had to be supercold. Medical researchers have applied the findings on freezing to the treatment of disease. A good example of this is the ice scalpel. This instrument is a probe about the size of a pencil through which supercold liquid nitrogen flows. The extreme cold can destroy tissue which is causing certain body disorders. This technique has been used successfully in treating victims of Parkinson's disease, certain cancers, a variety of visual disturbances, and tonsillectomies. It is hoped that cryogenics will also prove useful in treating burns and dental disorders by reducing pain.

Research is being conducted on the preservation of whole blood by this method. If successful, it may make it possible to store whole blood for indefinite periods of time without spoilage and waste.

Many new problems must continue to be investigated if space travel is to advance. Some authorities believe that doctors will be practicing in space in the 1980's. Consideration is being given to the feasibility of orbiting hospitals for the space traveler during the 1980's. Some of these ideas may seem extremely remote to you. It may, however, be possible to put to immediate use the knowledge gained from this basic research.

Synthetic Body Parts

Since the development of new synthetic materials, much progress has been made in replacing parts of the body that have been harmed or destroyed by disease. Artificial heart valves have been used successfully in the treatment of rheumatic heart disease. Many individuals have had damaged valves partially or completely replaced by the artificial valves. As a result, these individuals can expect to live many years longer in comparative good health.

Another example of progress is the work being done on the development of an artificial heart that can actually be implanted in an individual. Some success has already been achieved in this work.

Many other body parts may soon be produced to replace diseased areas.

Organ Transplants

The transplantation of living parts of the body from one person to another is an accomplished fact today. Many intricate surgical procedures have been developed to permit a variety of transplants.

The major obstacle to success still seems to be the rejection mechanism of the body itself, which is not very tolerant of anything that does not belong to the body. This is particularly true of areas of the body which involve a direct supply of blood. Whenever a foreign substance enters the body, elaborate defense mechanisms spring into action. Primary among the defense mechanisms is the action of the white blood cells. These cells seem to have a built-in ability to distinguish between what is foreign and what belongs to the body. Anything foreign is attacked and rejected unless something is done to reduce the action of the white blood cells.

Today, drugs have been developed which can suppress the action of the white blood cells. However, these drugs pose a potential problem in that the body is left vulnerable to infections that the white cells might normally handle. In spite of this problem, enough progress has been made in the application of the drugs to achieve great success in transplanting organs such as the kidney and heart.

Where these transplants seem to have failed, the failure is not usually due to surgery but to the inability of another part of the body to function properly with the new organ. Transplants of the liver have also been attempted but with little success. The rejection mechanism of the body has not been overcome in this type of transplant.

Great success has been achieved in the transplant of bones, cornea of the eyes, and hair. In each of these types of transplants the possibility of rejection is slight because of the lack of direct blood supply. As a result, the white blood cells cannot enter and cause rejection.

The art of transplanting human parts is well established today. Within your lifetime you may see even further progress in transplanting organs from human beings or from animals.

Acupuncture

Acupuncture as a means of treating disease has been practiced in China for hundreds of years. Charts related to the practice of acupuncture show 1,000 points where needles can be inserted into the body to treat illnesses and restore health. The practice of acupuncture involves the use of long, slender needles which are inserted into various parts of the body and twirled.

Chinese medical specialists have reported great success with acupuncture anesthesia. It is estimated that a significant percentage of medical operations in China are done with acupuncture anesthesia.

The Chinese cannot offer an explanation of why acupuncture works. Competent medical observers testify that the procedure seems to be a valid health treatment procedure. Acupuncture is being practiced on a limited basis in the United States, as well as in many other countries. Research teams throughout the world are working to find a scientific answer to the "why and how" of acupuncture.

International Health

Health is a worldwide concern. Because of the improvement in transportation, resulting in increased mobility of people, certain diseases can be spread rather quickly to every part of the world. As a result, all countries of the world need to cooperate in solving health problems. In addition, many people feel that the United States has an obligation to help other countries that have not yet achieved as high a level of health.

The United States makes significant contributions to international health in various ways. The U. S. participates in such organizations as the World Health Organization (WHO) and the United Nations Children's Fund (UNICEF) and also provides direct aid to individual countries.

The World Health Organization

WHO was organized in 1946 and is now composed of more than 100 member nations. It is concerned with improving medical education, raising the quality of a nation's health services, controlling outbreaks of communicable diseases, studying the occurrence and distribution of diseases on a worldwide basis, and standardizing the production of drugs used in medicine.

It was the original intent of WHO to try to control the major diseases and health problems affecting the world, such as malaria, tuberculosis, venereal diseases, inadequate rates of maternal and infant health, and low levels of nutrition. This approach has given way to a more general attitude of extending help, in any form, to improve the health of the nation requesting assistance. This includes emergency health programs.

WHO, at the request of any country, will provide various types of health experts and demonstration teams to assist in the control of disease and illness. The main goal of these professional experts is to help countries acquire the knowledge and skill to train their own personnel. In this way, the country can become more self-sufficient and less dependent on outside aid. Demonstration teams have gone into the most primitive areas of the world and shown native teams how to test for various diseases and how to treat these diseases.

WHO feels that no country can successfully fight against disease or promote health for its people without a well-organized program for administering health services. In this respect, much effort is expended to help countries plan for the services necessary for the prevention and cure of diseases.

The world is becoming healthier. While the World Health Organization cannot take all the credit for the advances that take place, it should get a major share.

Figure 17-4 ● WHO provides a variety of health services for people throughout the world.

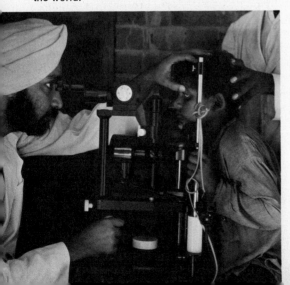
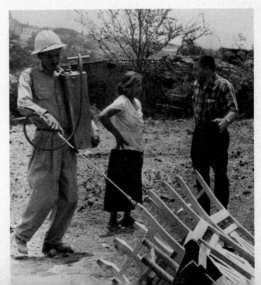

Direct Aid for Health

Many departments and agencies of the United States provide direct health aid to other countries of the world. The Agency for International Development (AID) is one such governmental agency. It helps other nations by providing military, economic, and technical assistance. A major part of the technical assistance is in the area of health.

Hundreds of health specialists work for AID in various parts of the world. A major role that these specialists have assumed is in training personnel in the countries that need help. Once again, the basic concept applied is that of helping people to help themselves.

Through AID, many persons from a number of countries have been able to come to the United States to receive professional training. They have returned home better equipped to solve the health problems of their own nations.

Efforts in the area of international health will continue to grow. The sincere desire of the people of one nation to assist people of other nations will do much to promote goodwill in this shrinking world, as well as to reduce human suffering.

The Future: The Decision Is Yours

What will your health status be tomorrow?

Do you have the knowledge to make intelligent decisions regarding the solution of health problems? Are you aware of your health assets and liabilities? Do you know how to select foods wisely? Do you know how to keep in good physical condition? Are you well-informed on reliable sources of health information? Do you select health products and services wisely? Are you aware of the dangers of self-medication? Do you recognize symptoms of disease and seek prompt medical care when they occur?

Only you can answer these and other questions about your health. It is your responsibility. Make the most of it.

in making health decisions . . .

Understand These Terms:

acupuncture
cryogenics
health personnel
medical technology

radioisotopes
therapist
urban design
WHO

Solve This Problem:

As a part of an interview related to an application for a health-related job, you have been asked to identify what you think was the most important advancement in medical technology during your lifetime, and give the reasons for your decision.

1. What would your decision be?
2. How would you support your decision?

Try These Activities:

1. If life expectancy is eventually extended to 100–125 years, what do you think some of the resultant problems might be? Would some of these problems be personal, social, or worldwide? Prepare a summary of your answers to present to the class.

2. Prepare a list of those health disorders which are genetically induced. Establish a priority ranking in terms of those that you would like to see solved first. Itemize the reasons for your priority ranking.

3. List what you think might be done to implement a valid health-care delivery system in your community within the next ten years.

Interpret These Concepts:

1. Health problems affect people without regard to political boundaries.

2. Health is a worldwide concern.

Explore These Readings:

Henry, James P., *Biomedical Aspects of Space Flight*. New York: Holt, Rinehart & Winston, Inc., 1965.

Irwin, Theodore, "Forecasting Your Future Health," *Today's Health,* Vol. 45 (May, 1967), pp. 25–29.

Lentz, John, "Super-Cold: The 'Hottest' Thing in Science," *Today's Health,* Vol. 45 (February, 1967), pp. 18, 82–88.

National Commission on Community Services, *Health Is a Community Affair.* Cambridge, Mass.: Harvard University Press, 1966.

Prehoda, Robert W., *Extended Youth: The Promise of Gerontology.* New York: G. P. Putnam's Sons, 1968.

Tressel, George W., "Nuclear Energy as a Medical Tool," *Today's Health,* Vol. 43 (May, 1965), pp. 50–55.

Zimmering, Stanley, "Pall Over America: Air Pollution Threatens Human Health," *Journal of Health, Physical Education, and Recreation,* November–December, 1969.

abnormal: deviating from the regular, normal, or average

abscess: a collection of pus localized in some part of the body

accident: an event occurring by chance, or from unknown causes

acidosis: an abnormal condition of lowered alkalinity in the blood and blood tissues

acne: a chronic skin condition characterized by pimples, blackheads, and blemishes, usually on the face, shoulders, or back

active immunity: commonly long-lasting immunity produced by antibodies caused either by infection by certain agents or disease or injection of these agents

adaptation: modification of structure, function, or behavior in meeting the requirements of the environment

addict: one who is physiologically and psychologically habituated to the compulsive use of narcotics, drugs, or alcohol

adjustment mechanism: the means by which persons become better adapted to their environment

adolescence: the growth stage between childhood and adulthood

adrenalin (adrenin): hormone produced by the adrenal glands

afterbirth: the placenta and that portion of the fetal membranes discharged from the uterus after the birth of a baby

agent of disease: organism capable of producing disease

aide: health worker with less than two years of specialized training beyond high school

alcoholism: a chronic illness that manifests itself as a disorder of behavior

alkali: a chemical compound that acts to neutralize acid

allergen: a substance capable of producing an allergy

allergy: an abnormal sensitivity to certain substances such as items of food, pollen, or dust

alleviation: the process of improving, correcting, or modifying

amnesia: complete or partial loss of memory

amnion: the membrane in which the embryo is enclosed, together with a saline liquid (**amniotic fluid**)

amoebic dysentery: a form of dysentery caused by a protozoan (amoeba)

amphetamine: a stimulant drug usually in tablet or capsule form

analgesic: a substance which tends to reduce pain

anemia: a condition in which there are too few red blood cells or too little hemoglobin, resulting in the reduction of the amount of oxygen carried by the blood

angina: a constricting pain

angina pectoris: a condition of the heart characterized by spasmodic, constricting pain, usually due to coronary artery disease, such as arteriosclerosis

antibiotic: a substance that destroys disease-producing organisms—usually produced from molds

antibody: a substance in the blood which destroys or reduces the effect of disease germs, their toxins, or other foreign substances

anticoagulant: a substance that reduces the clotting ability of the blood

antidote: a substance used to counteract a poison

antigen: an agent or substance which causes the production of an antibody

antihistamine: a substance used to treat allergies or allergy-type reactions

antiseptic: having the power to prevent development of bacteria; a drug with this power

antitoxin: a substance which neutralizes the effect of a toxin (poison)

anxiety: uneasiness or distress resulting from apprehension or uncertainty

aorta: the large artery that originates from the left ventricle of the heart; its branches carry blood to all parts of the body

appendicitis: inflammation of the appendix

appendix: a small bag or tube-like structure attached to the large intestine close to the point where the small intestine and the large intestine join

arteriosclerosis: hardening of the arteries; loss of elasticity

arthritis: a condition characterized by inflammation and/or swelling of the joints

aseptic: free of harmful organisms

aspirin: a derivative of salicylic acid, used as a medication in the relief of pain or fever

asthma: a condition resulting from contractions of the bronchi that causes shortness of breath, wheezing, and coughing; often caused by an allergic reaction

astigmatism: a condition resulting in impaired vision due to unequal curvatures of the cornea and/or lens

atherosclerosis: hardening of the inner lining of the arteries due to deposits such as cholesterol

athlete's foot: a fungus infection characterized by itching, redness, and cracking—usually between and around the toes

audiologist: one who is trained in measuring acuity of hearing

audiometer: an instrument used in measuring acuity of hearing

autopsy: a medical examination of a deceased person, usually to determine cause of death

bacteria (pl. form; sing. is **bacterium**): one-celled microscopic organisms some of which produce disease

barbiturate: a sedative-type drug usually in tablet or capsule form

basal metabolism: a measurement of the amount of energy used while the body is awake but at complete rest; minimum energy requirement expressed in kilocalories

benign: noncancerous abnormal cell growth which does not spread to or destroy adjoining tissue

beriberi: a deficiency disease that affects the nervous system; caused by lack of thiamine (vitamin B_1)

biochemical: involving chemical reactions in living organisms

biological: relating to life and living processes

biomedical engineer: a person who applies the principles of engineering to medical research and health care

biopsy: removal of a small piece of human tissue for microscopic examination

biostatistician: a person who specializes in working with health statistics

blackhead: a small, black-tipped fatty mass in a skin follicle

botulism: a disease of the nervous system produced by toxins of certain bacteria *(Clostridium botulinum)* which develops in spoiled foods; a type of food poisoning

bovine tuberculosis: a form of tuberculosis to which cattle are susceptible

bronchitis: an inflammation of the membrane lining of the bronchial tubes and windpipe

bubonic plague: a contagious disease spread by fleas from infected rats

Caesarean section: delivery of a baby as the result of surgery through the abdominal and uterine walls when birth through the natural passages is impossible or dangerous

calcium: a mineral element essential to proper bone and tooth development as well as blood clotting

calculus: hard mineral deposits which form on the teeth

calorie: the amount of heat (energy) required to raise the temperature of 1 kilogram of water 1 degree Centigrade

cancer: disorderly cell growth that is harmful to normal body cells and that may spread to other parts of the body

carbohydrate: a class of organic compounds containing carbon, hydrogen, and oxygen; a food high in calories, such as sugars and starches

cardiac: pertaining to the heart

cardiovascular: having to do with the heart and the blood vessels

caries: cavities in the teeth; tooth decay

carrier: person or animal with causative agents of disease in the body and capable of spreading the germs to others

casefinding: investigation or consideration of potential health problems in order to detect, treat, and bring under control at the earliest moment any disease which might be a threat to others

cataract: a condition that causes cloudiness of the lens of the eye; impairs vision: usually requires surgery for correction

causative agent: disease-producing organism

cementum: the hard outer covering of the root of the tooth between the dentin and the periodontal membrane

centigrade: a system of measuring temperature on a scale of 100 degrees, zero degrees representing the freezing point

cerebral palsy: term used to describe a group of conditions whose damage to the nervous system creates difficulty in movement

cervical: pertaining to the neck of the uterus **(cervix)**

chancre: a syphilitic sore resulting when the causative agent *Treponema pallidum* enters the body

chancroid: an ulcer-type sore on the reproductive organs as the result of infection by the organism *Haemophilus ducreyi*

chemotherapy: treatment of disease by use of drugs or chemicals

chiropody: the care and treatment of the foot in health and disease

chiropractic: a form of treatment that utilizes manipulation and specific adjustment of body structures, especially the spinal column

cholera: an infectious disease characterized by weakness, vomiting, and abnormal bowel movements; often contracted as the result of drinking impure water

cholesterol: a fatty, crystaline substance normally present in the blood plasma: saturated fats in the diet tend to increase cholesterol in the blood

chromosome: structure in the cell nucleus containing genes which determine inherited characteristics

chronic: of long duration; lasting, as in a long illness

cilia: tiny, living hairlike projections

circulatory: pertaining to circulation

coagulation: clotting, especially of blood

cocaine: a narcotic, with addicting qualities

coccidiodomycosis: a disease caused by infection of the lungs by the fungus *Coccidioides immitis;* commonly called valley fever

colitis: inflammation of the colon

compensation: an adjustment mechanism that enables a person to achieve satisfaction in an alternate way, a goal not easily achieved replaced by another goal

concave: hollow and curved; a lens that is narrowest in the middle and spreads light rays apart

conduction: the carrying of an impulse by a nerve or other tissue

congenital: existing at birth or dating from birth

conjunctiva: the outer membrane of the front of the eyeball and the lining membrane of the eyelids

conjunctivitis: an inflammation of the conjunctiva of the eyeball and eyelid

constipation: a condition in which the regular evacuation of the bowels is not carried out

contact lenses: small glass or plastic lenses that aid defective vision inconspicuously, and are held in place over the cornea by surface tension of the eye fluid

contagious: communicable; capable of being transmitted from one person to another directly or indirectly

contaminant: the agent of contamination; bacteria, other agent, or foreign substance

contamination: the entry into food, water, or other substances, of a contaminant which can cause disease

convex: bulging and curved; a lens that is thickest in the middle and brings light rays closer together

cornea: the transparent part of the outer layer of the eyeball through which light passes before entering the pupil

coronary: relating to the heart; arteries that supply the heart muscle with blood

coronary thrombosis: closing of a coronary artery by a clot which deprives heart muscle tissue of food and oxygen

cryogenics: branch of science that deals with the production and effects of very low temperatures

cyst: an abnormal pouch or sac containing fluid, semisolid material, or gas; usually found in a cavity or structure of the body

decibel: unit used to measure the relative loudness of sounds on a scale of 1 to 130

defense mechanism: an unconscious process of the mind that prevents the emergence into the consciousness of unacceptable or painful ideas and impulses

deficiency disease: disease resulting from lack or insufficiency of certain nutrients

degenerative: causing a change or breakdown of tissue that results in impairment of structure or function

delirium tremens: a violent mental disturbance caused by excessive and prolonged use of alcohol

delivery: the final stage in the birth of a child

dental hygienist: a dental worker who provides a variety of services under the supervision of the dentist

dentin: a hard substance that forms the greater part of a tooth under the enamel

deoxyribonucleic acid (DNA): a complex molecular structure in the genes, containing patterns of possible inherited characteristics

dependency: physiological and/or psychological habituation

depressant: a drug that reduces functional body activity, produces muscular relaxation, and slows down functions of the central nervous system

desalination: the removal of salts contained in solution; the treatment of sea water to make it suitable for commercial, industrial, or personal use

diabetes (diabetes mellitus): a health condition caused by an insufficient amount of insulin in the body and resulting in inability to burn sugar

diagnostician: a specialist who is trained to identify and interpret symptoms and test results and related material in detecting disease or health conditions requiring attention

diarrhea: increased frequency and liquid consistency of stools **(feces)**

dietitian: a specialist responsible for the nutritional care of people

digestion: the process by which food is broken up in the alimentary canal for absorption by the body, or into waste products

diphtheria: an infectious disease characterized by fever, sore throat, and the growth of a membrane in the throat

disease: a condition of the body in which there is incorrect function caused by heredity, infection, diet, or environment

dominant: a gene that causes a certain inherited trait to appear in a person whether or not an unlike gene for that trait is present

dormant: marked by a suspension of activity; not actively functioning

drug: substance used as medicine in treating disease

drug dependence: physiological and/or psychological habituation to and reliance upon the use of a narcotic or drug

dynamic: productive of activity; relating to expenditures of force or energy

dysentery: an intestinal disease causing severe diarrhea

dysmenorrhea: painful menstruation

ecology: the study of an organism's relationship to its total environment; in sociology, the spacing of people and institutions and their resulting interdependency

ejaculation: a sudden discharging of a fluid from a duct; the release of semen from the male body

embryo: a developing baby during the first few months of pregnancy

emphysema: a degenerative condition of the lungs characterized by changes in the lung tissue which make breathing very difficult and reduce the volume of oxygen available to the blood

enamel: hard outer covering of the tooth above the root

endocrine gland: a gland which secretes hormones into the bloodstream

endocrine system: a system of ductless glands which function in the production of internal secretions, particularly hormones

endodontist: a dentist who specializes in the treatment of diseases and injuries that affect the tooth pulp and periodontal tissues

endowment: a natural characteristic, ability, capacity, or trait inherited from parents

endurance: the ability to withstand physical or mental fatigue

enriched: having vitamins and minerals added (to food products)

environment: all of the external conditions and factors that affect the development and life of a person

environmental engineer: a person who applies engineering principles to environmental health problems

epidemic: an outbreak of an infectious disease which affects a large number of people at about the same time

epididymis: an elongated cordlike structure at the back of the testis; the tube in which spermatozoa are stored

epilepsy: a disease of the central nervous system characterized by loss of consciousness, convulsive movements, or temporarily reduced physical and mental efficiency

esophagus: the passageway for food from the mouth to the stomach

ethical drugs: drugs dispensed by prescription only, and advertised only in professional medical publications

eustachian tube: the tube which connects the middle ear with the throat

extrovert: one who is "outgoing": who tends to be more interested in working or being with people as compared to working or being alone

fad: a fashion, interest, or practice followed for a time with exaggerated zeal

fallacy: a false idea

fallopian tubes: slender tubes leading from the body cavity in the vicinity of the ovaries to the uterus

fantasy: an imaginative sequence fulfilling a psychological need; a daydream

fatality: death; cessation of life as the result of disease or accident

fats: a combination of fatty acids and glycerol which provide heat and energy for the body

fertilization: the biochemical combination of a sperm with an ovum (egg)

flagellum (pl. flagella): a whiplike tail or appendage projecting from a cell; primary organ of locomotion of sperm

fluoridation: the addition of controlled amounts of fluorides to the public water supply

follicle: a small sac, cavity, or receptacle

footcandle: a unit of lighting equal to the light produced by a standard candle at a distance of one foot

fraternal twins: twins resulting from the fertilization of two different ova by two different sperm at about the same time

fumigation: the process of applying smoke, vapor, or gas for the purpose of destroying agents of disease or pests

fungus (pl. fungi): simple nongreen plant such as mold and mildew; certain fungi are capable of producing disease

gamma globulin: a form of blood protein (globulin) which is used to prevent certain diseases

gene: the carrier of hereditary traits; part of the chromosomes

genital: pertaining to the sexual organs

genitalia: the organs of reproduction, especially the external organs

genitourinary system: pertaining to the organs of reproduction (genital) and the urinary organs

gestation: the process of development of young in the womb **(uterus);** pregnancy

gingivitis: an inflammation and swelling of the gums

gland: a cell, group of cells, or organ producing a secretion

glaucoma: a condition that results in intense pressure within the eyeball and often leads to blindness

gonads: male or female sex glands; glands which produce sperm, ova, and sex hormones

gonococcus: the bacterium causing gonorrhea

gonorrhea: a venereal disease; a communicable inflammation of mucous membrane lining of the genital tract, characterized in the male by pain, burning sensation upon urination, and discharge of pus; symptoms are less obvious in the female

gout: a disease characterized by painful inflammation of the joints

gram: a metric unit of weight measurement equal to one one-thousandth of a kilogram

granuloma inguinale: a venereal disease characterized by deep ulcerations of the skin in the vicinity of the external reproductive organs

hallucinogen: drug capable of producing illusions, fantasies, and hallucinations

hay fever: an allergic reaction to pollens; symptoms often resemble those of a cold

helminth: a parasitic intestinal worm

hemorrhage: excessive loss of blood

hemorrhoid: a dilation and engorgement of veins by blood in the anal region

hepatitis (infectious hepatitis): inflammation of the liver resulting from virus infection

hereditary: capable of being passed on from parents to offspring

hernia: a rupture; a condition which results when the intestine or another organ protrudes through the abdominal muscles

heroin: an addicting depressant narcotic made from opium; its possession or use is illegal

heterogeneous: dissimilar; mixed; not consisting of the same kind

heterosexual: relating to different sexes; consisting of both male and female

histamine: the chemical that produces allergy reactions

histoplasmosis: a disease caused by infection with a fungus, characterized by involvement of the lymph nodes of the trachea and bronchi

homogeneous: of uniform structure or composition; the same throughout

homosexual: pertaining to the same sex; also, a person attracted to members of the same sex

homosexuality: an attraction toward members of the same sex in preference to members of the opposite sex

hookworm: a parasitic worm which in the larva stage enters the body, usually through the skin of the feet, and eventually finds its way to the small intestine, where it matures

hormone: chemical substance secreted by the endocrine glands, regulating various body processes

host: living animal or plant from which a parasite or germ receives nutrition

hydrochloric acid: an acid found in the gastric juice of the stomach

hyperopia: farsightedness

hypertension: high blood pressure

hyperventilation: a condition in which there is an increased amount of air entering the pulmonary alveoli, resulting in a reduction of the necessary carbon dioxide level for normal function

hypnosis: the procedure of psychologically influencing a person to accept suggestions made during an induced trance, coma, or sleep; utilized, at times, in psychotherapy and the treatment of disease

hypochondriasis: a morbid anxiety about the health, often associated with a simulated disease

hypodermic: applied or administered beneath the skin; medication administered in this way

hysteria: a condition in which emotions become abnormally excited and in which certain motor functions are impaired

identical twins: twins resulting from one egg (ovum) fertilized by one sperm

identification: a mental adjustment mechanism whereby a person identifies himself with or patterns himself after someone else

immobilization: the act of rendering someone or something incapable of moving or being moved

immunity: the ability of the body (either with or without the help of an antigen) to form antibodies to counteract invading causative agents of disease

immunization: making the body immune to the causative agents of disease

implantation: the movement of cells to a new region, as fertilized ovum to uterus

incapacitation: to be made incapable of normal function; to be disabled

incidence: rate of occurrence or rate of influence

incubation period: the period of a disease between the time of infection and the beginning of specific visible symptoms

infancy: the period of early childhood (approximately one year)

infatuation: exaggerated or extravagant admiration, fondness, or love

infectious: communicable by infection; capable of being easily spread

infectious hepatitis: a disease caused by a virus; characterized by inflammation of the liver

infectious mononucleosis: a condition in which there is an abnormally large number of those white blood cells that contain a single nucleus (monocytes) in the blood; an acute infectious disease characterized by fever and swelling of the lymph nodes

inflammation: a diseased condition marked by swelling, heat, redness, and pain

influenza: a highly contagious disease caused by viruses; a respiratory disease, often reaching epidemic proportions

inguinal canal: a passage in the male through which the testis descends into the scrotum and in which the spermatic cord lies

inherent: present in the basic constitution or character of someone; inherited

insecticide: a chemical substance capable of controlling or destroying insects

insomnia: a condition characterized by the inability to sleep

insulin: a hormone produced by the Islands of Langerhans in the pancreas; lack of insulin causes diabetes

intern: an advanced or graduate student in medicine gaining supervised practical experience, as in a hospital

internist: specialist in internal medicine

introvert: a person who is not "outgoing"; one who usually prefers to be or to work by himself

inversion: a reversal of position, order, or relationship

iris: the colored portion of the eye surrounding the pupil

isolation: the process of separating a person with a disease from all other persons

isometric: relating to changes of pressure under conditions of controlled or constant changes in counter-pressure

jaundice: yellow color of skin resulting from bile pigments in the blood

kidneys: two bean-shaped, glandular organs in the rear of the upper abdominal cavity which remove water, urea, and other waste products from the blood to form urine

kilocalorie: the amount of heat required to raise the temperature of one kilogram of water one degree centigrade

kilogram: a metric unit of weight measurement; about 2.2 lbs.

labor: the physical activities involved in giving birth to offspring

latent: concealed; hidden; present, but not visible

laxative: a substance that speeds up peristalsis in the intestines; a substance that encourages bowel movement

lesion: a change of tissue structure as the result of disease or injury

leukemia: cancer of the blood-forming tissues; usually a great increase in white blood cells and decrease in red blood cells

LSD (LSD-25): d-lysergic acid diethylamid tartrate is a dangerous hallucinogenic drug; it is odorless, tasteless, and colorless

lymph glands: small glands located at numerous points along the lymphatic system; they are important in fighting infection

lymphogranuloma venereum: a specific venereal disease caused by a virus; primarily found in the tropics

maladjusted: lacking harmony with one's environment because of failure to reach a satisfactory adjustment between one's desires and the actual conditions of one's life

malalignment: improper or unbalanced alignment

malaria: a disease caused by microorganisms **(protozoa)** carried by the Anopheles mosquito; characterized by chills, fever, and sweating

malignancy: abnormal cell growth dangerous to life and destructive to adjoining tissue

malignant: tending to produce death or deterioration

malnutrition: a condition in which quantity or quality of food is inadequate or in which nutrients are not properly utilized by the body, resulting in lowered levels of health

malocclusion: a condition that prevents the teeth from fitting together properly

mammary glands: milk-producing glands of mammals including human beings; glands which produce and provide nourishment to infants

manic: highly excited, with disordered thinking and lack of self-control

manic-depressive: characterized by mania or psychotic depression or by alternating mania and depression

marijuana: an illegal narcotic derived from the leaves and flowering tops of the pistillate hemp plant

masturbation: self-manipulation of the genitals for personal gratification

maturation: the final stages of differentiation and refinement in process and function of cells, tissues, organs, systems, behavior, and judgment

maturity: the point of having developed to the maximum those traits and characteristics endowed through heredity as well as those acquired from infancy into adulthood

measles: a communicable disease usually contracted in childhood and characterized by fever, eruptions of red spots on the skin, and upper respiratory symptoms

membrane: a thin, soft, pliable sheet or layer of skin

menopause: cessation of ovulation and menstruation; the end of the child-bearing stage of life

menstruation: the process of releasing nutrient-rich blood from the walls of the uterus

metastasize: transfer a disease-producing agency from the site of the disease to another part of the body; form a secondary growth of a malignant tumor

microorganism: organism invisible to the unaided eye; requiring magnification of a microscope in order to be seen

migraine: a variety of severe headaches, usually localized and usually of allergic origin

minerals: inorganic compounds, many of which are required for normal growth, development, and health

molecule: the smallest particle of an element or compound capable of retaining chemical identity with the substance it represents

mononucleosis (infectious mononucleosis): a condition in which there is an abnormally large number of those white blood cells that contain a single nucleus (monocytes) in the blood; an acute infectious disease characterized by fever and swelling of the lymph nodes

morphine: a depressant narcotic derived from opium

mortality: the number of deaths in a given time or place; the proportion of deaths to population

mucous membrane: the membrane lining the inside of the mouth, the nose, all of the respiratory system, and the alimentary canal

multiphasic screening: mass screening technique, checking a variety of aspects or phases

multiple sclerosis: a nonremedial condition in which the myelin sheath of nerves is destroyed and replaced with scar tissue

muscular dystrophy: a group of diseases characterized by progressive muscular weakness due to the wasting away of the muscles

myopia: nearsightedness

mysticism: obscure or irrational speculation; the unfounded possibility of direct and intuitive acquisition of absolute knowledge or power

narcotic: inducing sleep

narcotic analgesic: any drug that relieves pain and induces sleep; when used other than as prescribed by a doctor they are very dangerous and often illegal

nausea: a sensation tending to cause vomiting

neoplasm: a new growth of tissue serving no physiological function; tumor

nephritis: inflammation of the kidneys

nephrosis: noninflammatory degeneration of the kidneys

neurological: having to do with the nervous system

neurosis: a mental disorder which usually does not involve loss of touch with reality

nicotine: a colorless and soluble alkaloid with a bitter taste, a poisonous drug found in tobacco

nocturnal emission: the involuntary discharge of semen during sleep

nutrient: chemical substance found in foods; it regulates body processes, repairs cells, promotes growth, and provides energy

obesity: the excessive accumulation of fat

obsession: persistent idea or impulse that one cannot get rid of by reasoning

obsessive habit: a compelling and persistent practice that one finds difficult to break

occlusion: proper alignment or fitting as in the relationship and position of the upper and lower teeth

oculist: a doctor who specializes in the structure, function, and diseases of the eyes; another name for **ophthalmologist**

ophthalmologist: another name for **oculist**

opiate: a preparation or derivative of opium; narcotic

opium: a depressant narcotic obtained from the unripe seeds of the opium poppy

optician: a person who grinds, prepares, or deals in lenses; not a physician

optimum: the most favorable conditions for growth and development; greatest degree attained under implied or specific conditions

optometrist: a person who tests vision and prescribes glasses; not a physician

oral: of, or relating to, the mouth

organic: pertaining to or derived from living organisms; exhibiting characteristics peculiar to living organisms

orgasm: a complex series of responses of the genital organs and skin at the culmination of a sexual act

orthodontist: a dentist who specializes in straightening teeth, correcting irregularities of alignment or spacing

osmosis: diffusion through a semipermeable membrane

osteopathic physician: a licensed physician trained in the use of all accepted diagnostic and therapeutic techniques in prevention and treatment of disease and injury, with special emphasis on the musculoskeletal system.

otitis media: inflammation of the middle ear

otolaryngologist: a doctor who specializes in diseases of the ear, nose, and throat

otologist: a doctor who specializes in disorders of the ear

otosclerosis: the formation of spongy bone in the inner ear which impairs hearing

outpatient: a person who is not confined to a hospital but who receives diagnosis or treatment in a clinic or dispensary connected with the hospital

ovaries: the organs which produce eggs **(ova)** and female sex hormones

ovulation: the process of an egg **(ovum)** being released from the ovary

ovum: egg, female sex cell

pandemic: a widespread epidemic

papilloma: benign tumor resembling a wart; caused by virus infection of the connective tissue of the skin, most frequently found on the soles of the feet

paramedical: of, or relating to the medical profession

paraplegic: a person with paralysis of the legs and lower part of the body, both motion and sensation being affected

parasite: an organism that lives on or in another living thing (the **host**) and obtains its food from the host

paresis: a brain disease caused by syphilis; a medical term for paralysis

Parkinson's disease (Parkinsonism): a nervous disease involving a shaking, rhythmic tremor of the body

passive immunity: immunity acquired by injection of serum from another individual or animal

pathogenic: capable of producing disease

pathological: pertaining to disease

pedodontist: a dentist who specializes in dental diseases of children

penicillin: an antibiotic extracted from mold

penis: male organ of copulation

peptic ulcer: ulceration of the mucous membrane of the esophagus, stomach, or small intestine caused by the action of acid gastric juice

periodontal disease: disease that affects the tissues that connect the cementum of the tooth to the gum and bone

periodontist: a dentist who specializes in diseases of the supporting tissues of the teeth

periodontitis: a disease of the supporting tissues of the teeth

peritonitis: an inflammation of the lining of the abdominal cavity; often in connection with a ruptured appendix

personality: the pattern or complex of characteristics that distinguishes an individual

pertussis: whooping cough

pesticide: a poison sprayed or dusted on crops in order to control or destroy insects

peyote: an illegal stimulating drug with no medicinal use

pharmacist: health worker who prepares and distributes medicinal products

phobia: a persistent, unreasonable fear of an object or situation

phosphorus: a mineral element essential in the formation of bone, muscles, blood, and nerves

photochemical: reactions which use the energy of light (or radiant energy) in producing chemical changes

physical dependency: dependency of or pertaining to the body, as for a drug or stimulant

physiological dependence: a condition in which the cells adjust and modify their normal function to accommodate the effect of a drug and, therefore, require the presence of the drug in order to function physiologically without pain; removal of the drug results in withdrawal symptoms

pituitary gland: a ductless gland located at the base of the brain; often called the "master" gland because it secretes hormones which control the functions of other ductless **(endocrine)** glands

placenta: the structure that unites the developing baby to the maternal uterus and functions in the provision of nutrients, oxygen, and the removal of waste products

plague: an epidemic-type disease caused by a bacterium; occurs in several forms

podiatry: the care and treatment of the human foot in conditions of health and disease

poliomyelitis: a virus disease which may kill motor nerve cells and cause paralysis; often called polio; sometimes called infantile paralysis

pollutants: substances that cause pollution, such as smoke, sewage, and garbage

pollution: contamination or impurity

preadolescence: the period preceding adolescence

precancerous: of a period preceding cancer

predisposition: being inclined toward or susceptible to a disease or health condition

prenatal: before birth

presbyopia: an impairment of vision in which near objects cannot be seen clearly; usually develops in later life

primitive: belonging to or characteristic of an early stage of development; relating to a relatively simple people or culture

projection: putting the blame for one's faults on someone else

proprietary drugs (formerly called **patent medicines):** drugs sold over the counter in pharmacies, supermarkets, etc., without prescription, and widely advertised via all the communications media

prostate gland: the gland which surrounds the base of the urethra in males

prosthodontist: a dentist who specializes in the artificial replacement of teeth

proteins: a group of organic compounds containing nitrogen, carbon, hydrogen, and oxygen; essential to growth, cell repair, and formation of new cells

protozoan (pl. **protozoa):** one-celled organism

psychiatrist: a doctor who specializes in the diagnosis and treatment of mental illness

psychodynamics: relating to mental or emotional forces or processes during early childhood and their effects on behavior and mental states

psychological dependency: an obsession based upon emotional and personality deficiencies which require the use of a drug in order to function at a self-defined level of normalcy

psychologist: a person with special training and skills who studies the mind and behavior

psychoneurosis: a condition based on emotional conflict in which an impulse that has been blocked seeks expression in a disguised response or symptom

psychosis: a mental condition characterized by loss of touch with reality

psychosomatic: pertaining to the effect of the mind upon the body; an illness which may show physical symptoms resulting from or aggravated by mental causes

psychotherapy: mental treatment of illness, especially nervous diseases and maladjustments

puberty: the stage of growth and development when one becomes capable of reproducing sexually

pubic: relating to the exterior area immediately surrounding the external reproductive organs

pyorrhea: a periodontal disease that affects the periodontal membrane and other supporting structures of the teeth

quackery: the practice of medicine, dentistry, or any other related health profession by a person who pretends medical skill and knowledge but who, in fact, is incompetent and unlicensed

quadruplets: multiple births consisting of four babies born at about the same time

quarantine: the limitation of freedom of movement of an ill person or one suspected of having a serious communicable disease

quinine: a drug used in the treatment of malaria as well as other diseases; obtained from the bark of a tropical tree

quintuplets: multiple births consisting of five babies born at about the same time

rabies: a virus-caused disease that attacks the central nervous system and is usually contracted through the bite of an animal that has the disease

radiation: sending forth of rays; also rays themselves as in radiation from splitting atoms

radioactive fallout: the descent through the atmosphere of radioactive particles, stirred up by, or resulting from, a nuclear explosion; also, these particles collectively

radioactivity: the ability of some elements (as uranium) of spontaneously emitting dangerous rays

radioisotope: unstable form of some elements (as radium) that give off radiation; some isotopes are extremely important in medical diagnosis and treatment

radiologist: one who practices the science of radioactive substances and X-rays and its application

radium: an element that continually gives off destructive radiation; used in some cases to treat cancer

rationalization: the process of giving oneself a reason other than the true reason for certain behavior in order to avoid facing the truth

recessive: a gene that causes a certain trait to appear only if another identical gene is present or if the dominant gene for the same trait is not present

reclamation: the process of restoring to use; recovering; reforming

rectum: the lower terminal section of the large intestine

refractive error: condition in the structure of the eye which causes entering light rays to reflect the visual image improperly, as in nearsightedness, farsightedness, and astigmatism

regression: the mental defense tactic in which one acts or thinks in a childish way

rehabilitation: the process of restoring to former capacity; restoring to a condition of health or useful and constructive activity

relaxation: a relaxing, or the state of being less firm or rigid

repression: the mental process of selectively and purposefully forgetting

reservoir of infection: the source of causative agents of disease

resistance: the ability of the body to withstand or resist infection

respiratory: of, or pertaining to the act or process of breathing

retina: the internal membrane of the eyeball which serves to receive visual images

Rh factor: a substance in the blood of most people; named after the experimental animal, Rhesus monkey; individuals are either Rh positive or Rh negative

rheumatic fever: an inflammation of the joints caused by certain bacteria and sometimes resulting in damage to the heart

rheumatoid arthritis: a constitutional disease of unknown cause, progressive in nature and characterized by inflammation and swelling of joints

rickets: a disease of the bones caused by lack of vitamin D

rickettsiae (pl.): microorganisms smaller than bacteria but larger than viruses; causative agents of disease transmitted by lice and ticks

ringworm: a contagious skin disease resulting from fungous infection and characterized by formation of ring-shaped patches

Rocky Mountain spotted fever: an infectious disease caused by rickettsiae; characterized by fever, body rash, and pains in joints, bones, and muscles

saliva: a digestive juice secreted by the salivary glands which open into the mouth

salivary glands: glands which open into the mouth and produce saliva

sanitarian: one especially interested or versed in sanitary measures

scarlet fever: an acute infectious disease caused by streptococci, characterized by fever and skin eruptions of a reddish color

schizophrenia: a mental condition in which there is a withdrawal from reality characterized by a "split," cleavage, or frustration of the mental processes; often classified as a psychosis

scrotum: the pouch of skin that contains the testicles

scurvy: a deficiency disease characterized by hemorrhage, especially into the skin and mucous membrane

sedative: a substance that quiets or reduces functional activity and nervousness

sedentary: inactive; passive

self-limited infection: an infection that runs its course and then subsides; a condition that does not perpetuate itself indefinitely

semen: a whitish fluid of the male reproductive system containing sperm suspended in secreted fluids

seminal vesicles: paired structures resembling small pouches through which stored sperm leave the **vas deferens**

serum hepatitis: a disease in which the symptoms resemble those of infectious hepatitis but which is caused by an entirely different virus; usually transmitted by inadequate sterilized syringes or needles, tattooing, and by administrations of infectious blood, blood plasma, or blood products

sexuality: the characteristics and role of femaleness and maleness in relationship to oneself and to others throughout life

shock: slowing down of the vital body functions and processes as the result of injury or loss of blood; in some cases, shock is the result of an emotional crisis rather than physical factors

Siamese twins: twins that are congenitally united in a physical manner; the name derived from the first widely reported case which happened to be Siamese children

sibling: one or two or more children of the same parents but not necessarily of the same birth

side effects: effects of a drug other than those the drug was intended to produce

silver nitrate: a chemical compound used in medicine as an antiseptic

sinusitis: an inflammation of the sinus

smallpox: an acute contagious virus disease characterized by skin eruptions and scar formations

smear test (Papanicolaou test): a diagnostic screening procedure used in the early detection of possible cervical cancer in women

sociologist: one who is trained in the science dealing with factors and problems of society, social institutions, and social relationships

specialist: one who is especially trained in a special field of knowledge or work

sperm (spermatozoan): male reproductive cell

spirochete: a spiral-shaped, one-celled organism which causes syphilis

sputum: saliva mixed with mucous and other secretions from the respiratory tract that is ejected from the mouth

stamina: endurance; staying power

staphylococcal infection: infection caused by certain round bacteria which often form clusters; boils and pimples are often staphylococcus infections; certain forms of this bacterium can contaminate food

sterile: free from microorganisms or other living things; unable to produce offspring

stimulant: a drug or other substance that speeds up the activity of the body

stimuli: any substances or conditions to which organisms react

strabismus: a condition in which the eye muscles are not properly balanced and the eyes do not work together; squinting or cross-eyedness

streptococcal organism: any of certain round bacteria that usually form chains, some of which cause infections of the respiratory system

stress: a physical, chemical, or emotional factor that causes physical or mental tension and which may be a factor in disease causation

stroke: paralysis, to different degrees, resulting from rupture of a blood vessel in the brain

stye: an inflamed swelling of a sebaceous gland at the margin of the eyelid

subclinical condition: an infection which is not severe enough to produce the typical symptoms of the disease

substitution: an adjustment mechanism that permits the replacement of an unrealistic goal or objective with one that is capable of being achieved

susceptible: not immune; capable of being infected

symbiotic condition: a condition in which dissimilar organisms live together, especially for their mutual benefit

symptoms: the observable signs and personal feelings which indicate the presence of a disease or health condition

Synanon: an organization in which members use mutual self-help in attempting to free themselves of drug use

syphilis: a communicable venereal disease caused by a spirochete organism

systemic: affecting the body generally

tapeworm: a long, flat worm that sometimes lives in the intestines as a parasite

tartar (calculus): a hard mineral deposit on the teeth near the gums; dental calculus

technician: a health worker in a variety of health areas who has two years of college or other formal training beyond high school

technology: advances or improvements in technical processes; improvement of methods of achieving practical purposes and goals

technologist: a health worker in a variety of health areas who has attained a college degree

telemetered: the process in which electrical apparatus measures various reactions such as pressure, radiation, intensity, speed, or temperature and transmits the results to an observation or recording station or point

tension: a state of mental unrest sometimes with signs of physical pain or discomfort; stress; pressure

testes: male organs that produce sperm and male hormones; **testicles**

testicles: the male sex glands; **testes**

tetanus: an infectious disease caused by tetanus bacilli which produces toxins that attack the central nervous system

Thalidomide: a drug used in Europe as a sedative during the early 1960's, discovered to be the cause of serious congenital deformities in the fetus when taken by women during early pregnancy

therapist: a person trained in methods of treatment and rehabilitation, usually in ways other than the use of drugs or surgery

therapy: the treatment of a disease or health condition

thiamine: vitamin B_1, formerly called vitamin B

thrombus: a blood clot

tolerance: the reduced effect that a person has from the same amount of a drug taken over a period of time; the need to take increased amounts of a drug to achieve the same results as formerly achieved from a smaller amount

tonsillitis: infection of the tonsils

topical application: designed for local application as in topical applications of fluorides to the teeth to prevent decay

toxic: having a poisonous effect

toxin: a poison produced by living organisms, usually bacteria

trachea: the windpipe

tranquil: free from agitation; quiet; calm, steady, or stable

tranquilizer: a drug used to reduce anxiety and tension

transfusion: a method of transferring blood from one person to another, or of injecting blood plasma or saline solution into the blood vessels

trauma: an injury or wound; a disorderly mental or behavioral state resulting from emotional stress or physical injury

traumatic: of, pertaining to, or resulting from a trauma, caused by a wound, injury, or shock

trichina (pl. trichinae): a small worm sometimes found in uncooked pork; a parasite that causes **trichinosis**

trimester: a term or period of three months

tuberculosis: a disease caused by the *tubercle bacillus;* usually affects the lungs but other tissues may also be infected

tumor: an abnormal growth of cells which may be either benign or malignant

typhoid fever: a disease caused by typhoid bacteria in water or food and affecting the intestinal tract

typhus: an acute infectious disease caused by rickettsial organisms and transmitted by infected lice and fleas

ulcer: an open sore on the skin or mucous membrane; often refers to ulcer of the stomach or intestine

umbilical cord: the cord that connects the fetus with the maternal placenta during the development of the baby

urban: relating to, characteristic of, or constituting a city

urethra: the tube that carries urine from the bladder to the exterior

urine: water and waste products which constitute that fluid collected by the kidneys

uterus: the female organ within which the baby develops before birth

vaccine: a preparation of dead or weakened germs or their toxins used to make a person produce his own antibodies against a certain disease

vagina: the passage leading from the uterus

to the external surface of the female reproductive system

valley fever: a fungus-produced infection of the respiratory system: **coccidiodomycosis**

varicose veins: swollen, enlarged, and sometimes twisted veins usually found in the legs

vas deferens: spermatic ducts leading from the male epididymis to the seminal vesicles

venereal disease: gonorrhea, syphilis, and other diseases transmitted primarily through sexual intercourse

viral infection: infection in which a virus is the causative agent

virulence: the disease-producing level or power of a germ

virus: one of a group of pathogenic agents smaller than bacteria

visual acuity: a measurement of the normalcy of sight

vitamin: an organic compound found in certain foods and necessary for normal growth, development, and metabolism

WHO (World Health Organization): a group of countries united together in the mutual interest of health

whooping cough: an acute infectious disease usually contracted during childhood, involving the mucous membrane of the respiratory tract; **pertussis**

withdrawal: the discontinuance of the administration or use of a drug

X-rays: short rays produced by special equipment for photographing and producing shadow pictures, used in diagnosis and treatment of disease

yellow fever: an acute infectious disease caused by a virus which is transmitted by a mosquito, characterized by fever, jaundice, and vomiting

Genes and chromosomes, 32–35
  dominant and recessive, 33
German measles, 194, 213
Gestation period, 36
Getting along with others, 16
Gingivitis, 88–89
Girls:
  early sex interest, 53
  energy needs, 73
  menstruation, 43–45
  ovulation process, 42–43
  physical changes in, 41–45
  secondary sex characteristics, 41, 54
Glasses (See Eyeglasses)
Glaucoma, 212
Glue sniffing, 153, 156
Gonads, 40
Gonorrhea, 180–182
  mode of transmission, 180
  treatment, 182
Gout, 206
Growth and development, 7, 30–51
  adolescence, 45–48
  adulthood and parenthood, 47, 48
  birth process, 36–38
  emotional maturity, 31
  infancy and early childhood, 38–39
  intellectual advancement, 31
  prenatal development, 31–38
    effects of environment, 35
    fertilization, 31–32
    gestation period, 35–36
    hereditary blueprint, 32–33
  puberty,
    effect of hormones, 40
  social responsibility, 31
Guilt feelings, 26, 27
Gumchewing, effect on teeth, 90
Gum diseases, 88–91
Guns, safety rules, 249

Handicapped persons:
  devices for, 307–308
  treatment and rehabilitation, 9
Halfway Houses:
  for alcoholics, 126
  for narcotic addicts, 159
Hallucinogens, 145, 149, 152, 155
Hay fever, 204–205
Headaches, migraine, 22
Health, 3–13, 303–311
  concepts, 3–13
  definition of, 5–6
  effect of religious beliefs, 3
  heredity, effects of, 6
  solving future problems, 303–311
Health Careers Guidebook, 281

Health Departments, local, 8–9
Health education, 304–305
  by voluntary health agencies, 9
Health educator, 296
Health information:
  evaluating, 10–11
  need for, 8
Health insurance programs, 274–275
  dental insurance, 275
  group plans, 274
  hospital insurance, 275
  major-medical, 274–275
  medical, 275
  Medicare, 276–277
  surgical-expense insurance, 275
Health personnel, 280–301
Health organizations, 9–10
  voluntary health agencies, 9–10
Health problems:
  future trends, 303–311
  national study, 303–311
  personal, 10–11
Health products, 259–263
  modern prescription drugs, 260–262
  importance of safeguards, 261–262
    indiscriminate use, 259–260
    side effects, 261
  selecting, 259–263
  self-medication, 259–260
Health programs:
  of industry and labor, 9–10
  of local service organizations, 10
Health services:
  choosing a doctor, 263–264
  comprehensive personal health services, 303
  future trends, 303–311
  international, 308–310
  organization for health, 303
  personal physician, 303–304
  selecting, 263–264
  technological developments, 305–308
    acupuncture, 308
    computers, 306
    electronic devices, 305
    organ transplants, 308
    radioisotopes, 306
    space medicine, 307
    synthetic body parts, 307
  voluntary participation, 304
Health statistician, 294
Hearing, 212–214
  disabilities, 212–214
  disorders, 212–214
    allergic reactions, 213
    central-neural defects, 214
    conduction defects, 213
    noise and, 213
    otosclerosis, 213

sensory-neural defects, 213
  effect of noise on, 213
  loss, 212
Heart disease, 193–198
  angina pectoris, 195
  anticoagulants, 195
  cholesterol and animal fats, 79
  congenital, 194
  coronary, 195–197
  effects of smoking, 134
  hypertension, 194–195
  physical activity and, 100
  rapid beating, 22
  reducing risk of, 197–198
  rheumatic, 195
  strokes, 198
  synthetic valves, 307
  transplants, 308
Helminths, 170
Hepatitis:
  infectious, 184
  serum, 184
Heredity:
  chromosomes and genes, 32–35
    transmission of characteristics, 33–35
  effect on health, 6
  effect on mental health, 16–18
  effect on tooth decay, 88
Hero worship, 26
Heroin, 149, 152, 156
High blood pressure, 22, 193–195
Hippocrates, 3
Histamines, 205
Histologic technician, 287
Home safety, 243–245
  checklist for, 244–245
Homosexuality, 59–60
Hookworms, 170
Hormones, 6
  effect on growth and development, 40
  pituitary glands, 41
Hospital administrator, 297
Hospital insurance, 275
  Medicare, 276–277
Hospitalization, for narcotic addicts, 157–158
Hoyman, Howard S., 5
Hyperopia (farsightedness), 210
Hypertension, 194–197
Hyperventilation, 22
Hypnosis, 209
Hysteria, conversion, 27

Identification, 26
Immunity to disease, 4, 175
  active, 175
  passive, 175

Transplantation of living parts, 308
  rejection mechanism, 308
Trichinosis, 170
Tuberculosis, 173
  detection of, 192
  examinations for, 9, 10
  skin test, 192
  X-ray tests, 192
Twins, 38
  identical and fraternal, 38
  Siamese, 38
Typhoid fever, 172

Ulcers of the stomach, 23
  effect of smoking, 135
Umbilical cord, 32, 36, 38
Unconsciousness, first aid treatment, 254
Underweight, 76–77
  dieting to gain weight, 76–77
UNICEF (United Nations Children's Fund), 309
United States:
  Agency for International Development, 310
  Food and Drug Administration, 77, 260, 271
  health aid to other countries, 308–310
Unknown, dread of, 22
Urban design, health services and, 304

Uterus, 32, 36, 38

Vagina, 31
Vas deferens, 40
Vegetables and fruits, need for, 65–66
Venereal diseases, 176–182
  blood tests for, 180
  gonorrhea, 180–182
  syphilis, 177–180
Veterinarian, 298
Viruses, 165, 169
  cancer and, 202
Vision, 210–212
  diseases of the eye, 212
    cataracts, 212
    glaucoma, 212
  disorders, 210–212
    astigmatism, 211
    hyperopia (farsightedness), 210
    myopia (nearsightedness), 210
    presbyopia, 211
    strabismus, 211
Visiting Nurse Association, 9
Vitality for living, 98–113
Vitamins, 67, 68, 69
  deficiency diseases, 67, 191
  fat-soluble, 67
  function in maintaining health, 67, 68
  use of supplements, 77
  water-soluble, 67, 77

Vocational counselors, 298
Vocational nurse, 286
Voluntary health agencies, 9

Walking, importance of, 102
Ward clerks, 286
Waste disposal, 6
Water:
  desalination plants, 227
  protection of supplies, 4
  purification of, 174
  reclamation, 226–227
  shortages, 225
Water pollution, 6, 225–227
  control of, 226–227
  extent of problem, 225
Weakness, 22
Weight control:
  basal metabolism, 73
  diet fads, 79
  overweight, 76
  physical activity and, 100
  underweight, 76–77
Welfare plans, 10
White blood cells, 168, 172, 173, 308
World Health Organization (WHO), 120, 150, 309
Worry, 22

Yellow fever, 174